D1521539

A Case a Week
Sleep Disorders from the Cleveland Clinic

A Case a Week
Sleep Disorders from the Cleveland Clinic

Nancy Foldvary-Schaefer, DO
Associate Professor of Medicine
Cleveland Clinic Lerner College of Medicine
Director, Sleep Disorders Center
Cleveland Clinic Neurological Institute
Cleveland, OH

Jyoti Krishna, MD
Head, Pediatric Sleep Medicine
Assistant Professor
Cleveland Clinic Lerner College of Medicine
Cleveland Clinic Sleep Disorders Center
Neurological Institute
Cleveland, OH

Kumar Budur, MD, MS
Assistant Professor
Cleveland Clinic Lerner College of Medicine
Cleveland Clinic Sleep Disorders Center
Medical Director, Neuroscience (Current)
Takeda Global Research and Development
Lake Forest, IL

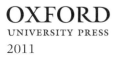
OXFORD
UNIVERSITY PRESS
2011

OXFORD
UNIVERSITY PRESS

Oxford University Press, Inc., publishes works that further
Oxford University's objective of excellence
in research, scholarship, and education.

Oxford   New York
Auckland   Cape Town   Dar es Salaam   Hong Kong   Karachi
Kuala Lumpur   Madrid   Melbourne   Mexico City   Nairobi
New Delhi   Shanghai   Taipei   Toronto

With offices in
Argentina   Austria   Brazil   Chile   Czech Republic   France   Greece
Guatemala   Hungary   Italy   Japan   Poland   Portugal   Singapore
South Korea   Switzerland   Thailand   Turkey Ukraine   Vietnam

Copyright © 2011 by Oxford University Press, Inc.

Published by Oxford University Press, Inc.
198 Madison Avenue, New York, New York 10016
www.oup.com

Oxford is a registered trademark of Oxford University Press

All rights reserved. No part of this publication may be reproduced,
stored in a retrieval system, or transmitted, in any form or by any means,
electronic, mechanical, photocopying, recording, or otherwise,
without the prior permission of Oxford University Press.

Library of Congress Cataloging-in-Publication Data

A case a week: sleep disorders from the Cleveland Clinic/[edited by] Nancy Foldvary-Schaefer,
Jyoti Krishna, Kumar Budur.
     p.; cm.
  Includes bibliographical references and index.
  ISBN 978-0-19-537772-9 (alk. paper)
1. Sleep disorders— Case studies. I. Foldvary-Schaefer, Nancy, 1962- II. Krishna, Jyoti. III. Budur, Kumar.
IV. Cleveland Clinic Sleep Disorders Center.
  [DNLM: 1. Sleep Disorders — diagnosis. 2. Sleep Disorders — therapy. 3. Case Reports. WM 188 C3366
2010]
  RC547.C373 2010
  616.8'498–dc22   2009053339

Printed in the United States of America
on acid-free paper

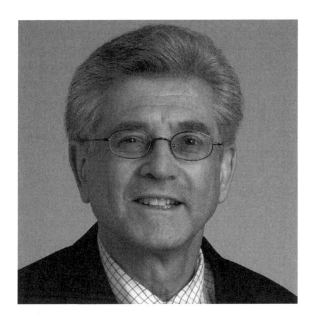

This book is dedicated to the memory of Dudley S. Dinner, MD, founder of the Cleveland Clinic Sleep Disorders Center. Dudley was introduced to Sleep during his clinical neurophysiology fellowship at the Cleveland Clinic in 1979. In the years that followed, he developed a state-of-the-art sleep laboratory and instructed hundreds of residents and fellows on polysomnography and clinical sleep medicine. A selfless mentor and friend, he will be forever missed by those of us in the sleep medicine community who had the privilege of knowing him.

To my husband, Errol; my daughter, Isabela; and my father, Eugene—*NF*

To the three generations of my family for the triple blessing of life, love, and laughter!—*JK*

To my brother Dhanunjaya—*KB*

Preface

It is an exciting time for sleep medicine! Today we know that sleep affects virtually every aspect of life and interrelates with most medical disciplines. Being one of the body's basic needs, sleep is critical for restoring and preserving good health. In recent years, the field has grown into an established medical specialty, and more people than ever before are turning to sleep specialists and sleep disorders centers for answers to heretofore unaddressed questions. Many of these questions are now being raised by doctors at health clinics, and media attention to the pervasive sleep related problems in society has raised the awareness of the average person enough to trigger these questions for themselves.

In these pages, we introduce you to clinical and laboratory sleep medicine through actual case histories of patients evaluated and treated in the Cleveland Clinic Sleep Disorders Center. The patients we have selected to highlight are reflective of a broad spectrum of sleep and wake disorders, ranging from the most ordinary to some of the more exceptional, even bizarre, presentations. In keeping with current standards, we have classified disorders after the second edition of the International Classification of Sleep Disorders (ICSD-2) and highlighted the accepted diagnostic criteria accordingly. While these cases represent true patient stories, as in so many instances in clinical medicine, the evaluation and management may not be "by the book." Rather, these cases are examples of practical challenges encountered by sleep professionals—some with favorable outcomes, and others not necessarily so. The style of presentation, evaluation, discussion, and interpretation of data is our own and should not be interpreted as a guideline or consensus. While permission was obtained from the American Academy of Sleep Medicine (AASM) to reproduce tables from the ICSD-2, this work has not been reviewed or approved by the AASM.

Over the past 20 years, we have had the privilege of working with hundreds of physicians, nurses, technicians, administrative professionals, and other staff in the Cleveland Clinic Sleep Disorders Center. All of these professionals have been dedicated to improving the lives of our patients. We would like to thank them for their contributions and extend a special thanks to three individuals without whom this work would not have been possible. Shirlontae Moss, sleep fellowship education coordinator, served as our administrative assistant and worked diligently to compile and organize materials. Zahr Alsheikhtaha, MD, RPSGT provided extensive support in graphics preparation. Nengah Hariadi, biomedical engineer, assisted in the production of hypnograms and video clips. Finally, we would like to acknowledge the thousands of men, women, and children we have had the privilege to treat over the years. By entrusting us with their care, they have taught us so much about the fascinating field of sleep.

To appeal to generalists, specialists, and trainees alike, we have written this volume in a simple, informal style, and avoided jargon. We hope the glossary at the end will serve as a handy reference and allow you to open the book at any case and begin reading. We hope this effort increases your interest and understanding of sleep medicine and serves as a resource in your encounters with patients with sleep and wake complaints. We trust this work will supplement the several more excellent and authoritative texts on the subject and serve as a springboard to further reading, because, as we say here at the Cleveland Clinic, *every life deserves a good night's sleep*!

Nancy Foldvary-Schaefer, DO
Jyoti Krishna, MD
Kumar Budur, MD, MS

Contents

Abbreviations   xvii
Contributor List   xxi
Ancillary Videos   xxvii

Introduction to the Sleep Clinic   3
Kumar Budur, Nancy Foldvary-Schaefer, and Jyoti Krishna

Introduction to the Sleep Laboratory   14
Jyoti Krishna, Nancy Foldvary-Schaefer, and Kumar Budur

Insomnias

1. A Car Dealer Who Could Not Get His Mind Out of Top Gear   27
   Psychophysiological Insomnia—Diagnosis and Pharmacological Management
   Victoria Luppa and Kumar Budur

2. Teaching the Teacher How to Sleep   34
   Psychophysiological Insomnia—Non-Pharmacological Management
   Michelle Drerup

3. Scared to Sleep: A Hurricane Katrina Survivor   43
   Depression, Anxiety, and Insomnia
   Kathleen Ashton and Kumar Budur

4. Rock a Bye Baby: The Case of the Midnight Crier   49
   Behavioral Insomnia of Childhood
   Margaret Richards

5. 45 Days Awake and Counting   56
   Paradoxical Insomnia
   Mia Zaharna and Kumar Budur

6. Alpha Delta: One Sorority You Don't Want to Join!   64
   Chronic Pain and Insomnia
   Kamala Adury and Kumar Budur

Sleep Related Breathing Disorders

7. The Case of the Sleepless Insurance Agent   70
   Primary Central Sleep Apnea
   Haralabos Mermigis and Zahr Alsheikhtaha

8. Out of Sight, Out of Mind   78
   Central Sleep Apnea Due to Cheyne Stokes Breathing
   Inga Sriubiene, Stella Baccaray, and Nancy Foldvary-Schaefer

9. Can't Breathe or Won't Breathe: How Would I Know if I Am Asleep?   85
   Central Sleep Apnea Due to Brainstem Glioma
   Bruce Cohen and Jyoti Krishna

10. Three's a Charm   92
    Complex Sleep Apnea
    Haralabos Mermigis and Zahr Alsheikhtaha

11. Ahhh... The Comforts of Home   100
    Obstructive Sleep Apnea in Adults—Diagnostic Criteria, Use of Portable Monitoring and Screening Tools
    Stella Baccaray, Noah Andrews, and Nancy Foldvary-Schaefer

12. Teaching Tommy How to Breathe   109
    Challenges with Positive Airway Pressure Therapy—Role of Behavioral Strategies
    William Novak and Julianne Sliwinski

13. When Weight Loss Is Not Enough   115
    Obstructive Sleep Apnea and Bariatric Surgery
    Roop Kaw and Charles Bae

14. "Advancing" the Treatment of Obstructive Sleep Apnea   123
    Mandibular Advancement Surgery for Obstructive Sleep Apnea
    Sally Ibrahim and Robert Armstrong

15. The Case of the Windblown Bus Driver   130
    Upper Airway Surgery in Adults with Obstructive Sleep Apnea
    Alan Kominsky

16. No Sleep for the Squeaky Infant   136
    Laryngomalacia as a Cause of Obstructive Sleep Apnea
    Rahul Seth, Jyoti Krishna, and Paul Krakovitz

17. For this Teen, Life Begins after OSA!   144
Pediatric Obstructive Sleep Apnea—Diagnostic Criteria, Identification and Treatment of High Risk Patients
Jennifer Sciuva and Jyoti Krishna

18. This Thing Is Impossible!   151
Positive Airway Pressure Troubleshooting in Adults with Sleep Apnea
Loutfi Aboussouan, Zakk Zahand, and Petra Podmore

19. Of Broken Homes, Chocolate, and Apnea   160
Pediatric Obstructive Sleep Apnea and Obesity
Jennifer Sciuva and Jyoti Krishna

20. Oral Appliance Lets Teen Sleep Easy   165
Oral Appliances for the Treatment of Obstructive Sleep Apnea
Flavia Sreshta

21. Desaturating, but Why?   173
Sleep Related Hypoxemia Due to Pulmonary Arterial Hypertension
Nattapong Jaimchariyatam and Omar Minai

22. Keeping Up with the 20-Somethings   180
Sleep Related Hypoxemia Due to Chronic Obstructive Pulmonary Disease and Obstructive Sleep Apnea
Nattapong Jaimchariyatam and Omar Minai

23. A Teen with Sleep Apnea sans Acid Maltase: A Tale with a Twist   186
Obstructive Sleep Apnea and Pompe Disease
Nattapong Jaimchariyatam, Loutfi Aboussouan, and Jyoti Krishna

Hypersomnias

24. It's No Joking Matter   191
Narcolepsy with Cataplexy
Catherine Griffin, Silvia Neme-Mercante, and Nancy Foldvary-Schaefer

25. When Dormant Issues Awaken, Waking Patients Sleep!   203
Narcolepsy Due to Brain Neoplasm: Craniopharyngioma
Roxanne Valentino and Farid Talih

26. Basic Instincts: Hungry, Sleepy, and Misbehaving   209
Klein-Levin Syndrome
Craig Brooker and Prakash Kotagal

27. An Over-the-Counter Recipe for Getting through Medical School   215
Idiopathic Hypersomnia with Long Sleep Time
Nattapong Jaimchariyatam and Kumar Budur

28. Another Cup of Joe for Jacquie   221
    Behaviorally Induced Insufficient Sleep Syndrome
    Nattapong Jaimchariyatam and Kumar Budur

29. Tackling Teenage Hypersomnia: "Joint" Partners Required   227
    Hypersomnia Due to Drug Use
    Jennifer Sciuva, Kumar Budur, and Jyoti Krishna

Circadian Rhythm Sleep Disorders

30. More Stimulants, Please   233
    Delayed Sleep Phase Disorder—Evaluation of Hypersomnia
    Carlos Rodriguez

31. How Shall I Wake? Let Me Count the Alarms   239
    Delayed Sleep Phase Disorder—Diagnosis and Management
    William Novak

32. A Machinist Who Could Not Take Shift Work Anymore   246
    Shift Work Disorder
    Kumar Budur

33. Why Humans Don't Have Wings   252
    Jet Lag
    William Novak

Parasomnias

34. The Case of Hobbling José   257
    Confusional Arousals and Sleepwalking
    Asim Roy, Silvia Neme-Mercante, and Nancy Foldvary-Schaefer

35. Young, Terrified, and Does Not Even Know It!   266
    Sleep Terrors
    Anna Irwin and Jyoti Krishna

36. Catch Me if You Can   272
    REM Sleep Behavior Disorder
    Silvia Neme-Mercante and Alon Avidan

37. Peter and the Wolf   278
    Obstructive Sleep Apnea Mimicking REM Sleep Behavior Disorder—
    "Pseudo RBD"
    Carlos Rodriguez

38. Why Can't John Go to a Slumber Party?   283
    Sleep Enuresis
    Jennifer Sciuva and Jyoti Krishna

39. Not Tonight, Dear   287
    Sexsomnia
    Craig Brooker and Nancy Foldvary-Schaefer

40. The Midnight Raider   293
    Sleep Related Eating Disorder
    Stella Baccaray and Nancy Foldvary-Schaefer

41. The Case of the Sick Coyote   299
    Sleep Related Groaning (Catathrenia)
    Madeleine Grigg-Damberger and Nancy Foldvary-Schaefer

Sleep Related Movement Disorders

42. When More Is Less   304
    Restless Legs Syndrome—Diagnosis and Treatment
    Joyce Lee-Iannotti and Charles Bae

43. They Call Me "Twinkle Toes"   311
    Secondary Restless Legs Syndrome
    Ai Ping Chua, Li Ling Lim, and Nancy Foldvary-Schaefer

44. A 52-Year-Old Man with Flying Legs at Night   320
    Periodic Limb Movement Disorder
    Fahd Zarrouf and Kumar Budur

45. The Woman Who Moved Her Feet with a Beat   325
    Hypnogenic Foot Tremor and Alternating Leg Muscle Activation
    Sally Ibrahim and Roxanne Valentino

Sleep Disorders Associated with Other Conditions

46. Sleepless in Kalamazoo   330
    Nocturnal Frontal Lobe Epilepsy
    Silvia Neme-Mercante and Nancy Foldvary-Schaefer

47. Seizures and Stimulators and Sleep, Oh My!   339
    Temporal Lobe Epilepsy and Vagus Nerve Stimulation
    Joanna Fong, Charles Bae, Kwang Ik Yang, and Nancy Foldvary-Schaefer

48. The Boy Who Seized Every Time He Slept   349
    Continuous Spike Waves during NREM Sleep (CSWS)
    Tobias Loddenkemper and Prakash Kotagal

49. The Case of the "Sleepy Stiff"   357
    Sleep Disturbances in Parkinson's Disease
    Jessica Vensel-Rundo and Carlos Rodriguez

50. It's Never Too Late, or Is It?   365
    Sleep and Dementia
    William Novak

51. "Mom, I Have a Bad Headache, I'm Tired, and I Can't Go to School"   369
    Sleep and Headache
    David Rothner

52. A Stroke of Bad Luck   375
    Sleep Disorders in Stroke Patients
    Maha Alattar and Joyce Lee-Iannotti

Appendices   381
Glossary   397
Index   403

Abbreviations

AED	Antiepileptic drug
AF	Atrial fibrillation
AHI	Apnea-hypopnea index
ALMA	Alternating leg muscle activation
ANA	Antinuclear antibody
ASV	Adaptive servo-ventilation
BDI	Beck Depression Inventory
BMI	Body mass index
BNP	Brain natriuretic peptide
CBC	Complete blood count
CBTi	Cognitive behavioral therapy for insomnia
CMP	Complete metabolic panel
CPAP	Continuous positive airway pressure
CSA	Central sleep apnea
CSF	Cerebrospinal fluid
CSR	Cheyne Stokes respiration
CT	Computerized tomography
DLMO	Dim light melatonin onset
DSPD	Delayed sleep phase disorder
ECG	Electrocardiogram
ECHO	Echocardiogram
EDS	Excessive daytime sleepiness
EEG	Electroencephalogram
EMG	Electromyogram
EPAP	Expiratory positive airway pressure
ESR	Erythrocyte sedimentation rate
ESS	Epworth Sleepiness Scale
$EtCO_2$	End tidal carbon dioxide

FDA	U.S. Food and Drug Administration
FFL	Flexible fiberoptic laryngoscopy
FSS	Fatigue Severity Scale
GABA-BDZ	Gamma-amino butyric acid, benzodiazepine
HF	Heart failure
HFT	Hypnagogic foot tremor
ICD	Implantable cardioverter defibrillator
ICSD-2	The International Classification of Sleep Disorders: 2nd edition
IPAP	Inspiratory positive airway pressure
IRLS rating scale	International Restless Leg Syndrome Study Group rating scale
ISI	Insomnia Severity Index
LVEF	Left ventricle ejection fraction
MI	Myocardial infarction
min	Minutes
MMA	Maxillomandibular advancement
MMSE	Mini Mental Status Examination
mPAP	Mean pulmonary arterial pressure
MRA	Mandibular repositioning appliance
mRAP	Mean right atrial pressure
MRI	Magnetic resonance imaging
MSA	Mixed sleep apnea
MSLT	Multiple sleep latency test
MVO^2	Mixed venous oxygen saturation
N-CPAP	Nasal continuous positive airway pressure
NCS	Nerve conduction study
NIDDM	Non-insulin dependent diabetes mellitus
NPPV	Noninvasive positive pressure ventilation
NREM	Non-rapid eye movement
NYHA FC	New York Heart Association Functional Class
OSA	Obstructive sleep apnea
OSAS	Obstructive sleep apnea syndrome
PAP	Positive airway pressure
PET	Positron emission tomography
PLMAI	Periodic limb movement arousal index
PLMD	Periodic limb movement disorder
PLMI	Periodic limb movement index
PLMS	Periodic limb movements in sleep
PSG	Polysomnogram
PTSD	Post traumatic stress disorder
PVR	Pulmonary vascular resistance
RBD	REM behavior disorder

REM	Rapid eye movement
RLS	Restless legs syndrome
RPR	Rapid plasma reagin test
SE	Sleep efficiency
SL	Sleep latency
SOREMPs	Sleep onset REM periods
SPECT	Single photon emission computed tomography
SpO$_2$	Oxygen saturation via pulse oximetry
SRBD	Sleep related breathing disorder
SSRI	Selective serotonin reuptake inhibitor
TCA	Tricyclic antidepressant
TIB	Time in bed
TMJ	Temporomandibular joint
TRT	Total record time
TSH	Thyroid stimulating hormone
TST	Total sleep time
VEEG	Video electroencephalography
WASO	Wake after sleep onset

Contributor List

Loutfi Aboussouan, MD
Respiratory and Neurological Institutes
Cleveland Clinic Sleep Disorders Center
Beachwood, OH

Kamala Adury, MD, FAASM
Summit Behavioral Health Group
Akron, OH

Maha Alattar, MD
Director of the Stroke Program
Sleep and Wake Disorders Center of Fredericksburg
Mary Washington Healthcare
Fredericksburg, VA

Zahr Alsheikhtaha, MD, RPSGT
Cleveland Clinic Sleep Disorders Center
Cleveland, OH

Noah Andrews, RPSGT
Cleveland Clinic Sleep Disorders Center
Cleveland, OH

Robert Armstrong, DMD
Eastern Carolina Oral & Maxillofacial Surgery
Jacksonville, NC

Kathleen Ashton, PhD
Cleveland Clinic Sleep Disorders Center
Cleveland, OH

Alon Avidan MD, MPH
Associate Professor of Neurology
Neurology Residency Program Director
Director, UCLA Neurology Clinic
Associate Director, Sleep Disorders Center
UCLA, Department of Neurology
Los Angeles, CA

Stella Baccaray, RN
Cleveland Clinic Sleep Disorders Center
Cleveland, OH

Charles Bae, MD
Assistant Professor of Medicine, Cleveland Clinic Lerner College of Medicine
Cleveland Clinic Sleep Disorders Center
Neurological Institute
Cleveland, OH

Craig Brooker, MD
Cleveland Clinic Neurological Institute
Department of Neurology
Cleveland, OH

Kumar Budur, MD, MS
Assistant Professor, Cleveland Clinic Lerner College of Medicine
Cleveland Clinic Sleep Disorders Center
Medical Director: Neuroscience (Current)
Takeda Global Research and Development
Lake Forest, IL

Ai Ping Chua, MD
Cleveland Clinic Sleep Disorders Center
Department of Pulmonary, Allergy, and Critical Care Medicine
Cleveland, OH

Bruce Cohen, MD
Professor of Medicine, Cleveland Clinic Lerner College of Medicine
Center for Pediatric Neurology
Cleveland, OH

Michelle Drerup, Psy.D., C.BSM
Clinical Assistant Professor of Medicine, Cleveland Clinic Lerner College of Medicine
Cleveland Clinic Sleep Disorders Center
Cleveland, OH

Nancy Foldvary-Schaefer, DO
Associate Professor of Medicine, Cleveland Clinic Lerner College of Medicine
Director, Sleep Disorders Center
Cleveland Clinic Neurological Institute
Cleveland, OH

Joanna Fong, MD
Department of Neurology
Cleveland Clinic Epilepsy Center
Cleveland, OH

Catherine Griffin, MD
Cleveland Clinic Sleep Disorders Center
Department of Neurology
Cleveland, OH

Madeleine Grigg-Damberger, MD
Professor of Neurology
Department of Neurology
University of New Mexico
Albuquerque, NM

Sally Ibrahim, MD
Cleveland Sleep Disorders Center
Neurological Institute
Cleveland, OH

Anna Irwin, MD
Cleveland Clinic Neurological Institute
Department of Neurology
Cleveland, OH

Nattapong Jaimchariyatam, MD, MSc
Clinical and Research Instructor
Division of Pulmonary and Critical Care Medicine
Chulalongkorn University
Excellent Center for Sleep Disorders, King Chulalongkorn Memorial Hospital
Lumpini, Pathumwan, Bangkok, Thailand

Roop Kaw, MD
Assistant Professor of Medicine, Cleveland Clinic Lerner College of Medicine
Departments of Hospital Medicine (Medicine Institute) and Outcomes Research
(Anesthesiology Institute)
Cleveland Clinic
Cleveland, OH

Alan H. Kominsky, MD, FACS
Head and Neck Institute
Cleveland Clinic Sleep Disorders Center
Cleveland, OH

Prakash Kotagal, MD
Section Head, Pediatric Epilepsy
Cleveland Clinic Neurological Institute
Cleveland, OH

Paul Krakovitz, MD
Assistant Professor of Surgery, Cleveland Clinic Lerner College of Medicine
Section Head of Pediatric Otolaryngology
Cleveland Clinic
Cleveland, OH

Jyoti Krishna, MD
Head, Pediatric Sleep Medicine
Assistant Professor, Cleveland Clinic Lerner College of Medicine
Cleveland Clinic Sleep Disorders Center
Neurological Institute
Cleveland, OH

Joyce Lee-Iannotti, MD
Cleveland Clinic Sleep Disorders Center
Department of Neurology
Cleveland, OH

Li Ling Lim, MBBS, MRCP, MPH
Medical Director & Consultant Neurologist
Singapore Neurology & Sleep Centre
Gleneagles Medical Centre
Singapore

Tobias Loddenkemper, MD
Assistant Professor of Neurology, Harvard Medical School
Division of Epilepsy and Clinical Neurophysiology
Children's Hospital Boston
Boston, MA

Vicky Luppa, APN
Cleveland Clinic Sleep Disorders Center
Cleveland, OH

Haralobos Mermigis, MD
General Army Hospital Sleep Disorders Center
Athens, Greece

Omar A. Minai, MD, FCCP
Department of Pulmonary, Allergy, and Critical Care Medicine
Cleveland Clinic Sleep Disorders Center
Cleveland, OH

Silvia Neme-Mercante, MD
Cleveland Clinic Sleep Disorders Center and Epilepsy Center
Cleveland Clinic Neurological Institute
Cleveland, OH

William Novak, MD
Akron Neurology, Inc.
Akron, OH

Petra Podmore, REEGT, RPSGT
Laboratory Manager, Cleveland Clinic Sleep Disorders Center
Department of Neurology
Cleveland, OH

Margaret Mary Richards, PhD, ABPP
Cleveland Clinic Children's Hospital
Center for Pediatric Behavioral Health
Cleveland, OH

Carlos Rodriguez, MD
Program Director, Sleep Medicine Fellowship
Cleveland Clinic Sleep Disorders Center
Department of Neurology
Cleveland, OH

A. David Rothner, MD
Center for Pediatric Neurology
Cleveland Clinic Neurological Institute
Cleveland, OH

Asim Roy, MD
Assistant Clinical Professor
Division of Neurology and Sleep Medicine
University of Pittsburgh Physicians
Pittsburgh, PA

Jennifer Sciuva, MSN, PNP
Cleveland Clinic Sleep Disorders Center
Cleveland, OH

Rahul Seth, MD
Cleveland Clinic, Head and Neck Institute
Cleveland, OH

Julianne Sliwinski, RPSGT
Cleveland Clinic Sleep Disorders Center
Cleveland, OH

Flavia Sreshta, DDS
Assistant Professor of Comprehensive Care
Case Western Reserve University School of Dentistry
Marymount Hospital
Garfield Heights, OH

Inga Sriubiene, MD
Sleep Medicine of Lakeland
St. Joseph, MI

Farid Talih, MD
Co-Director of Psychiatry and Sleep Disorders
Ashtabula County Medical Center
Ashtabula, OH

Roxanne Valentino, MD
Medical Director, St. Thomas Health Services Center for Sleep
Tennessee Neurology Specialists
Nashville, TN

Jessica Vensel-Rundo, MD
Cleveland Clinic Sleep Disorders Center
Department of Neurology
Cleveland, OH

Kwang Ik Yang, MD
Associate Professor of Neurology
Department of Neurology, College of Medicine
Soonchunhyang University Cheonan Hospital
Cheonan, Korea

Zakk Zahand, RPSGT
Cleveland Clinic Sleep Disorders Center
Cleveland, OH

Mia Zaharna, MD
Stanford University School of Medicine
Redwood City, CA

Fahd Zarrouf, MD
AnMed Health
Lung and Sleep Center
Anderson, SC

Ancillary Videos

The following videos, as referenced throughout the text as "(see video 1)," for example, can be found at www.oup.com/us/sleepdisordersccf

1. **Chapter 15 Video 1:** This video shows an almost complete collapse, in a sphincter-like fashion, of the patient's airway on videolaryngoscopy.
2. **Chapter 15 Video 2:** This video shows complete obstruction of the patient's airway due to enlarged tonsils.
3. **Chapter 16 Video 1:** Video showing laryngomalacia on laryngoscopy.
4. **Chapter 24 Video 1:** The video illustrates a cataplexy attack in a woman with narcolepsy that occurred in between naps of an MSLT.
5. **Chapter 35 Video 1:** All three videos show a variety of brief parasomnia events in a child admitted for PSG and seizure monitoring. Video 1 shows an abrupt arousal from sleep and further perpetuation with maternal stimulus.
6. **Chapter 35 Video 2:** Video 2 shows an abrupt arousal apparently precipitated by the stimulus of touch as the mother reaches across the sleeping child to place her glasses on the table. Note the resumption of sleep after the brief confused agitation.
7. **Chapter 35 Video 3:** Video 3 shows abrupt spontaneous sleep terror from deep sleep and resumption of sleep afterward.
8. **Chapter 36 Video 1:** Representative episode of dream enactment in an elderly male with RBD and sleep apnea (note he was using continuous positive airway pressure therapy).
9. **Chapter 41 Video 1:** The video shows a one-minute tracing from the polysomnogram accompanied by audio. Note the groaning and moaning coinciding with chin and snore artifact on the tracing characteristic of catathrenia.
10. **Chapter 43 Video 1:** Restless legs recorded during PSG in a female patient. Note the repetitive repositioning and leg movements as well as

rubbing of the thighs, a form of counterstimulation. The patient appears frustrated and sleepy.

11. **Chapter 43 Video 2:** Periodic jerks of the legs, arm and trunk during stage N2 sleep in a patient with RLS. The movements are stereotyped and the inter-jerk interval is stable in the range of 22 to 25 second intervals.

12. **Chapter 44 Video 1:** Video clip showing frequent, periodic limb movements during sleep.

13. **Chapter 45 Video 1:** Video during PSG demonstrating repetitive foot movements alternating from left to right prior to sleep onset.

14. **Chapter 45 Video 2:** Hypnagogic foot tremor and alternating leg muscle activation. Note the repetitive, rhythmic movements alternating from left to right.

15. **Chapter 46 Video 1:** Typical seizure recorded during the non-invasive VEEG evaluation. Note the patient arouses from sleep and within a few seconds exhibits body shifting followed by turning to the left and pronation. She holds the bed rail and seems to shake. She then assumes her previous body position in bed and is hyperventilating. She responds immediately after the end of the seizure and recalls the word given to her during the seizure.

16. **Chapter 46 Video 2:** Typical seizure recorded during the invasive VEEG evaluation. Note that the seizure semiology is nearly identical to that of the non-invasive evaluation. At the end of the seizure, there are subtle clonic movements of the right hand supporting left hemisphere seizure origin. This degree of stereotypy between events is strongly supportive of epilepsy.

17. **Chapter 47 Video 1:** Temporal lobe seizure arising from the left hippocampal formation. Within a few seconds of arousal, the patient begins to exhibit audible oral automatisms (lip smacking). When the technologist enters the room, he is staring and unresponsive and does not follow commands. At the end of the seizure, he returns to sleep. The ictal EEG is shown in Figure 47.4.

18. **Chapter 48 Video 1:** The video clip shows a representative myoclonic seizure involving the axial musculature. The child becomes unresponsive and has a blank stare during the event. Repetitive jerks of the trunk are observed.

A Case a Week
Sleep Disorders from the Cleveland Clinic

Introduction to the Sleep Clinic

KUMAR BUDUR, MD, MS
NANCY FOLDVARY-SCHAEFER, DO
JYOTI KRISHNA, MD

As far as medical specialties are concerned, sleep medicine is the new kid on the block! Perhaps more than any other, sleep medicine is based on a multidisciplinary approach, routinely interfacing with neurology, pulmonology, psychiatry, psychology, internal medicine, pediatrics, otolaryngology, dentistry, and maxillofacial surgery. Each subspecialty brings its own perspective and adds its unique flavor to the evaluation and treatment of patients with sleep disorders.

Over the past 4 decades, sleep medicine has made significant advances. Indeed, culminating years of research and consensus refinement, the American Academy of Sleep Medicine (AASM) has recently published the second edition of the International Classification of Sleep Disorders (ICSD-2), which describes epidemiology, pathophysiology, and diagnostic criteria of more than 80 sleep disorders. Concomitantly, training in sleep medicine has undergone a transformation—from a loosely organized curriculum to highly structured fellowship programs that are now defined and monitored by the Accreditation Council for Graduate Medical Education (ACGME). Together, this evolution has resulted in the recognition of sleep medicine as a discipline in its own right by the American Board of Medical Specialties (ABMS).

The goals of this chapter are:

A. To overview clinical evaluation, including history taking and examination of patients with sleep complaints.
B. To discuss the most commonly used screening tools in the sleep clinic, and
C. To introduce the reader to the classification of sleep disorders.

The reader is cautioned that the clinical methods and assessment tools described herein, though commonly used, reflect our own perspective. As such, this chapter is not intended to serve as an unequivocal blueprint of clinical sleep practice. Rather, it is our hope that readers will be encouraged to explore information from other comprehensive resources and customize their method in the context of their own unique clinical setting and the demographic peculiarities of the populations they serve.

Clinical Evaluation

A detailed sleep history is the most important initial step in the evaluation of sleep disorders. If possible, the assessment should begin even before the patient is seen in the clinic with the help of a sleep log maintained for a period of time prior to the initial visit. In comparison to a retrospective history in the clinic, this method offers an insight into typical sleep-wake patterns in a prospective, and likely more representative manner.

Patients with sleep disorders usually present with the complaints of inability to get adequate quantity or quality of sleep and/or excessive daytime sleepiness. A detailed history regarding symptom onset, duration, course, precipitants, relieving factors, impact on daytime functioning, and social implications is *sine qua non* for further direction in the evaluation process. It is vital to elicit the patient's attitudes and beliefs about "normal" sleep, obtain a description of the sleeping environment, and gather relevant information about past medical, surgical, family, and social history. Analysis of current medications is pertinent since, unbeknownst to the patient or his primary care physician, pharmaceuticals may influence sleep patterns as well as impact the planning and interpretation of sleep testing. Many of these issues are expanded below and in the case discussions in the ensuing pages.

Sleep History

The sleep history includes a review of sleep habits, nighttime behaviors, and daytime functioning.

Sleep Habits   Pertinent information in this category includes habitual sleep and wake times during workdays and non-workdays, ideal (i.e., patient's preferred) sleep-wake schedule, preferred sleeping position, activities prior to going to bed (reading, writing, watching TV, eating), and the length of time taken to fall asleep. The number and cause of awakenings during the major sleep period, time taken to return to sleep after awakening, and average number of sleep hours per night should be recorded. The sleep history should address psychological factors such as tension, anxiety, racing thoughts, worries, and feelings of depression that may interfere with sleep onset or continuity. It is useful to know if sleep is improved in alternative sleeping environments (say, on vacation), by use of relaxation techniques or other interventions. A survey of the sleep environment, including ambient light, temperature, electronic devices, and bedroom comfort, is important. Focused questioning sometimes reveals that the patient is sleeping on a couch, sharing the bed with pets, or simply has no "real bedroom" due to socio-economic constraints or poor sleep habits.

Nighttime Behaviors Although sleep is assumed to be a time of rest with relatively few physical movements, this is not necessarily true in patients with sleep disorders. Useful information in this context includes a history of snoring, shallow breathing, or respiratory pauses during sleep. There may be complaints of awakening from snorting, choking or gasping for air; morning headaches, sore throat or dry mouth may accompany. Other nighttime symptoms worth inquiring about include an urge to move the legs either before falling asleep or during awakenings at night, leg jerks, or kicking during sleep. Pertinent details of unusual behaviors during sleep such as sleepwalking, sleep talking, sleep related eating, seizures or potentially injurious dream enactment should be sought. Attention to the timing of events relative to sleep onset, as well as event description, frequency and stereotypy are important factors to elicit.

Daytime Functioning Information on daytime consequences and impairment is critical in establishing the diagnosis of some sleep disorders as well as assessing their impact on social, academic and occupational functioning. This includes an evaluation of excessive sleepiness or fatigue, daytime naps including the frequency, timing, and duration on workdays and non-workdays, and whether naps are refreshing. Further, a history of sleepiness leading to motor vehicle accidents or near-miss incidents, occupational injury, and impaired work or academic performance is important to elicit, as is the use of caffeine, and illicit drugs. A history of sudden weakness with laughter, surprise, or anger (cataplexy), feeling paralyzed whilst falling asleep or upon waking up (sleep paralysis), or hallucinations at sleep onset or offset (hypnagogic or hypnopompic hallucinations) are vital to diagnose narcolepsy. Since some disorders of sleepiness are cyclical or secondary to central nervous system disorders including trauma, it is important to elicit these details. Frequently, sleepiness emerges with the development of snoring or weight gain, and this may heighten suspicion of sleep related breathing disorders.

Medical and Surgical History

A general history, with special focus on disorders that are relevant to sleep, is required. This includes an assessment of cardiovascular disease (hypertension, angina, heart failure), pulmonary disorders (asthma, emphysema, chronic bronchitis), otolaryngological problems (sinus diseases, nasal fracture, deviated nasal septum, tonsillomegaly, nasal allergies), metabolic disorders (obesity, diabetes, hypercholesterolemia, hypothyroidism) and gastrointestinal disorders (heartburn, gastroesophageal reflux). Screening for neurological disorders (headaches, degenerative disorders, epilepsy, cerebrovascular disease, multiple sclerosis, peripheral nerve disorders) and psychiatric illnesses (depression, anxiety, panic disorder, bipolar disorder) is also recommended. A psychological assessment may be required to assess for common psychological disorders that often co-exist with sleep disorders, including mood disorders, anxiety disorders, adjustment disorders, and substance abuse. Pertinent surgical history may include questions regarding upper airway interventions, including but not limited to nasal surgery, adeno-tonsillectomy or uvulopalatopharyngoplasty (UPPP).

Medication History

Careful attention to medications, including prescription and over-the-counter products as well as herbal supplements is a vital part of the sleep history. Many medications cause or exacerbate sleep disturbances. Drugs such as beta blockers, serotonin re-uptake inhibitors, dopamine re-uptake inhibitors, thyroid supplements, and corticosteroids can cause or worsen insomnia. Similarly, medications such as tricyclic antidepressants, serotonin re-uptake inhibitors, and diphenhydramine can trigger or worsen symptoms of restless legs syndrome. Some medications like sedating antidepressants, anti-epileptics, muscle relaxants, or antihistamines contribute to daytime sleepiness.

Family History

A focused family sleep history is an important part of the sleep history, since many sleep disorders are believed to have a genetic basis. Further, due to similarities in body habitus, dietary and psychosocial factors, many sleep disorders cluster in families. In general, it is also useful to elicit a history of significant medical or psychiatric disorders in family members.

Social History

Knowledge of the nature and hours of occupation, including shift work, use of tobacco, caffeine, alcohol, illicit drugs, special diets, and exercise (when, how long, and how often) helps in better understanding a patient's sleep complaints. Marital status, relationship history, and psychosocial stressors should also be elicited.

Physical Examination

A general physical examination and focused upper airway, neck, cardiac, pulmonary, and neurologic examination should be performed in all patients presenting to the sleep clinic. Patients with sleep disorders who are regularly deprived of adequate sleep often appear irritable, tired or sleepy, and they may yawn or even doze off in the exam room. Severe sleep deprivation can cause gait disturbances, ptosis and dysarthria.

Vital signs including pulse rate, blood pressure, respiratory rate and oxygen saturation, as well as anthropometric measurements including height, weight and neck circumference should be recorded and body mass index (BMI) should be derived. Some disorders, such as sleep apnea and restless legs syndrome, may be associated with hypertension, while patients with insomnia due to anxiety disorder may present with elevated heart rate, blood pressure, and respiratory rate. BMI and neck circumference are particularly important in patients with sleep related breathing disorders since elevated BMI ($>25 \, \text{kg/m}^2$) and large neck girth (≥ 16 inches in women and ≥ 18 inches in men) are often seen in patients with obstructive sleep apnea (OSA).

A detailed upper airway examination is important in patients with suspected sleep apnea. The exam begins with inspection of the exterior of the nose (signs of fracture, deformity) and nasal cavity (septal deviation, polyps, turbinate hypertrophy). The oral examination is conducted with the patient's mouth wide open and the tongue resting inside the mouth in normal position. The tongue position relative to the palate and the tonsils is graded and the posterior pharyngeal space is staged based on the combination of findings (refer to Chapter 15 for details).

Clues to cardiopulmonary disorders include dyspnea, orthopnea, abnormal oximetry, tachycardia, abnormal peripheral pulses, pedal edema, basal pulmonary rales, wheezing, barrel-shaped chest, cyanosis, and digital clubbing. These are more often seen in patients with sleep apnea. It is not uncommon, however, to see patients with heart failure presenting to the sleep clinic with a complaint of insomnia.

Since sleep disorders are commonly encountered in patients with a range of neurologic disorders, an assessment of mental status, cranial nerves, motor and sensory function, deep tendon reflexes, and coordination including gait is suggested. For the sleep clinic patient without a history of neurologic disease, these domains can be readily assessed (e.g. a patient who provides a detailed history and interacts appropriately has demonstrated himself to be oriented, with largely intact attention and concentration, good fund of knowledge and memory and intact speech and language.) Of particular importance is to assess for disorders compromising facial, pharyngeal and tongue strength and mobility, general muscle strength, tone and coordination, sensory or motor loss in the distal extremities suggestive of a peripheral neuropathy, adventitious motor activity (tremor, abnormal movements) as seen in patients with neurodegenerative disorders, and focal or localized neurological deficits suspicious for stroke or other central nervous system dysfunction.

Evaluating Children

It often comes as a surprise to many that children may suffer from a wide range of sleep disorders similar to adults. Therefore, much of what has been said above also applies to children. A few disorders are unique to childhood and deserve special attention. Other conditions deserve mention due to peculiarities that may be important to bear in mind at the time of a sleep-focused evaluation of a child or teen.

Behavioral insomnia of childhood comes in the form of the sleep onset association type and the limit-setting type. In the former, the child has inappropriate and strong reliance on routines and processes that help with sleep initiation. These are generally also required to be present at the time of any nocturnal awakenings in order to help resume sleep (i.e., bottle feeding, rocking to sleep, co-sleeping). In the latter, the major disrupter of smooth bedtime routines is the stalling behavior exhibited by the child with regard to bedtime rules (i.e., more TV, one more story, one more drink). These behaviors are disruptive for the parent and the child. The history should therefore focus on the details of the behavior and parental responses to the behavior, as well as a sense of how problematic the issue is. This should be placed in the context of reasonable, age-appropriate expectations. A sense of the family's social structure is essential to any intervention. One cannot, for instance, suggest behavioral changes to only one parent if the child shares time with parents who are separated. Nor is it feasible to use "cry-it-out" techniques in a household in which 5 people share 2 bedrooms and one parent is a shift worker. A grasp of why the sleep association came to be established in the first place may identify the precipitant, such as a hospital admission. Daytime temperament and behavior often feed into the limit-setting issues at night and have to be carefully elicited. Oppositional behaviors are often seen with one, but not another, caretaker (e.g. the child goes right to bed at nap time at daycare but never does this for the parents at home). The interventional path thus clarifies itself after a thorough social history.

Pediatric OSA is similar in concept to its adult counterpart, but some patterns of breathing (prolonged hypoventilation) and preservation of sleep architecture are unique. Children, moreover, have faster respiratory rates and different pulmonary dynamics, and thus a greater propensity to desaturate. They may exhibit paradoxical rib cage movements due to increased rib cage compliance or sleep in odd postures (hyperextended neck) to protect the airway. Large adenoids and tonsils, odd facial structure (Pierre Robin sequence, cleft palate, Down syndrome), gastroesophageal reflux (GER), metabolic disorders (hypothyroidism, mucopolysaccharidoses), obesity, prematurity at birth, and neuromuscular disorders all may predispose a child to OSA. Associated with childhood OSA may be failure to thrive, cardiovascular complications such as pulmonary hypertension, sleep enuresis, hyperactive behaviors, and decline in school performance. Thus, the history and exam should elicit the predisposing factors, as well as the complications associated with pediatric OSA.

Other disorders of respiration presenting in childhood include primary sleep apnea of infancy and the rare congenital central alveolar hypoventilation syndrome (CCHS). Primary sleep apnea of infancy is characterized by central, obstructive, or mixed apneas or hypopneas. Predisposing factors include prematurity, anemia, sepsis, GER, cardiopulmonary diseases, central nervous system (CNS) or metabolic disorders, and medications. The patient may present with an apparent life-threatening events (ALTE). Frequently, apnea of prematurity resolves by 40 to 44 weeks postconceptional age. CCHS is a rare disorder of central control of breathing, often associated with alterations in the PHOX2B gene. It usually presents in infancy, with or without apnea, and results in hypoventilation that is worse during sleep. A high index of suspicion is needed after metabolic, neuromuscular, and pulmonary disorders have been considered. Ventilatory support is commonly required. Associated features include Hirschsprung's disease, ocular abnormalities, autonomic instability, and neural crest tumors. The history and exam in an infant with sleep related breathing disorder therefore should, among other things, focus on the pregnancy, its complications, association of apneas with feeding, and infant neuromotor development in relation to post-conceptional age, as well as the baby's physical well-being and parenting environment, in order to try and elicit risks that may predispose to apnea. A high index of suspicion may lead to a diagnosis of child abuse.

Several other disorders of sleep present commonly, but not exclusively, in childhood, and some caveats are worth considering during the clinical interview. Pediatric restless legs syndrome (RLS) is similar to its adult counterpart, although young children often cannot describe their symptoms. In this event, a family history of RLS may lend support to the diagnosis. Importantly, sleep enuresis is not a consideration until the expected age of bladder maturity (5 years). It should be distinguished by history into the primary type (never achieved bladder control) or the secondary type (regression after achieving bladder control for at least 6 months), since etiologies of secondary enuresis including endocrine (diabetes insipidus), metabolic (diabetes mellitus), dietary (caffeine), respiratory (OSA), renal (conditions of hyposthenuria), or psychological (stress, child neglect) disorders must be excluded. Narcolepsy often begins in the second or third decade of life, but it has been reported as early as the first decade. It may be "monosymptomatic," presenting only with daytime sleepiness without cataplexy or hypnagogic phenomena. Narcolepsy may be associated with Prader-Willi syndrome and Neiman Pick disease Type C. Other disorders of sleepiness presenting in adolescence result from insufficient sleep, substance abuse, circadian phase delay, and Kleine-Levin syndrome. Several genetic and neurodevelopmental disorders have strong associations with a variety of sleep problems. Examples include the autism spectrum disorders (insomnia), attention deficit hyperactivity disorder (insomnia, OSA, periodic limb movements in sleep [PLMS]), Smith Magenis syndrome (inverted melatonin rhythm), achondroplasia (OSA), and William syndrome (PLMS). The history and examination should be judiciously tailored in this context.

Assessment Tools Commonly Used in the Sleep Clinic

Several questionnaires are used in sleep clinics to estimate the severity of sleepiness (Epworth Sleepiness Scale), fatigue (Fatigue Severity Scale), insomnia (Insomnia Severity Index), restless legs (International Restless Legs Syndrome Study Group Rating Scale), circadian preference (Horne-Ostberg Morningness-Eveningness Scale), and to monitor outcomes (Functional Outcome Sleep Questionnaire). These are but adjuncts to the sleep history. Sleep apnea screening tools, such as the Berlin and STOP questionnaires, are generally used by health care providers outside the sleep clinic setting. There are several validated pediatric instruments available, including some that are modified versions of adult questionnaires. Many of them are used primarily for research. For the interested reader an excellent discussion has been published by Luginbuehl and Bradley-Klug.

Epworth Sleepiness Scale (ESS)

The ESS is an 8-item, self-administered questionnaire that rates the chances of dozing off in 8 common situations of daily life. The patient is asked to estimate his/her chance of dozing on 8 items on a scale of 0 to 3; the higher the score, the sleepier the subject (Appendix I). While the ESS is widely used and well-validated, it is still a subjective assessment and some patients overestimate or underestimate the severity of daytime sleepiness. The ESS and the Multiple Sleep Latency Test (MSLT), the gold standard test to objectively assess daytime sleepiness in patients with narcolepsy, correlate though inconsistently.

Insomnia Severity Index (ISI)

The ISI is a 5-item, subjective survey used in screening and measuring treatment outcomes in patients with insomnia. It is a valid and reliable method of quantifying perceived difficulties with sleep (Appendix II).

Fatigue Severity Scale (FSS)

The FSS is a 9-item, subjective assessment that measures a subject's perceived level of fatigue and its impact on daily functioning. Although the FSS is not specifically validated in patients with sleep disorders, it is often used in sleep clinics to measure fatigue and monitor treatment effects (Appendix III).

Horne-Ostberg Morningness-Eveningness Scale

The Horne-Ostberg Morningness-Eveningness Scale is a 7-item, self-administered questionnaire that assesses circadian rhythms. The relative propensity of morningness-eveningness is used to identify patients with advanced phase or delayed phase tendencies (Appendix IV).

Functional Outcome Sleep Questionnaire (FOSQ)

The FOSQ is a 30-item, self-administered questionnaire designed to measure the impact of disorders of excessive sleepiness on activities of daily living by assessing the extent to which feeling sleepy or tired affects one's ability to carry out certain activities. This scale is also used to determine the extent to which these abilities improve after treatment. In validation studies, the FOSQ was able to discriminate between normal subjects and those seeking medical attention for a sleep problem.

The FOSQ comprises 5 dimensions: activity level, vigilance, intimacy and sexual relationships, general productivity, and social outcome. The responses are numbered from 0 to 4 (0: I don't do this activity for other reasons; 1: Yes, extreme difficulty; 2: Yes, moderate difficulty; 3: Yes, a little difficulty; and 4: No difficulty). The mean-weighted item score for each subscale is calculated and the subscale scores are totaled to produce a global score. Lower scores indicate greater dysfunction.

Patient Health Questionnaire-9 (PHQ-9)

The PHQ-9 is a 9-item, self-administered questionnaire used to screen for depression and monitor progress after treatment initiation. Depression-screening questionnaires (PHQ, Beck Depression Inventory, Hamilton Rating Scale for Depression) are often used in sleep clinics because of the significant co-morbidity of depression with sleep disorders such as insomnia and sleep apnea. The PHQ-9 is based on the diagnostic criteria for major depressive disorder in the Diagnostic and Statistical Manual of Mental Disorders, Fourth Edition (DSM-IV). Each item is scored on a scale of 0 to 3 and the total score ranges from 0 to 27 (Appendix V).

International Restless Legs Syndrome Study Group
Rating Scale (IRLS)

The IRLS Rating Scale is a validated, subjective scale used to rate the severity of restless legs symptoms. Each of the 10 items has 4 possible responses, with scores ranging from 0 to 4. The total score ranges from 0 to 40 (Appendix VI).

Classification of Sleep Disorders

The ICSD-2, published by the AASM in 2005, classifies disorders into 8 categories based on presenting symptoms (i.e., the hypersomnias), presumed etiology (i.e., circadian rhythm disorders), or the organ system(s) from which the primary problem originates (i.e., sleep related breathing disorders). Both adult and pediatric disorders are included; in the vast majority of the cases, the pediatric presentation is described within the general discussion of the disorder. Four pediatric-specific diagnoses are categorized separately, however, including behavioral insomnia of childhood, pediatric OSA, CCHS, and primary sleep apnea of infancy.

The major categories of the ICSD-2 are: (1) insomnias; (2) sleep related breathing disorders; (3) hypersomnias of central origin: not due to a circadian rhythm sleep disorder, sleep related breathing disorder, or other cause of disturbed nocturnal sleep; (4) circadian rhythm sleep disorders; (5) parasomnias; (6) sleep related movement disorders; (7) isolated symptoms, apparently normal variants and unresolved issues; and (8) other sleep disorders. The disorders within each of these categories are listed in Appendix VII.

Bibliography

Bastien CH, Vallieres A, Morin CM. Validation of the Insomnia Severity Index as an outcome measure for insomnia research. *Sleep Med.* 2001;2:297–307.

Friedman M, Ibrahim H, Lee G, Joseph NJ. Combined uvulopalatopharyngoplasty and radiofrequency tongue base reduction for treatment of obstructive sleep apnea/hypopnea syndrome. *Otolaryngol Head Neck Surg.* 2003;129(6):611–621.

Horne JA, Ostberg O. A self-assessment questionnaire to determine morningness-eveningness in human circadian rhythms. *Int J Chronobiol.* 1976;4:97–110.

Johns MW. A new method for measuring daytime sleepiness: the Epworth Sleepiness Scale. *SLEEP.* 1991;14 (6):540–545.

Krupp LB, LaRocca NG, Muir-Nash J, et al. The fatigue severity scale. Application to patients with multiple sclerosis and systemic lupus erythematous. *Arch Neurol.* 1989;46:1121–1123.

Luginbuehl M, Bradley-Klug KL. Assessment of sleep problems in a school setting or private practice. In: Ivanenko A, ed. Sleep and psychiatric disorders in children and adolescents. New York: NYL Informa Healthcare, 2008:109–138.

Netzer NC, Stoohs RA, Netzer CM, Clark K, Strohl KP. Using the Berlin Questionnaire to identify patients at risk for the sleep apnea syndrome. *Ann Intern Med.* 1999. Oct 5;131(7):485–491.

Spitzer R, Kroenke K, Williams J. Validation and utility of a self-report version of PRIME-MD: the PHQ Primary Care Study. *JAMA.* 1999; 282:1737–1744.

Walters AS, LeBrocq C, Dhar A, Hening W, Rosen R, Allen RP, Trenkwalder C; International Restless Legs Syndrome Study Group. Validation of the International Restless Legs Syndrome Study Group rating scale for restless legs syndrome. *Sleep Med.* 2003 Mar;4(2):121–132.

Weaver TE, Laizner AM, Evans LK, et al. An instrument to measure functional status outcomes for disorders of excessive sleepiness. *SLEEP.* 1997;30:835–843.

Introduction to the Sleep Laboratory

JYOTI KRISHNA, MD
NANCY FOLDVARY-SCHAEFER, DO
KUMAR BUDUR, MD, MS

The enigma of the phenomenon we know as "sleep" notwithstanding, standardization of how its normalcy or aberration can be measured is as important as the ensuing clinical question of how it may be intervened upon. To the lay person, nothing is more synonymous with a "sleep study" than the nocturnal polysomnogram (PSG). The PSG has come a long way since the first scalp EEG recordings were acquired in the earlier part of the last century. With humble beginnings of what can generally be termed the "bedroom observations" of relatively few physiological phenomena, the PSG has now blossomed into a complex technological marvel that measures a variety of neurophysiologic signals utilizing increasingly sophisticated means. Due to miniaturization and portability of equipment, it is now possible to do studies at the hospital bedside and even at the patient's home.

As of 2007, new guidelines for acquisition, scoring, and reporting of polysomnography data have been published by the American Academy of Sleep Medicine (AASM). These provide a reference point for quality standards based upon the latest scientific evidence and expert consensus, and they also allow for better comparison of data from one laboratory to another. While the intent of this chapter is not to discuss the detailed requirements for an accredited laboratory, certain technical specifications are now expected of commercially available polysomnography acquisition systems. Current models are capable of meeting all, or virtually all, of these standards. Similarly, scoring criteria for sleep staging, limb movements, hypoventilation, and respiratory events are now updated, and adherence to these revised standards is a requirement for accredited laboratories. In this chapter, we will briefly overview some of the common sleep tests. While a detailed discussion of the technique of polysomnography and other sleep testing procedures is beyond the scope of this chapter, certain basic points are highlighted for the benefit of the unfamiliar reader.

The Polysomnogram

The Basics

The PSG is useful for diagnosis of sleep related breathing disorders, unexplained nocturnal awakenings, unusual behavioral events in sleep, and excessive day-time sleepiness, and to assess efficacy of treatments for various sleep disorders. Polysomnography is not routinely indicated in patients with the primary insomnias or restless legs syndrome (RLS). However, sleep testing may be considered in patients with insomnia or RLS who fail to respond to conventional therapy when other co-morbid sleep disorders, such as sleep apnea, are suspected.

Traditionally, this is a multihour procedure that is performed in the sleep laboratory by a trained technologist. The "bedrooms" are designed to be comfortable and need to meet specifications set by the AASM for accredited facilities. The PSG typically is run overnight, usually for 6 to 8 hours or longer. It comprises an abbreviated electroencephalogram (EEG), electro-oculogram (EOG), and electromyogram (EMG) for the definition of wakefulness and various sleep stages. The recommended EMG derivations include 3 chin electrodes (middle, right, and left) and limb EMG (right and left anterior tibialis). The EKG consists of a single pair of electrodes (Lead II). It is recommended that abdomino-thoracic respiratory efforts be measured using calibrated or uncalibrated respiratory inductance plethsmography (RIP belts). Other physiologic parameters measured include oro-nasal airflow (via a thermistor and nasal pressure transducer), pulse oximetry, and body position monitoring, as well as snoring sounds and vocalizations (via microphone). Video monitoring (infra-red camera) in real time accompanies the recording (Figure I2.1).

While most of the "PSG hook-up" mentioned above is easy to conceptualize for the reader not trained in sleep medicine, the EEG may require some elaboration. The internationally accepted 10–20 system of electrode placement has long been used for EEG. The numbers "10" and "20" in this system allude to the measurements depicted as percentages of the circular arcs formed when imagining lines connecting bony landmarks such as the tip of the left mastoid (M1) through the vertex (Cz) to the opposite mastoid (M2), or the horizontal circle drawn to connect the nasion anteriorly and the inion posteriorly. Letters denote the area of the brain underlying (F = frontal; C = central; O = occipital). Odd numbers are used for the left and even numbers for the right side, while the letter "z" is used for saggital placements. An imaginary grid can thus be made and standard EEG placement points may be defined using letters and numbers (Figure I2.2). Stated simplistically, the EEG signal is essentially the digitally subtracted sum of

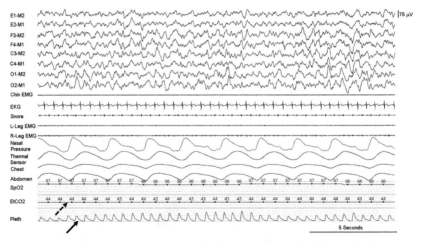

Figure I2.1 Typical 30 s epoch of a PSG showing recommended channels to measure eye movements, EEG, EMG, airflow, respiratory effort, and gas exchange. Note the end-tidal CO_2 (broken arrow) and plethysmogram from the pulse-oximeter (solid arrow). See text for discussion.

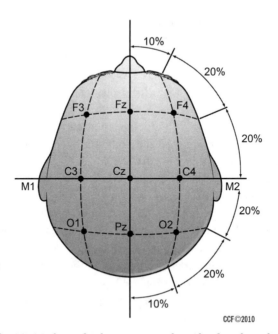

CCF©2010

Figure I2.2 The 10–20 electrode placement uses bony landmarks to form an imaginary grid on the skull to standardize electrode placement. Reprinted with permission, Cleveland Clinic Center for Art and Photography © 2010. All rights reserved.

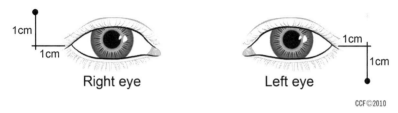

CCF©2010

Figure I2.3 The standard placement of the ocular leads is based on distance from the outer canthii. Reprinted with permission, Cleveland Clinic Center for Art and Photography © 2010. All rights reserved.

2 electrodes. By convention these "derivations" are defined by paired letters denoting the position of the electrode on the 10–20 grid. Thus, an EEG channel labeled "C3-M2" is the signal derived by subtracting the electrophysiologic signal recorded by the M2 from the C3 electrode. This pair of electrodes then results in one channel on the PSG labeled as C3-M2 by convention.

For most sleep laboratories dealing primarily with adult sleep related breathing disorders, the recommended EEG derivations include F4-M1, C4-M1 and O2-M1. Mirror image "back-up" electrodes (F3-M2, C3-M2 an O1-M2) are suggested to minimize interventions needed to "repair" fouled electrodes once the study is initiated. Alternate derivations have been suggested utilizing saggital placements. The recommended ocular channels utilize left-lower-lateral and right-upper-lateral positioning (Figure I2.3). The AASM recommends as an alternate a right and left lower-lateral placement for better delineation of the direction of eye movements.

Event Scoring in Polysomnography

The purpose of the PSG is to score nocturnal phenomena using the physiological data acquired during the study and to interpret these in relation to the patient's symptoms. The study is scored to delineate the sleep stages Wake (W), Rapid eye movement (REM), and the three nonrapid eye movement (NREM) stages N1, N2, and N3. Each of these stages is characterized by specific EEG, EOG, and EMG criteria (Table I2.1 and Figure I2.4).

Respiratory events are scored as primarily apneas or hypopneas. An apnea is scored if there is a 90% or greater reduction of the thermal sensor signal as compared to baseline for 10 seconds or longer. It is classified as obstructive if respiratory effort (RIP belts) continues during the cessation of oro-nasal airflow. An apnea is classified as central if there is a cessation of both airflow and respiratory effort. Mixed apneas have both central and obstructive components. In the recently revised AASM scoring guidelines, hypopneas are defined in one of 2 ways. A hypopnea is scored if the nasal pressure transducer signal decreases by 30% or more from baseline for at least 10 seconds accompanied by a desaturation that is at least 4% from baseline. Alternatively, a hypopnea is scored if the

Table I2.1 Polysomnographic characteristics of sleep stages seen in older children and adults (see also Figure I2.4)

Sleep Stage	Characteristic features
Wake	Alpha rhythm appears with eyes closed and is seen as trains of sinusoidal 8–13 Hz EEG waves over occipital leads that disappears with eye opening. Chin EMG is elevated and eye movements are rapid with blinks and reading/scanning activity.
N1	Slow sinusoidal eye movements on EOG (initial deflection >500 msecs) with low amplitude mixed frequency EEG activity in theta (4–7 Hz) range. Chin EMG varies but may be lower than wake. Vertex sharp waves may be seen in central leads but are not essential.
N2	K-complexes lasting at least 0.5 seconds comprising a sharp upward (negative) and immediate downward (positive) EEG deflection, most prominent over frontal and central areas of the head. These waves stand out from the background that is otherwise similar to theta activity of N1. Alternatively, sleep spindles (11–16 Hz) of distinct morphology lasting at least 0.5 seconds may be seen. Chin EMG is variable but usually lower than wake.
N3	Frontal dominant slow-wave EEG activity (0.5–2 Hz) with high amplitude (>75 microvolts) occupying more than 20% of the 30 second epoch. Chin EMG variable but usually lower than wake.
REM	Sharply peaked conjugate rapid eye movements on EOG (initial deflection <500 msecs). Chin EMG is the lowest among all stages for the entire recording (REM atonia). EEG background is mixed frequency and low amplitude with superimposed trains of 2–6 Hz irregular bursts of sharply serrated, "sawtooth" waves.

nasal pressure signal decreases by 50% or more from the baseline for at least 10 seconds and is associated with either a desaturation of at least 3% or an EEG arousal (illustrated in Chapters 10 and 17).

An arousal is scored in any stage of sleep when there is an abrupt change in EEG frequency including alpha, theta, or frequencies higher than 16 Hz. This definition excludes spindles and requires the frequency shift to persist for at least 3 seconds. For an arousal to be scored in stage REM, however, a concomitant increase in chin EMG is also required. To differentiate one arousal from another, a 10 second interval between 2 arousals is required.

Another commonly scored phenomenon is the periodic limb movement (PLM). A qualifying limb movement is scored when the limb EMG (most commonly anterior tibialis) amplitude increases by 8 microvolts over baseline for at least 0.5 seconds but no longer than 10 seconds. A PLM series is scored if 4 such movements occur in a row, provided each component LM occurs within 5 to 90 seconds of its neighbor (illustrated in Chapter 44).

By convention, the various events defined above are totaled once they have been scored throughout the PSG recording. The total occurrences are then

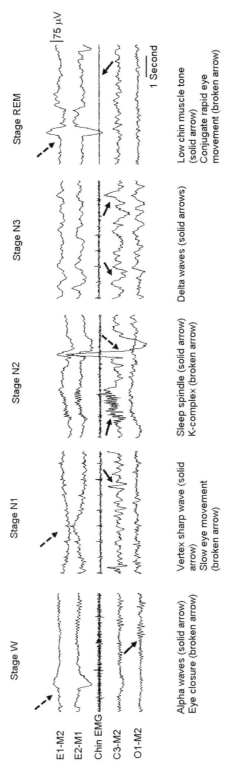

Figure 12.4 Collage of characteristic findings in various sleep stages seen beyond early infancy (See also Table 1).

averaged over the night to calculate the respective index. Thus, the apnea-hypopnea index (AHI) denotes the apneas and hypopneas per hour of the total sleep time recorded. The arousal and PLM indices are similarly reported in the data summary.

Most of the data can be reported in tabular form or it may also be displayed pictorially as a hypnogram (illustrated in Chapter 7).

Polysomnography in Special Situations

While detailed discussion of special cases is beyond the scope of this chapter, it is worthwhile to briefly mention that laboratories doing more sophisticated testing routinely make modifications to the "basic hook-up." For instance, respiratory parameters in children or patients with suspected hypoventilation (i.e. associated with obesity or neuromuscular disorders), are best studied with capnometry in place (end-tidal and/or transcutaneous CO_2).

Patients with unusual nocturnal behaviors may require specialized overnight PSGs to differentiate seizures and parasomnias. In such cases, expansion to an 18-channel EEG (full 10-20 system electrode placement) montage with the addition of extra limb leads may be required. Should unusual motor phenomena occur, trained staff should be at hand to perform immediate and appropriate intervention during the event to help delineate and appropriately document event semiology. Safety protocols have to be in place for complex potentially injurious behaviors. As a corollary, this also implies that the data acquisition equipment must be versatile enough to handle the demand for a substantially expanded montage with extra AC and DC channels.

In other instances, esophageal pH channel for suspected co-morbid reflux may be useful. Esophageal manometry may detect the presence of intermittent cycles of negative intrathoracic pressures for several successive breaths followed by relief of the negativity after an arousal as normal breathing resumes. These respiratory effort related arousal (RERA) events are the hallmark of upper airway resistance syndrome (UARS) wherein the classic apneas and hypopneas are absent in a patient otherwise symptomatic for obstructive sleep apnea (OSA).

Daytime studies often test the flexibility of staffing a busy sleep laboratory. Often, the timing of a sleep study in a person with circadian or shift work-related sleep disorder raises such challenges. Accommodating these needs with unconventional PSG start times may be key to a successful diagnostic outcome.

Portable Polysomnography

Sleep monitoring has been categorized into 4 types based upon the sophistication of data acquired. The Type-1 study described above refers to a PSG with 7 or more channels that is fully attended by a trained technologist in the laboratory setting. A similar but unattended study is termed Type-2 and such devices are now becoming available for home monitoring. The other so-called "portable studies" are unattended Type-3 studies with 4–7 channels including respiratory effort, airflow, heart rate, and oxygen saturation monitoring. Type-4 refers to unattended 1-or 2-channel studies, which usually include overnight oximetry. The Centers for Medicare and Medicaid Services (CMS) defines the Type 4 category a little differently, requiring a minimum of 3 channels that would allow direct or indirect measurement of the AHI or respiratory disturbance index (RDI). While accredited sleep centers have historically performed Type-1 studies, as a result of the 2008 CMS decision approving portable studies for the diagnosis of OSA, increasingly centers are incorporating Type 2 or 3 studies into their repertoire of services offered, as discussed in Chapter 11.

The Positive Airway Pressure (PAP) Titration Study

Aside from a diagnostic PSG, the second most common nighttime test is the positive airway pressure (PAP) titration study. The titration itself may be performed once the diagnostic PSG shows evidence of significant sleep apnea during the night. From here there are generally 2 choices. Often, one choice is to "split the night." This means that the second part of the PSG study is converted into a therapeutic trial of PAP. Certain criteria need to be met for the split-night study to be allowed. These criteria have been set forth by the Centers for Medicare and Medicaid Services (CMS) and can be accessed at http://www.cms.hhs.gov/mcd/search.asp. The guidelines state there should be sufficient sleep time and respiratory event frequency to convincingly diagnose sleep apnea. Further, there should be sufficient time left in the remainder of the night (typically 3 hours) to allow for a reasonable attempt at PAP titration. If these criteria are not met but sleep apnea is diagnosed, the alternate choice is to subsequently run a full-night titration study on a different night. As a corollary, the decision to do a split-night study requires that the nighttime technologist is vigilant in scoring the respiratory events as they happen and make the decision once criteria are met.

Successful PAP therapy requires optimal mask fitting and consideration of choice of pressure delivery modalities which may include continuous, bi-level or auto-adjusting positive airway pressure (CPAP, Bi-level PAP, Auto-PAP) as well as adaptive servo-ventilation (ASV) with or without supplemental oxygen. The titration of pressure settings during a study is both an art and a science. The experienced technologist should be able to titrate pressures up or down depending on the patient's response and is mindful of the effect of sleep stages as well as body position as titration progresses. He/she should thus be vigilant for mask leaks and intervene appropriately by adjusting the mask/interface, be ready to utilize a chin strap for mouth leaks, as well as encourage supine body position if possible. All this is done while minimizing sleep disruption and scoring for respiratory events in real time to help decision making for pressure changes. By no measure is this an easy task!

While a discussion of titration technique is beyond the scope of the chapter, the reader is directed to a recent publication describing this in detail (see references). With recognition of complex sleep apnea and availability of a multitude of oro-nasal interfaces and pressure delivery systems, a variety of therapeutic options are available to the patient with sleep related breathing disorders. These are discussed in the ensuing chapters of this book.

MSLT and MWT

Aside from overnight sleep studies, the accredited sleep laboratory is also equipped to run the multiple sleep latency test (MSLT) and often times the related maintenance of wakefulness test (MWT). These tests respectively measure tendency to sleep or ability to stay awake during the subjective daytime. Normative data are available for interpretation. The tests will be briefly overviewed here to familiarize the reader. Pitfalls and drawbacks of these tests are not discussed.

The MSLT and the MWT are daytime studies performed over several hours in the sleep laboratory with a trained technologist in attendance. The MSLT comprises 5 nap trials that are separated by 2-hour intervals, beginning 1.5 to 3 hours after the final morning awakening. It is usually preceded by an overnight PSG to ensure sufficient sleep time is documented and that no sleep related disorders such as sleep apnea syndromes are present to influence the daytime test results. Drug screens and sleep diaries are helpful as well. The MWT comprises four 40-minute trials that are separated by 2-hour intervals, also starting between 1.5–3 hours after waking up.

Since the purpose is simply to measure sleep onset and to define sleep stages, especially looking for REM onset in the case of MSLT, the montage is significantly truncated compared to the full PSG hook-up described earlier. Thus, only EEG, EOG, chin EMG and EKG are used during these tests.

For each of the 5 nap trials during the MSLT, the patient rests fully clothed in a bed in a quiet, darkened room and is instructed to try fall asleep. If the allotted 20 minutes are exhausted before any sleep is recorded, that particular nap opportunity is terminated and lights are turned back on. However, if sleep is recorded within the allotted time, the subject is allowed to sleep for a further 15 minutes to see if REM sleep can be recorded. For the period in between naps, there are specific standardized rules of conduct including limiting stimulating activity, smoking, and caffeine consumption.

Each trial of the MWT lasts for 40 minutes, during which time the patient is asked to try and remain awake while seated in a dimly lit room. The trials are ended if the patient does not fall asleep in 40 minutes, or if unequivocal sleep is recorded. Similar rules for patient activity and conduct apply between naps and the technologist is required to be vigilant that the test conditions are not compromised.

The sleep latency (measured from lights-out to first epoch of sleep) is calculated for each nap and then averaged over 5 naps (MSLT) or 4 naps (MWT) to give the mean sleep latency (MSL). REM sleep within 15 minutes of sleep onset in any nap is noted as a sleep onset REM period (SOREMP). Thus, in regard to the MSLT, a MSL less than 5 minutes is abnormal, 5 to 10 minutes is borderline, and more than 10 minutes is considered normal. Presence of 2 or more SOREMPs is supportive of the diagnosis of narcolepsy. Normative data are less robust for the MWT. In this case, MSL less than 8 minutes is generally considered abnormal and the ability to stay awake is best supported by absence of sleep in any of the 4 trials.

Actigraphy

Outside of traditional laboratory monitoring, the actigraph is an instrument that is now increasingly used in the characterization and diagnosis of sleep disorders. In the simplest sense, the actigraph is a motion sensor that monitors rest-activity data over prolonged periods of time, typically ranging between 3 to 14 days. As such, its accelerometer generated output can serve as a surrogate for the subject's sleep-wake cycle. Typically, the actigraph is used to study sleep patterns in normal individuals as well as patients with circadian rhythm disorders. It also finds use in monitoring response to therapy for insomnia and hypersomnia disorders. Usually a sleep log is simultaneously maintained by the patient and helps with analysis of the data, since actigraphy may overestimate sleep time and underestimate wake time. A complete discussion of evidence based indications for actigraphy was recently published by the AASM and its clinical application is further illustrated in some of the cases in this book (see Chapter 31).

Studying Children and Special Needs Patients

It is important to underscore the expertise needed for studying children and patients with special needs. While patience and understanding during hook-up is paramount, it is just as important that education and desensitization to a novel, and conceivably intimidating, sleep environment is offered during a clinic visit prior to the study itself. This generally requires significant planning and cooperation between daytime and nighttime staff. The décor of the clinic and sleep laboratory should be child oriented, with age-appropriate distractions and entertainment. The child's own teddy bear or familiar bed sheet may be invaluable items to bring along. It goes without saying that the technologist requires friendliness and foresight to allay the nervous child's anxiety or to gain the cooperation of the very hyperactive toddler. Often the hook-up needs to be "turned into a game." The technologist should be aware that the "face is hooked up last," and often this means saving the flow transducer until the child is in deep sleep. This may be helpful, too, for the special needs adult.

Children also are prone to generate more movement associated artifact than adults. Hence, redundancy in electrodes is a sine qua non of EEG lead placement, since extra leads are almost always useful in the smaller child. Similarly, a concurrent plethysmography signal with the oximetry is beneficial in "artifacting out bad data" before a significant desaturation is ascribed to a genuine physiological event (Figure I2.1).

Furthermore, children with sleep apnea tend to preserve their sleep architecture in comparison to adults. Not infrequently, they may exhibit obstructive-hypoventilation instead of the classical recurrent pattern of desaturations and arousals following airflow reductions as seen in adult sleep apnea. It is therefore recommended that children be studied with capnometry in place (Figure I2.1). The traditional scoring method for sleep stages needs modification in the case of neonates and infants. In neonates, typically the staging terms "active," "quiet," and "indeterminate" sleep are used, with active sleep being the equivalent of traditional REM sleep. Beyond the age of 2 months, the use of N1, N2, and N3 is encouraged if the usual criteria for these stages are met. However, if adequate slow waves, K-complexes or spindles are not seen, the generic terms Stage N and Stage R may simply be used to distinguish NREM and REM sleep from Stage W.

Other Tests

Innovative tools that will find increasing clinical application in the future include pulse transit time (PTT) and peripheral arterial tonometry (PAT). Sophisticated analyses of EEG including spectral distribution and cyclic alternating pattern (CAP) are primarily used in sleep research at this time. The nocturnal penile tumescence test (NPT) as well as the suggested immobilization test (SIT) may be used for testing impotence and restless legs syndrome, respectively. However, these are again more commonly used in the research setting.

Sleep Testing as a Tool

It is important to emphasize that the PSG, MSLT, actigraphy, and other sleep tests described above are but tools, and they should be used judiciously to answer a clinical question with adequate foresight and preparation. The clichéd phrase "garbage-in, garbage-out" applies just as much to sleep testing as it does to any bio-behavioral test. For example, if the snoring patient is suspected to have sleep apnea but happens also to be a shift worker, the PSG should be run at a time that matches the patient's usual sleep period. Otherwise, one runs the risk of not capturing enough sleep data to make a diagnosis. A neuromuscular patient with questionable lung function and declining daytime alertness may benefit from addition of overnight capnography to screen for hypoventilation. If there is suspicion of unusual sleep related motor phenomena such as dream enactment behavior, extra limb leads and perhaps, extra EEG leads should be requested.

Drugs often confound results of testing. The MSLT for example, should be planned after adequate period of withdrawal from REM-suppressing drugs and adequate attention to ensure any sleep debt from insufficient sleep in the near past is addressed. Selective serotonin re-uptake inhibitors (SSRIs) may increase limb movements in sleep and bias the scoring of REM sleep in a critical MSLT due to their effect in enhancing eye movements. These so-called "Prozac eyes" are well known in the sleep laboratory. Thus, many medications affect sleep architecture and may interfere with testing. It is optimal if the tests are run after discontinuation of as many medications as far in advance of testing as is safely possible after considering the time it may take to wash out their active metabolites. In the case of some SSRIs, this may mean weaning should begin weeks in advance.

Normative data for various sleep related parameters must take into consideration the patient's age. For instance, an apnea index greater than 1 may be abnormal in the younger child, but not in an adult. Similarly, it is essential to interpret the MSLT results in light of the Tanner stages of sexual maturity in children and adolescents.

The reader will find many more examples of such technicalities in the ensuing chapters. The point here is simply to acquaint the reader with the complexity of the process of appropriately preparing for, running, and interpreting a sleep study. The sleep test is relatively expensive and time consuming both for the patient and the laboratory. As such, before ordering the test, the physician should consider the impact of any medical, psychological or environmental factors on the study itself. While for the usual case of "suspected sleep apnea" a direct referral to a sleep laboratory for a PSG may suffice, a sleep-medicine consultation should be considered for the more complex case to increase diagnostic yield and efficiency of the process.

Bibliography

Collop NA, Anderson WM, Boehlecke B, Claman D, Goldberg R, Gottlieb DJ, Hudgel D, Sateia M, Schwab R. Clinical guidelines for the use of unattended portable monitors in the diagnosis of obstructive sleep apnea in adult patients. *J Clin Sleep Med.* 2007;3(7):737–747.

Iber C, Ancoli-Israel S, Chesson A, Quan SF, for the American Academy of Sleep Medicine. The AASM manual for the scoring of sleep and associated events:

Rules, terminology and technical specifications. 1st ed. Westchester, Ill: American Academy of Sleep Medicine; 2007.

Kushida CA, Chediak A, Berry RB, Brown LK, Gozal D, Iber C, Parthasarathy S, Quan SF, Rowley JA. Positive airway pressure titration task force of the American Academy of Sleep Medicine. Clinical guidelines for the manual titration of positive airway pressure in patients with obstructive sleep apnea. *J Clin Sleep Med.* 2008;4:157–171.

Kushida CA, Littner MR, Morgenthaler T, et al. Practice parameters for the indications for polysomnography and related procedures: An update for 2005. SLEEP. 2005;28:499–521.

Littner MR, Kushida C, Wise M, et al. Practice parameters for clinical use of the multiple sleep latency test and the maintenance of wakefulness test. SLEEP. 2005;28(1):113–121.

Morgenthaler T, Alessi C, Friedman L, Owens J, Kapur V, et al. Practice parameters for the use of actigraphy in the assessment of sleep and sleep disorders: An update for 2007. SLEEP. 2007; 30(4): 519–529.

Zaremba EK, Barkey ME, Mesa C, Sanniti K, Rosen C. Making polysomnography more "child friendly": A family-centered care approach. *J Clin Sleep Med.* 2005;1(2):189–198.

1

A Car Dealer Who Could Not Get His Mind Out of Top Gear

VICTORIA LUPPA, APN
KUMAR BUDUR, MD, MS

Case History

Robert was a 39-year-old man who presented to the sleep center with excessive daytime sleepiness (EDS) for the last 5 to 6 months. He had had difficulty falling asleep, and sometimes staying asleep, on and off for as long as he could remember. However, the recent development of EDS worried him, as it had begun to affect his functioning at work. He went to bed at 10 p.m and woke up at 6 a.m. Before going to bed, he read books to help him relax. It typically took him 1 hour to fall asleep. He generally felt sleepy when he went to bed, but once he got there, he just could not sleep. He felt alert and nervous. His mind would "race like a car in top gear." He worried about his business' recent expansion and its impact on the employees and finances. However, invariably, these thoughts were replaced by fears of not sleeping for the night and how the lack of sleep would affect him the next day. He sometimes felt angry that his wife could sleep like a baby while he was awake during the night. He would watch the clock and find himself doing the "countdown to alarm." After falling asleep, he would wake up for no apparent reason once or twice during the night and have difficulty getting back to sleep. Sometimes, he would lie awake for up to 1 hour, feeling tense and worrying about the next day's activities. When the alarm went off at 6 a.m., he felt tired and unrefreshed. He sometimes would doze off at work, especially while working on the computer or reviewing accounts. On weekends, he tried to catch up with an afternoon nap, but he was never able to fall asleep, despite the opportunity. His wife had found him to be more irritable in recent months, though he denied depression, daytime anxiety, and panic attacks. On a recent family vacation to Florida, he was pleasantly surprised to have not had any problems falling asleep or staying asleep during the entire trip. He slept an uninterrupted 7 hours each night and felt refreshed on awakening. This reassured him and made him feel that with help he might sleep well again. He usually slept in the side position, and he denied snoring, witnessed apnea, and symptoms of narcolepsy, restless legs syndrome, and parasomnias.

Robert was otherwise healthy with no significant medical history. He denied using alcohol or tobacco, and he consumed one or two 8-oz cups of coffee each morning. He made sure to avoid all caffeinated foods and beverages after noon each day. He took aspirin and glucosamine-chondroitin supplements daily but denied over-the-counter or prescription sleep aids. His family history was notable for a mother with Alzheimer's disease. He was happily married for 12 years and had 3 children, aged 12, 9, and 8 years. He owned a successful car dealership and financing company for the past 8 years.

Evaluation

Robert completed a sleep log for 2 weeks prior to his first visit to the sleep center (Figure 1.1).

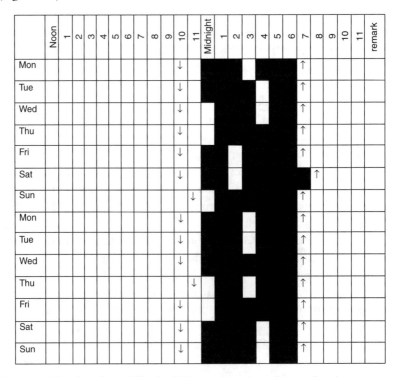

Figure 1.1 Sleep log shows difficulty falling and staying asleep and early morning awakenings. The black shaded area represents patients self-reported sleep period.

Physical Examination

On examination, Robert was of normal weight with a body mass index of $24\,kg/m^2$. His oropharyngeal exam showed Grade I tonsils and a Freidman tongue position Grade II. His general and neurological examinations were otherwise unremarkable.

Diagnosis

Psychophysiological insomnia.

Outcome

Robert received a thorough explanation of his diagnosis and treatment options (which included pharmacological therapy; cognitive behavioral therapy for insomnia, or CBTi; or a combination) and the relative advantages of each of the therapies. He was motivated to try CBTi. However, since insomnia was affecting his ability to function at home and work, a 1-month trial of extended release zolpidem (Ambien CR) was prescribed to help him sleep until he learned the skills to relax on his own. He was advised to avoid going to bed unless he was sleepy, lying in bed for extended periods of time (i.e., no more than 20 minutes) awake, and watching the clock at night (he was told to set the alarm and turn the clock away). If he was unable to sleep within 20 minutes, he was advised, he should get out of bed and engage in something relaxing. He was educated on normal sleep requirements in healthy adults and advised not to "overvalue" sleep. He was referred to a sleep psychologist for CBTi.

At his 4-week follow-up, Robert reported that he was sleeping 7 hours per night, and felt refreshed in the morning. He still woke up during the night on occasion, but he was able to get back to sleep within minutes. He was no longer getting into bed before feeling sleepy, and he stopped focusing on the clock during the night. On one occasion when he had difficulty going back to sleep, he got out of bed and read a novel; that helped him relax. He had seen the sleep psychologist twice in the interim, and he liked the deep-breathing exercises and progressive muscle relaxation. He practiced them regularly and felt that they not only helped him relax at night, but also allowed him to better manage stress at work. He was encouraged to continue to practice good sleep hygiene, follow up with the sleep psychologist, and use the sleep medication only if absolutely necessary, such as if he were to have important engagements the next day and was unable to sleep on his own even 1 to 2 hours past his usual sleep time.

At his 8-week return visit, Robert continued to do well and reported using Ambien CR only once, on a night before he had an important meeting with his employees. He completed 5 sessions with the sleep psychologist, and he felt that his insomnia was much improved.

Discussion

Although Robert presented to the sleep disorders center with a complaint of EDS, his main problem was insomnia. He met the general criteria for insomnia (Table 1.1). He had difficulty falling asleep and staying asleep, and he woke up unrefreshed despite having an adequate opportunity to sleep. Furthermore, he had daytime impairments secondary to his sleep problems, including irritability and feeling tired during the day.

Robert also met the ICSD-2 diagnostic criteria for psychophysiological insomnia (Table 1.2). He had conditioned difficulty falling asleep in his bed at a desired time. He had heightened mental and somatic tension at night and excessively focused on sleep. When he slept at a different place, away from the conditioned sleep environment, (in this case, on vacation in Florida), he slept better.

The differential diagnosis in Robert's case includes several other types of insomnia, including paradoxical insomnia, previously known as sleep misperception disorder. Patients with paradoxical insomnia generally present with dramatic complaints of not being able to sleep at all for days or longer. This was ruled out by Robert's history and sleep log, which supported one another. Actigraphy can be a useful tool in subjects suspected to have paradoxical insomnia. Since Robert has some symptoms of anxiety, insomnia due to mental disorder is another differential diagnosis that should be considered. Insomnia commonly is associated with mental disorders (and vice versa), primarily with

---

Table 1.1 ICSD-2 general criteria for Insomnia

A. Difficulty initiating sleep, maintaining sleep, early awakening or sleep that is chronically non-restorative or poor in quality.
B. The above sleep difficulty occurs despite adequate opportunity and circumstances for sleep
C. At least one of the following forms of daytime impairment related to the night time sleep difficulty is reported by the patient:
Fatigue or daytime sleepiness
Attention, concentration or memory impairment
Poor social, occupational or academic performance
Mood disturbance or irritability
Reduction in motivation, energy or initiative
Errors/accidents at work or while driving
Tension, Headaches, GI distress
Worries about sleep.

---

depression and anxiety disorders. Although Robert had heightened mental and somatic tension at night, mainly around bedtime, he did not have any symptoms suggestive of generalized anxiety disorder (such as pervasive free-floating anxiety, persistent inability to relax or stop thinking, or muscle tension). He also denied symptoms suggestive of major depressive disorder, such as depressed mood or lack of interests. Idiopathic insomnia is another consideration. This is a chronic condition, with onset in infancy or childhood and no identifiable precipitant or cause, in which insomnia persists without sustained remission. Robert had transient periods of difficulty sleeping on and off all his life not associated with any significant daytime impairment. Finally, another consideration, although low on the list, is adjustment insomnia. It is temporally associated with an identifiable stress, is expected to resolve once that stress is eliminated or the individual adjusts to the situation, and it does not last for more than 3 months. Although stress at work was a factor for Robert, it was not associated with the onset of his symptoms, and his insomnia clearly lasted for more than 3 months.

Robert's case illustrates the importance of a detailed history in the diagnosis and management of patients with insomnia. Although he presented with EDS, the fact that he was not able to nap during the day, intentionally or unintentionally, despite inadequate nocturnal sleep suggested the diagnosis of psychophysiological insomnia. This is explained by the fact that affected individuals are hyperarousable. It is not uncommon for insomnia patients to misconstrue fatigue as EDS.

The management of insomnia can be broadly classified into 2 main categories: psychological (primarily CBTi) and pharmacological. Psychological treatments

Table 1.2 ICSD-2 criteria for psychophysiological insomnia

A. The patient's symptoms meet the criteria for insomnia.
B. The insomnia is present for at least 1 month.
C. The patient has evidence of conditioned sleep difficulty and/or heightened arousal in bed as indicated by 1 or more of the following:
   i. Excessive focus on, and heightened anxiety about sleep.
   ii. Difficulty falling asleep in bed at desired bedtime or during planned naps, but no difficulty falling asleep during other monotonous activities when not intending to sleep.
   iii. Ability to sleep better away from home than at home.
   iv. Mental arousal in bed characterized either by intrusive thoughts or a perceived inability to volitionally cease sleep-preventing mental activity.
   v. Heightened somatic tension in bed reflected by perceived inability to relax the body sufficiently to allow the onset of sleep.
D. The sleep disturbance is not better explained by another sleep disorder, medical or neurological disorder, mental disorder, medication use, or substance use disorder.

are discussed in Chapter 2. The pharmacological treatments of insomnia are broadly classified into benzodiazepines, benzodiazepine receptor agonists (also known as BZRAs), and miscellaneous agents.

Benzodiazepines were the treatment of choice until the early 1990s, when the first BZRA was introduced in the form of zolpidem. Benzodiazepines were superior to their predecessors, the barbiturates, from the safety standpoint. They act primarily at the gamma-aminobutyric acid-benzodiazepine (GABA-BDZ) complex. The U.S. Food and Drug Administration (FDA)has approved 5 benzodiazepines for the treatment of insomnia: triazolam, temazepam, estazolam, quazepam, and flurazepam. Although the benzodiazepines are highly effective in the treatment of insomnia, they are associated with tolerance, dependence, abuse, hypotension, and risk of falls, especially in the elderly. Also, many of the benzodiazepines have a long half life that can cause daytime sleepiness and impairment of cognitive and motor skills, including driving, during the day. Because of these limitations, and also the availability of better drugs, benzodiazepines are no longer commonly used to treat insomnia.

The BZRAs are seen as good alternatives to benzodiazepines due to their select action at the alpha1 subunit of GABA-BDZ, which has specific hypnotic properties. This action does not result in the anxiolytic or muscle-relaxant properties

Table 1.3 Drugs approved by the FDA that are commonly used in the treatment of insomnia

Drug	Brand name	Dosage (mg)	Onset of action	Halflife (h)	Metabolism (substrate of)	Useful in patients with	Common adverse effects
Zolpidem	Ambien Generic	5–10	Rapid	1–2.5	CYP3A4, CYP2C9 and CYP1A2	Sleep onset insomnia	Dizziness, drowsiness, headaches
Zolpidem ER	Ambien CR	6.25–12.5	Biphasic	1.6–4	CYP3A4, CYP2C9 and CYP1A2	Sleep onset/ maintenance insomnia	Dizziness, residual effects during the next day
Zaleplon	Sonata	5–10	Rapid	1	Aldehyde oxidase, CYP3A4	Sleep onset insomnia	Dizziness, drowsiness
Eszopiclone	Lunesta	1–3	Rapid	6	CYP3A4 and CYP2E1	Sleep onset/ maintenance insomnia	Headaches, "metallic" after-taste
Ramelteon	Rozerem	8	Rapid	1–2.6	CYP1A2 and CYP3A4	Sleep onset insomnia	Fatigue, drowsiness

seen with benzodiazepines. The 4 BZRAs approved by the FDA for the treatment of insomnia are zolpidem (Ambien), extended-release zolpidem (Ambien CR), zaleplon (Sonata), and eszopiclone (Lunesta). The major differentiating factor among these agents is the half life (Table 1.3). The BZRAs are thought to be relatively safe for long-term use, although the potential for tolerance and dependence still exists.

A variety of other agents have been used in the treatment of insomnia. Ramelteon (Rozerem) is a novel hypnotic agent that interacts with melatonin 1 and melatonin 2 receptors. Since ramelteon has no interaction with GABA-BDZ receptors, it is a nonscheduled drug and has no abuse or dependence potential. Other drugs that are not approved by the FDA specifically for insomnia, but that are nevertheless used off-label, include: (1) antidepressants such as mirtazapine, trazodone, and amytriptyline; (2) antipsychotics such as olanzapine, quetiapine, and risperidone; (3) anticonvulsants such as gabapentin and pregabalin; (4) antihistamines such as diphenhydramine hydrochloride, doxylamine succinate, and doxylamine citrate; and (5) melatonin. None of these drugs has been studied systematically, and hence their efficacy and safety in the treatment of insomnia is not established.

Bibliography

Bonnet MH, Arand DL. 24-hour metabolic rate in insomniacs and matched normal sleepers. *Sleep*. 1995;18:581–588.

Pavlova M, Berg O, Gleason R, Walker F, Roberts S, Regestein Q. Self-reported hyperarousal traits among insomnia patients. *J Psychosom Res*. 2001;51:435–441.

2

Teaching the Teacher How to Sleep

MICHELLE DRERUP, Psy.D., C.BSM

Case History

Karen, a 51-year-old married woman who worked as a gifted-education teacher presented to the Cleveland Clinic Sleep Disorders Center with a chief complaint of insomnia. Her main concerns were difficulty staying asleep and feeling tired during the daytime.

She noted her sleep problems started about 21 years prior. She was undergoing significant stress at the time and realized that her perfectionistic tendencies were causing distress to not only herself, but to her daughter as well. She did not have much difficulty with sleep onset; her main problems were with sleep maintenance. Associated symptoms included fatigue, depression, and anxiety. When these symptoms began, about 21 years ago, she started seeing both a psychologist and a psychiatrist for her depression and anxiety issues. Her psychiatrist started her on bupropion 100 mg TID. After a few months, Karen felt that although her depression and anxiety symptoms had improved, her sleep problems actually worsened with this medication. Her psychiatrist therefore prescribed zolpidem 5 mg and trazodone 50 mg to deal with the worsening sleep issues. She was on this combination of medications for several years and had no problems sleeping. However after many years of treatment she decided to discontinue taking all the medications, only to experience a recurrence of the insomnia. Five years ago, she was prescribed gabapentin 300 mg QHS for headaches by her primary care physician, and the dose was increased to 1600 mg over time. She benefited in terms of both her headaches and her sleep with this medication, but she again tapered herself off the prescription after about a year and started having recurrent problems with insomnia as a result.

After this recurrence, her primary care provider referred her to the Sleep Disorders Center, where she was diagnosed with psychophysiological insomnia.

Her treatment plan involved discussing elements of good sleep hygiene and relaxation as well as a referral to a sleep psychologist for cognitive-behavioral therapy for insomnia (CBTi). A self-help book was recommended for additional reading about insomnia. She was to follow up in 6 weeks, after her evaluation with the sleep psychologist.

The next contact with the patient was more than 2 years after her initial visit, when she returned to see the neurologist for insomnia and chronic headaches. She reported that after her first visit she had read the self-help book for insomnia and made sleep hygiene changes, including eliminating caffeine and trying to relax before bedtime. These changes led to slight improvement in her insomnia for a few months. She noted that she did not follow up with the sleep psychologist because she thought it would be too inconvenient. As her insomnia issues re-emerged, she started taking over-the-counter sleep aids, mainly antihistamines, about 4 nights a week. These sleep aids helped her to some extent but left her very tired during the day. She was again referred to the sleep psychologist, but she did not follow up.

Four years after her initial referral to see the behavioral sleep specialist, Karen was finally scheduled for an appointment with behavioral sleep medicine services. Unlike the past 2 psychology referrals, this referral actually was initiated by Karen, because she felt this was her last glimmer of hope that her sleep problems could be resolved.

At her initial evaluation with the behavioral sleep psychologist, Karen reported that she dreaded going to bed at night due to fear of not sleeping. She noted that as soon as it started getting dark outside she would start to worry about not being able to sleep through the night. Karen reported that she typically would go to bed between 10:30 and 11 p.m. with minimal problems falling asleep. Her average sleep latency was 10 to 15 minutes. She noted that she would wake up 3 to 5 times a night, taking anywhere from 15 to 30 minutes to go back to sleep each time. Occasionally, she would have to go to the restroom, but otherwise she had no idea what was waking her. At times she would be awake for as long as an hour or more, and she would tend to stay in bed, tossing and turning, worrying about how lack of sleep would affect her functioning at work the next day. Her final awakening would be around 6:15 a.m., and she did not feel refreshed upon awakening. She estimated that on average she was sleeping 4 to 5 hours per night of the 7 to 8 hours she was in bed. Thus, her estimated sleep efficiency (SE), which is calculated as total time asleep divided by total time in bed expressed as a percentage, was 50%–60%. She had continued many good sleep hygiene habits, including reading before bed in a quiet room, avoiding caffeine, wearing ear plugs and an eye mask, and using relaxation strategies before bedtime. However, she did tend to take a brief nap after school every day, to stay in bed when not sleeping, and to watch TV in bed. She reported having problems relaxing at nighttime and admitted to numerous negative thoughts about sleep, including, "Here we go again; it's going to be another bad night," and, "How am I going to make it through work tomorrow if I don't sleep?" She noted significant distress related to her sleep and reported that she was not functioning well because of her fatigue. She complained that the most distressing part of her insomnia was that it significantly impacted her ability to teach and dampened her enthusiasm and creativity during the work day.

Karen denied insomnia or hypersomnia problems in childhood or adolescence, nor did she have any symptoms or signs suggestive of other sleep disorders, such as obstructive sleep apnea, restless legs syndrome, periodic limb movement disorder, narcolepsy, or parasomnias.

Karen's only other medical problem was migraine headaches, for which she was taking venlafaxine XR 150 mg and eletriptan 40 mg. Her review of systems was otherwise unremarkable. She reported occasional social alcohol consumption (1 to 2 glasses of wine per month) and denied any history of tobacco use. There was no significant family medical or psychiatric history.

Karen had been married to her second husband for the past 2 years. She had two daughters, aged 27 and 24, from her first marriage. She obtained a master's degree in education and worked as a gifted-education teacher. In terms of recent stress, she had experienced several recent deaths among family and friends, but, overall, things were going well in her life. Despite her history of depression, she denied any current symptoms. She did admit that she continued to be an anxious-type person, but she denied symptoms of generalized anxiety disorder, post traumatic stress disorder, panic disorder, or obsessive compulsive disorder.

Physical Examination

On examination, Karen had a body mass index (BMI) of 27.2 kg/m^2. Her neck circumference was 32 cm. She had a blood pressure of 136/82 mmHg, a heart rate of 88 bpm, and a respiratory rate of 14 bpm. She appeared tired but not sleepy. Her upper-airway examination was normal, with Grade I tonsils and a Friedman tongue position Grade I. The rest of the physical examination was normal.

Evaluation

Karen scored a high 27 of a possible 28 on a 5-item Insomnia Severity Index Scale (ISI), indicating severe insomnia. Her Epworth Sleepiness Scale score was 5/24 and her Fatigue Severity Scale score was 45/63.

Diagnosis

Psychophysiological insomnia (Table 2.1).

Table 2.1 ICSD-2 diagnostic criteria: Psychophysiological insomnia

A. The patient's symptoms meet the criteria for insomnia.
B. The insomnia is present for at least 1 month.
C. The patient has evidence of conditioned sleep difficulty and/or heightened arousal in bed as indicated by one or more of the following:
   i. Excessive focus on and heightened anxiety about sleep.
   ii. Difficulty falling asleep in bed at the desired bedtime or during planned naps, but no difficulty falling asleep during other monotonous activities when not intending to sleep.
   iii. Ability to sleep better away from home than at home.
   iv. Mental arousal in bed characterized either by intrusive thoughts or a perceived inability to volitionally cease sleep-preventing mental activity.
   v. Heightened somatic tension in bed reflected by a perceived inability to relax the body sufficiently to allow the onset of sleep.
D. The sleep disturbance is not better explained by another sleep disorder, medical or neurological disorder, mental disorder, medication use, or substance use disorder.

Outcome

Based on the evaluation, it was determined that CBTi would be the treatment of choice due to diagnosis of psychophysiological insomnia. The rationale and typical course of CBTi was discussed, and Karen was somewhat skeptical about its effectiveness but willing to give it a try since nothing else had been helpful long-term.

At the end of the initial session, Karen was provided education about sleep hygiene with a review of the rationale behind various behavioral changes. The most difficult change for Karen to make was avoidance of naps during the daytime. After a stressful day teaching, she would typically come home and take a 15- to 30-minute nap. She felt that she would not be productive in the evening without one. Explanation was provided that avoiding naps would provide better preparation for a continuous, longer sleep period at night, as well as strengthen the connection between nighttime sleep and the bed. Providing the rationale behind this change allowed her to feel more comfortable and more likely to follow through with guidelines. Karen was also oriented to keeping a sleep log as an essential component of CBTi.

At the beginning of the second session, her sleep diary was reviewed and sleep variables were calculated, including sleep latency (SL), wake after sleep onset time (WASO), total sleep time (TST), and time in bed (TIB). Over the course of the previous 2 weeks, Karen averaged 6 hours of sleep per night. However, she was spending an average of 8 hours in bed. Her sleep efficiency average was 75% (Table 2.2). A sleep-restriction plan was developed for Karen to stay awake until 1 a.m. and wake up at 7 a.m. The guidelines were discussed; the most

Table 2.2 Karen's sleep log, week 1

Calendar date	Day 1	Day 2	Day 3	Day 4	Day 5	Day 6	Day 7
Daytime naps	3:15 p.m.	None	None	None	None	3–3:30 p.m.	3–3:15 p.m.
Medication for sleep or alcohol use	None	None	None	None	None	None	None
Time attempted to fall asleep	10 p.m.	10:30 p.m.	10 p.m.	10:30 p.m.	10:30 p.m.	10:30 p.m.	11:30 p.m.
Sleep onset latency	20 min	20 min	4 hours	15 min	30 min	10 min	2 hours
# of awakenings	3	4	0	2	3	3	2
Length of each awakening	20 min, 5 min, 15 min	10 min, 5 min, 10 min, 25 min		10 min, 5 min	15 min, 5 min, 10 min	5 min, 5 min, 10 min	10 min, 20 min
Final awakening	7:15 a.m.	7 a.m.	7 a.m.	5 a.m.	6:30 a.m.	7 a.m.	6:30 a.m.
Time out of bed	7:15 a.m.	7:15 a.m.	7:15 a.m.	5 a.m	7 a.m.	7:30 a.m.	6:30 a.m.
Quality of sleep 1 = very poor, 2 = poor, 3 = fair, 4 = good, 5 = excellent	3	2	1	3	3	4	2
When I awoke today I felt: 1 = not at all rested 2 = slightly rested 3 = somewhat rested 4 = rested 5 = well rested	3	2	1	4	2	4	2
Sleep efficiency	77%	79%	55%	91%	82%	88%	64%

important were to avoid naps and to get up every morning at the same time, even on weekends. Possible barriers for implementing the plan were identified and discussed. Karen also was instructed not to spend more than 15 to 20 minutes in bed trying to fall asleep; if still awake, she was to go into another room and read a magazine or listen to music until she felt sleepy. Her negative automatic thoughts about sleep were identified and coping thoughts were developed, such as, "I have been able to function rather well even on nights that I don't sleep well." Her instructions for the next week were to complete the sleep logs, follow the sleep restriction plan, and practice relaxation techniques.

At the third session, review of her sleep log indicated that Karen was doing well with the sleep-restriction plan. Her sleep efficiency was above 95% every night; she was now going to bed at midnight and waking up at 7 a.m. Sleep latency was 5 to 10 minutes, and she reported minimal awakenings in the middle of the night. She noted that she started to have negative thoughts about sleep some nights (i.e., "It's worked 3 days in a row; it's not going to work tonight"), but she was able to engage in cognitive restructuring techniques that were discussed at session 2 in order to decrease anxiety and tension related to these thoughts. Karen was implementing relaxation-training techniques, as well, to help her wind down at night. A sleep-restriction plan was therefore developed. She was to begin going to bed at 11:30 p.m., provided sleep efficiency remained above 90% for 2 to 3 days in a row. She would then advance bedtime by 15 minutes earlier until she found the right length of sleep for her.

A month later, at her last session, the first thing that Karen stated as she entered the office was "You saved my life." Review of sleep logs (Table 2.3) indicated that her sleep efficiency never fell below 95% over the previous month. She had been falling asleep within 5 to 10 minutes of going to bed, with minimal awakenings in the middle of the night. Her ISI score at our final session was 2, which was normal. She noted some anxiety about starting the new school year and how this would affect her sleep, but she was able to utilize cognitive therapy strategies to think about this situation in a more positive light. Relapse-prevention strategies were discussed in case she noticed any changes in her sleep patterns, and she was offered the option of returning for a "booster session" of CBTi, if necessary, in the future.

Discussion

Karen met criteria for psychophysiological insomnia (Table 2.1), which is described as a disorder of somatized tension and learned sleep preventing associations that results in a complaint of insomnia and associated decreased functioning during wakefulness. In terms of general insomnia symptoms, she complained of difficulty maintaining sleep (Criterion A). This sleep difficulty occurred despite adequate opportunity for sleep. She also reported numerous

Table 2.3 Karen's sleep log, week 7

Calendar date	Day 1	Day 2	Day 3	Day 4	Day 5	Day 6	Day 7
Daytime naps							
Medication for sleep or alcohol use	None	None	None	None	None	None	None
Time attempted to fall asleep	11:30 p.m.	10:30 p.m.	10:30 p.m.	10:15 p.m.	11:30 p.m.	10:30 p.m.	10:125 p.m.
Sleep onset latency	10 min	5 min	5 min	5 min	5 min	5 min	2 min
# of awakenings	2	1	1	1	1	1	1
Length of each awakening	5 min 5 min	5 min	15 min	5 min	5 min	5 min	3 min
Final awakening	6:30 a.m.	6:00 a.m.	6:30 a.m.	5:45 a.m.	6:30 a.m.	6:00 a.m.	5:30 a.m.
Time out of bed	6:30 a.m.	6:00 a.m.	6:30 a.m.	6:00 a.m.	6:30 a.m.	6:00 a.m.	5:30 a.m.
Quality of sleep 1 = very poor, 2 = poor, 3 = fair, 4 = good, 5 = excellent	4	5	4	5	5	5	5
When I awoke today I felt: 1 = not at all rested, 2 = slightly rested, 3 = somewhat rested, 4 = rested, 5 = well rested	4	5	4	5	5	5	5
Sleep efficiency	95%	97%	95.8%	97.7%	97.6%	97.7%	98.3%

daytime impairments associated with the sleep difficulty, including difficulties with concentration and memory, disruption of her performance at work, daytime sleepiness, decreased motivation, and worries about sleep. Her insomnia complaints had been present for more than 20 years (Criterion B). In terms of the psychophysiological component, Karen demonstrated excessive focus and worry about sleep, racing thoughts, mental arousal in bed, and difficulty relaxing physically at bedtime (Criterion C). Finally, there were no other sleep disorders, medical or mental disorders, or medication/substance use issues that could explain her symptoms (Criterion D).

One possible differential diagnosis for Karen would be insomnia due to mental disorder. Although initially, at the onset of her insomnia 21 years ago, she was diagnosed with depression, she denied any current symptoms of depression or anxiety. Insomnia due to mental disorder may have been a more relevant diagnosis at the onset of her insomnia symptoms; however this was not a factor in her current sleep problems. Another differential diagnosis for Karen would be insomnia due to drug, alcohol, or substance. This would be a diagnostic consideration, since a worsening of the insomnia was initially associated with starting on the medication bupropion. Bupropion has been found to cause insomnia because of its alerting effects; however her insomnia persisted even when this medication was discontinued, making it an unlikely cause of insomnia.

CBTi is a multicomponent therapy that typically includes sleep-hygiene education, stimulus control, sleep-restriction therapy, relaxation training, and cognitive therapy. CBTi has been proven to be as effective as sedative hypnotics during short-term treatment and more effective in the long-term following treatment intervention. This case study specifically illustrates this point. When Karen was on medications for her insomnia, she would do well, but as soon as she discontinued medications she would experience a recurrence of the insomnia. This case also supports previous research suggesting sleep hygiene education does not work as a stand-alone treatment for chronic insomnia. Although it is often incorporated into CBTi treatment, sleep hygiene alone has been demonstrated to have little benefit. This patient had read a self-help book on her own and implemented many sleep hygiene changes, but she did not experience long-term benefits in resolution of the insomnia with these lifestyle and behavioral changes.

One essential component of CBTi is having patients keep sleep logs. There are 3 main purposes for utilizing a sleep log. First, sleep logs allow for relatively more accurate and reliable estimates of sleep variables. Second, sleep logs allow the provider to determine where to intervene and which components of CBTi most likely would be effective. Third, and perhaps most important, sleep logs allow for assessment of treatment outcomes and efficacy.

Several times during the course of CBTi treatment, Karen demonstrated some opposition to the treatment plan. There was some initial resistance to the sleep restriction plan, but discussion of the detriments of staying in bed when not sleeping helped her to feel more comfortable with and confident about these changes. These initial difficulties in acceptance of the treatment strategies support the importance of describing the rationale and discussing these issues with patients. When just given a list of sleep-hygiene guidelines or a self-help book to read, patients are unlikely to change long-standing patterns and habits unless they know the reasons why and are able to discuss these issues with their providers.

Despite having problems with insomnia for more than 20 years, Karen had significant improvement in her sleep quality, total sleep time, and daytime functioning after only 4 sessions of CBTi. At the time of the last telephone contact with Karen, she was doing well and had actually referred several of her friends and co-workers to the Sleep Disorders Center for help with their insomnia. Karen noted that her only regret was that she did not follow through with CBTi the first time around.

Bibliography

Bastien C, Vallieres A, Morin CM. Validation of the insomnia severity index as an outcome measure for insomnia research. *Sleep Medicine*. 2001;2:297–307.

Morin CM, Colecchi C, Stone J, Sood R, Brink D. Behavioral and pharmacological therapies for late-life insomnia: a randomized controlled trial. *JAMA*. 1999;281(11):991–999.

Morin CM, Hauri PJ, Espie CA, Spielman AJ, Buysee DJ, Bootzin RR. Nonpharmacological treatment of chronic insomnia. *SLEEP*. 1999;22(8):1134–1156.

3

Scared to Sleep: A Hurricane Katrina Survivor

KATHLEEN ASHTON, PhD
KUMAR BUDUR, MD, MS

Case History

Trisha, a 46-year-old African-American woman, following a referral from her psychiatrist, scheduled an appointment at the sleep clinic for a complaint of insomnia. Other presenting symptoms included anxious mood and trauma memories. The patient related these symptoms to stress because of being a Hurricane Katrina survivor.

She noted that her sleep had significantly worsened since she moved to Cleveland after losing her home in Hurricane Katrina. She reported problems falling asleep and staying asleep. Associated symptoms included fatigue and daytime sleepiness. She approached her primary care physician, who prescribed zolpidem for sleep and bupropion for mood. Trisha had been taking zolpidem for the past month with mixed results, and she had recently stopped the medications due to their high cost. She estimated her sleep time to be about 4 hours per night.

She saw a new psychiatrist after moving to Cleveland, and he switched her from bupropion to sertraline after diagnosing her with post traumatic stress disorder (PTSD), major depressive disorder (MDD), and generalized anxiety disorder (GAD). Her insomnia symptoms persisted despite treatment of the psychiatric disorders. She was then referred to a psychologist at the sleep center who specialized in behavioral sleep medicine for insomnia.

During the initial visit, Trisha reported dreading going to bed at night due to fear of nightmares. She typically waited until she was exhausted before going into her bedroom, usually around 11 p.m. She estimated that she took up to 3 hours to fall asleep. During this time she tried to listen to jazz, which typically relaxed her, but she often would have intrusive thoughts about Hurricane Katrina. She noted difficulty avoiding these thoughts, and feeling tense in bed. She typically would wake at least once per night, triggered by nightmares about the hurricane. The nightmares often involved seeing dead bodies floating in the water, running from a monster through the wind and rain, or being stranded on an island in a storm. After she woke at night, it would take up to an hour to fall back asleep. She woke at 7 a.m. daily. Her estimated sleep efficiency was 50%. Trisha also would have negative thoughts during the day about whether she would have another nightmare. Her score on the Insomnia Severity Index (ISI), a measure of insomnia severity, was 20, indicating moderately severe insomnia. She noted significant distress related to her sleep and reported that she was not functioning well because of her fatigue. She denied a prior history of sleep or wakefulness disturbance in childhood or adolescence. She reported that she never had insomnia until after the hurricane and the subsequent nightmares.

Trisha was tearful during the evaluation when discussing her experiences in Louisiana. She noted that beyond having difficulty sleeping, she also felt anxious. She was finding it hard to relax and felt like she was having some anxiety "all the time." It got significantly worse at night. She felt restless and irritable, and found herself constantly worrying. She felt tremulous and shaky. She denied ever having had a panic attack.

She also felt "depressed" in her mood and had no interest in her usual activities. She reported spontaneous crying spells, and she felt helpless and worthless. She felt guilty and worried she had become a burden to her son, with whom she was living, since relocating to Cleveland. Her self-esteem was low, and she sometimes felt hopeless. However, she denied any thoughts, plans, or intent to harm herself or others.

She complained of vivid nightmares of Hurricane Katrina and felt like she was "there again, every night." She feared for her life during the hurricane and believed that she was lucky to have escaped death. She felt "on the edge" and had become "jumpy" around noise. She avoided watching TV programs that featured hurricanes, earthquakes, or other natural disasters. She noted that these symptoms were worse around the anniversary of the hurricane.

Trisha did not have any symptoms or signs suggestive of other sleep disorders, such as restless legs syndrome, periodic limb movement disorder, narcolepsy, or parasomnias. Trisha had a prior diagnosis of obstructive sleep apnea (OSA) and had been treated successfully with continuous positive airway pressure (CPAP) for the past 4 years. She was using her CPAP nightly for 4 to 5 hours. A recent polysomnogram (PSG) confirmed severe OSA, and the CPAP setting she was on was found to be appropriate.

Trisha's only other medical problems were osteoarthritis and chronic back pain. Her review of systems was unremarkable. There was no significant family medical or psychiatric history. She was taking sertraline 50 mg, and the goal was to titrate the dose to 150 mg. She denied consuming any caffeine or alcohol, and at the time of evaluation she had recently stopped smoking.

Trisha was born and raised in Louisiana and was the fifth of 11 children. Her parents were both deceased, and 3 of her siblings were deceased. She had 3 children and was living with her oldest son after relocating to Cleveland. She had been married twice and was divorced 6 years ago. She had a GED education, and her achievement in school was average. She had been receiving disability compensation for back problems since past 12 years. Her daily activities included cooking, cleaning, doing needlework, and taking care of her grandchildren. She noted she had been avoiding leaving the house and was spending more time sitting in front of the TV lately. Her main coping strategies included spirituality and music.

Physical Examination

On examination, Trisha was obese, with a body mass index of 32 kg/m^2. Her oropharyngeal exam showed Grade I tonsils and a Freidman tongue position Grade II. Her general and neurological examinations were otherwise unremarkable.

Diagnosis

Insomnia due to mental disorder.

Outcome

Based on the evaluation, Trisha was given the following recommendations: (1) continue treatment with her psychiatrist for psychiatric illness; (2) cognitive behavioral treatment for insomnia (CBTi), including relaxation training, attention to cognitions related to sleep, and sleep restriction, and (3) imagery rehearsal therapy for coping with traumatic nightmares. Imagery rehearsal is a brief treatment that appears to decrease chronic nightmares, improve sleep quality, and decrease PTSD symptoms.

The first CBTi session focused on relaxation training, sleep restriction, and coping with cognitive distortions about sleep. Trisha was instructed not to spend more than 15 minutes in bed trying to fall asleep; if still awake, she was to go into another room and read the Bible until she felt sleepy. She found reading the Bible relaxing. Her negative cognitions about sleep also were discussed, and it was highlighted how they would increase her anxiety, resulting in conditioned emotional arousal in her bedroom. Coping thoughts, including that she was working on skills such as relaxation to help her sleep, were developed. Trisha was taught diaphragmatic breathing and a relaxation exercise involving imagery. She was found to have a good aptitude for visual imagery during the exercise and was quickly responsive to relaxation. Her instructions for the next week were to practice the relaxation daily, utilize sleep restriction, and write down the details of at least 1 nightmare when it occurred.

Trisha came to the second session noting significant improvement in sleep efficiency with a total sleep time estimated at 5 hours. She attributed the improvements to sleep restriction and relaxation training. The next step in treatment was to employ imagery rehearsal. She shared a nightmare: "I am alone in bed, in dark, when I hear a noise like a train coming through the wind and rain outside. I know it's a monster that is coming to get me and my family. I start to try to get my family to get away but everyone is moving slowly. I know I will not be able to get away and feel terrified." The dream was typical of her nightmares and had recurred many times.

Trisha was able to recreate the dream in good detail for the session. The psychologist then focused on helping Trisha "rewrite" the dream to be less threatening. She noted, "I will think of the monster shrinking and dying as the rain and wind calm, the sun coming up, and the water all around becoming peaceful." The psychologist then led her through the relaxation imagery she typically used and had her rehearse the dream, both the nightmare and then her re-imagining session. She was instructed to practice the imagery daily for 15 minutes until the next session.

At the third session, Trisha noted further improvement in both time to sleep onset and sleep quality. She noted that she had used imagery rehearsal daily as discussed, and her nightmare had become much less frightening. She no longer dreaded going to sleep and noted feeling more in control of her sleep and dreams. At this session, the psychologist again engaged the patient in imagery rehearsal for another recurrent dream, which involved seeing her parents in caskets floating out of the graveyard after the hurricane. She was able to effectively visualize changing the dream to involve seeing them as angels floating in a boat instead of in caskets. Trisha also shared some of her memories of Hurricane Katrina, including being stranded alone in her home for 9 days, as part of this session.

By the fourth session, Trisha noted she no longer feared going to sleep. She estimated her sleep time at 6 hours and her sleep efficiency was 85%. She continued to use the relaxation training daily and had also increased using prayer and music as coping strategies at night. She was interested in increasing psychotherapy sessions for trauma and continued to see her psychiatrist for medication, who optimized the dose of sertraline. She continued using her CPAP for 6 hours per night.

Trisha's insomnia improved after 4 sessions of CBTi and imagery rehearsal. Her sleep latency improved to less than 20 minutes and her sleep efficiency to 85%. Her ISI score was in the subthreshold insomnia range (9) following treatment. In addition, Trisha's PTSD symptoms showed significant improvement. This was consistent with other research suggesting imagery rehearsal may improve both sleep quality and PTSD symptoms. She was able to use the imagery rehearsal to provide exposure to trauma material while using relaxation strategies to reduce psychophysiological arousal. She specifically noted reductions in daytime memories of trauma, increased social functioning, increased concentration, and decreased irritability, which she attributed to the CBTI treatment. She had recurrent acute insomnia during anniversary dates of trauma, but she was able to utilize the techniques learned to prevent the return of more chronic insomnia.

Discussion

Insomnia often is associated with psychiatric conditions, and more often than not it is challenging to determine the cause-and-effect relationship. Trisha clearly met the diagnostic criteria for insomnia due to mental disorder. She had insomnia that was temporally associated with mental disorder, and the complaint of insomnia was more prominent than it is when seen with other typical mental illnesses (Table 3.1).

However, Trisha also met the diagnostic criteria for other psychiatric disorders, including:

(1) Post traumatic stress disorder, chronic: Trisha had all the core features of PTSD, such as exposure to a traumatic event that involved a threat to the physical integrity of self that resulted in intense fear and horror, re-experiencing the event in the form of nightmares, avoidance of thoughts and activities that would remind her of the traumatic experience, and symptoms of hyperarousal.

Table 3.1 ICSD-2 criteria for insomnia due to mental disorder

A. The patient's symptoms meet the criteria for insomnia.
B. The insomnia is present for at least 1 month.
C. A mental disorder has been diagnosed according to standard criteria (i.e., formal criteria as provided in the Diagnostic and Statistical Manual of Mental Disorders).
D. The insomnia is temporally associated with mental disorder; however, in some cases, insomnia may appear a few days or weeks before the emergence of the underlying mental disorder.
E. The insomnia is more prominent than that typically associated with the mental disorders, as indicated by causing marked distress or constituting an independent focus of treatment.
F. The sleep disturbance is not better explained by another sleep disorder, medical or neurological disorder, medication use, or substance abuse disorder.

(2) Generalized anxiety disorder: Trisha had excessive anxiety occurring on most days for more than 6 months, and this was associated with restlessness, irritability, fatigue, and sleep disturbances.

(3) Major depressive disorder: The complaint of feeling depressed and lack of interests (essential symptoms), along with symptoms of sleep disturbances; lack of energy; feelings of inappropriate guilt, helplessness and worthlessness; and problems with concentration fulfill the diagnostic criteria for major depressive disorder.

Other diagnostic considerations include adjustment insomnia, since the insomnia was associated with a significant stressor (the hurricane). However, adjustment insomnia, by definition, lasts for less than 3 months. One other diagnostic category that should invariably be considered in patients with chronic mental disorders is insomnia secondary to drug or substance abuse. Patients with psychiatric illness, especially PTSD, are at a higher risk for substance abuse. Trisha denied substance abuse, and since she presented as a trustworthy and reliable historian, urine toxicology screening was not done. Bupropion causing insomnia is a possibility because of its known alerting effects, but her insomnia persisted even after she was switched to sertraline, which she took in the morning.

A more accurate way to classify Trisha's insomnia may be co-morbid insomnia. In fact, one of the major advances in the past decade in the field of insomnia is elevating insomnia from a symptom status to a disease status. The National Institutes of Health (NIH) confirmed insomnia as a chronic disorder with significant morbidity that requires specific treatment. Rather than considering her insomnia as secondary to her PTSD and depression/anxiety, it should be conceptualized as a co-morbid issue and as important as her psychiatric issues. Traditional recommendations to treat the primary disorder may ignore benefits of CBTi treatment for a large segment of the population. Only a small percentage of patients have true primary insomnia, and recent research suggests that simultaneous treatment of insomnia and co-morbid psychiatric condition is highly effective.

Bibliography

Krakow B, et al. Imagery rehearsal therapy for chronic nightmares in sexual assault survivors with posttraumatic stress disorder. *JAMA*. 2001; 286:5,537–545.

Lichstein KL, McCrae CS, Wilson NM. Secondary Insomnia: Diagnostic issues, cognitive-behavioral treatment, and future directions. In: Perlis ML, Lichstein ML, eds. *Treating Sleep Disorders: Principles and Practice of Behavioral Sleep Medicine*. NJ: John Wiley & Sons, 2003:286–304.

4

Rock a Bye Baby: The Case of the Midnight Crier

MARGARET RICHARDS, PhD

Case History

Zachary was a 12-month-old Caucasian boy initially seen by a sleep physician due to frequent nighttime wakings and disrupted sleep. He was living with his biological parents and was their only child. His parents brought him to the sleep clinic due to concerns that he rarely slept through the night. While Zack typically fell asleep easily, he woke every 1 to 2 hours and could not return to sleep until held or rocked by his parents. His parents reported that when Zack was born, he had an underdeveloped diaphragm and cow's milk protein allergy. As an infant, Zack had significant colic and reportedly often cried for more than 15 hours at a time.

Due to his underdeveloped diaphragm, he experienced frequent vomiting, particularly when lying down. Zack was followed by a pediatric gastroenterologist and placed on medication to manage his reflux. Initially, he was placed on H2 blockers, followed by lansaprozole. Unfortunately, these did not improve his symptoms, so he was switched to omeprazole liquid and then to omeprazole/sodium bicarbonate powder. His symptoms improved significantly on the powder combination. Prior to effective medical management of his symptoms, when his parents were able to get him to sleep, he would frequently vomit upon being placed in his crib or upon lying down. Consequently, Zack learned to sleep sitting up, either in his car seat or in a reclining swing. He slept in his swing until he was approximately 10 months old, at which point his parents were able to transition him into a crib. After initial evaluation, the sleep specialist determined that Zack's nighttime behaviors were a reflection of his inability to self-soothe, rather than related to physical difficulties, and the specialist referred the family to a pediatric psychologist.

Evaluation

Given Zack's age at the time of the referral, his initial evaluation with the psychologist comprised a detailed clinical interview with his parents as well as interactions with Zack to assess his current development. The clinical interview included a detailed account of the current sleep problems, focusing on the pattern of sleep, duration of the sleep problems, frequency and duration of naps and nighttime wakings, reviewing additional sleep difficulties that may have been present, and reviewing previous attempts to remedy these problems, including a review of past and current medications. Specific focus was also placed on the bedtime rituals, identifying what patterns had developed and identifying what Zack "needed" to have in order to sleep (i.e., a bottle, music, being held, etc.).

During this diagnostic interview, it became apparent that Zack's sleep was quite disrupted. His parents noted he typically took 2 naps per day, but each lasted only 30 to 40 minutes. He returned to sleep if his parents held and rocked him, but he began crying as soon as he was returned to his crib. Additionally, nighttime sleep was extremely difficult. His parents described Zack as screaming to the point of vomiting when put to bed at night. They also noted that Zack would often begin to cry just being carried into his room at night. In order to help Zack sleep better, his parents began rocking him in a rocking chair until he fell asleep, prior to transferring him to his crib. He would then sleep for approximately 45 minutes before waking and beginning to scream. Given his history of reflux and nighttime emesis, his parents were appropriately concerned about letting him cry. If they were able to get Zack back to sleep (typically accomplished by holding and rocking him), he would often wake in the night and cry, again to the point of vomiting. They described a typical night of "good sleep" as:

6:45 p.m.	Bath time.
7 p.m.	Play time with Mom and Dad.
7:45 p.m.	Rocked in rocking chair until he falls asleep.
8 p.m.	Placed in crib, already sleeping.
10 p.m.	Wakes in crib, crying. If parents do not pick him up within 10 to 30 minutes, he will cry until he vomits. Parents then change him, comfort him, and return him to his crib once he is asleep.
2 a.m.	Zack wakes in crib, crying. Receives a bottle and is rocked in rocking chair until asleep. Above cycle begins again.
3 a.m.	Zack placed in crib, already sleeping. Typically wakes within 30 minutes and above interventions are implemented.
6:30 a.m.	Wakes for the day, appearing refreshed.

Daytime naps followed a similar pattern, but with sleep cycles lasting only 30 minutes. If held the entire time, he would sleep for 90 minutes. Thus, Zack typically slept approximately 8 to 9 hours per night, albeit disrupted, with an additional hour of napping during the day, for a total of 10 to 11 hours of sleep per 24-hour day. In comparison, the average 1-year-old typically requires 13 hours of sleep per day, including 2 naps totaling 2 to 2.5 hours.

During the initial evaluation, Zack was playful and interactive. He demonstrated appropriate attachment with his parents, and they were both attentive to his needs. His parents described him as achieving developmental milestones within normal limits.

Diagnosis

Behavioral insomnia of childhood.

Outcome

To assist his parents in managing Zack's sleep difficulties, the first step was to help Zack fall asleep independently. Indicators of sleepiness were reviewed (i.e., rubbing his eyes, slower sucking, drooping eyelids, etc.), and his parents were encouraged to place Zack in his crib when he was drowsy but still awake. Education was provided about sleep associations and how these related to Zack's condition. Because Zack was in the habit of falling asleep while being held and rocked, when he woke in the night and his situation was different, he was unable to return to sleep. Thus, he would cry until these conditions were reinstated. If allowed to cry long enough, he would become exhausted and stressed, resulting in greater difficulty soothing and in vomiting.

Addressing these concerns required 2 levels of intervention. Because his parents reported that Zack would often begin crying when entering his room, it was recommended that parents spend part of the day playing or engaging in positive activities in Zack's room, separate from his sleep routine. This was designed to allow Zack to develop some positive associations with his bedroom, rather than associating it primarily with bedtime and his associated distress. Second, it was recommended that his parents place Zack in his crib when he was drowsy but not yet asleep. Alternative ways to soothe besides picking him up were discussed (i.e., patting or rubbing his back, speaking softly to him, transitional objects) with a focus on helping parents to slowly limit their interventions with him over time so that he would be able to fall asleep and return to sleep independently. More specifically, work with his parents focused on helping them to decrease their involvement with Zack when he woke during the night. Due to his parents' anxiety about Zack's nighttime wakings, a very gradual approach was developed.

His parents were encouraged to wait progressively longer intervals prior to entering his room when Zack awoke., They were encouraged to limit their interactions upon entering the room. So instead of picking him up, they were asked to begin by rubbing his back or speaking quietly with Zack to soothe him, but were to stop before he was asleep. These interventions were gradually limited until Zack was able to fall asleep independently.

Regular follow-up was initiated with the family, with appointments occurring every 2 to 3 weeks to assist them in maintaining progress and to troubleshoot any issues that might arise. The parents were encouraged to contact the psychologist by phone between sessions for any additional problem solving or support required. Approximately 2 months after the initial consultation and regular follow up, Zack was successfully sleeping through the night and sleeping for approximately 90 minutes each day during his daytime naps.

Discussion

In order to clarify how to diagnose Zack's constellation of symptoms, a brief review of the diagnostic criteria is necessary (Table 4.1). The ICSD-2 criteria nicely delineate Zack's sleep difficulties. Based on the reports from his parents,

---

Table 4.1 ICSD-2 criteria for behavioral insomnia of childhood

A. A child's symptoms meet the criteria for insomnia based upon reports of parents or other adult caregivers.
B. The child shows a pattern consistent with either the sleep-onset association or limit-setting type of insomnia described below:
   a. Sleep-onset association type includes each of the following:
     i. Falling asleep is an extended process that requires special conditions.
     ii. Sleep-onset associations are highly problematic or demanding.
     iii. In the absence of the associated conditions, sleep onset is significantly delayed or sleep is otherwise disrupted.
     iv. Nighttime awakenings require caregiver intervention for the child to return to sleep.
   b. Limit-setting type includes each of the following:
     i. The individual has difficulty initiating or maintaining sleep.
     ii. The individual stalls or refuses to go to bed at an appropriate time or refuses to return to bed following a nighttime awakening.
     iii. The caregiver demonstrates insufficient or inappropriate limit setting to establish appropriate sleeping behavior in the child.
C. The sleep disturbance is not better explained by another sleep disorder, medical or neurological disorder, mental disorder, or medication use.

Zack had a pattern of falling asleep through an extended process, requiring special conditions (i.e., sitting up in a chair or in his car seat). Though initially these conditions were based on his reflux and medical complications, as these symptoms became more manageable, Zack learned to fall asleep while being rocked and held by his parents. In the absence of this assistance, Zack's sleep was significantly delayed and disrupted (Criterion B. a. iii). Because of this, when Zack woke in the night, he required his parents to soothe him so he could return to sleep (Criterion B. a. iv).

While the ICSD-2 criteria are used by pediatricians and medical doctors to diagnose Zack's sleep problems, psychologists diagnose sleep disorders based on the *Diagnostic and Statistical Manual of Mental Health Disorders 4th Edition, Text Revision* (DSM-IV-TR). Since Zack was evaluated by a pediatric psychologist, a review of the DSM-IV criteria is necessary. The DSM-IV classifies sleep disorders according to similar categories as the ICSD-2: dyssomnias, parasomnias, sleep disorders related to another mental disorder (i.e., anxiety, depression), and other sleep disorders (i.e., substance-induced or medically induced sleep disorders). A review of the DSM-IV diagnostic criteria indicates that the criteria for insomnia from a psychological perspective are similar to those identified by the ICSD-2. Specifically, certain criteria are required for a diagnosis of primary insomnia (Table 4.2). In Zack's case, he clearly had difficulty initiating and maintaining sleep for more than 1 month. However, while he became upset to the point of vomiting when waking during the night, his level of distress was not related to the sleep disturbance itself but rather to his inability to return to sleep without parental comfort. His distress appeared to be more a reflection of his wanting to be hugged and rocked by his parents than distress related to his inability to sleep. At the time of evaluation, his sleep difficulties were not related to an underlying sleep disorder (as indicated in C) or related to a mental disorder (Criterion D). While initially his sleep problems could be attributed to his reflux and colic, those were being managed medically, and so Criterion E no

---

Table 4.2 DSM-IV diagnostic criteria for primary insomnia

A. The predominant complaint is difficulty initiating or maintaining sleep, or nonrestorative sleep, for at least 1 month.

B. The sleep disturbance (or associated daytime fatigue) causes clinically significant distress or impairment in social, occupational, or other important areas of functioning.

C. The sleep disturbance does not occur exclusively during the course of narcolepsy, breathing-related sleep disorder, circadian rhythm sleep disorder, or parasomnias.

D. The disturbance does not occur exclusively during the course of another mental disorder (i.e., major depressive disorder, generalized anxiety disorder, a delirium).

E. The disturbance is not due to the direct physiological effects of a substance (i.e., a drug of abuse, a medication) or a general medical condition.

longer applies. However, an argument could be made that Zack meets criteria for an insomnia based primarily on behavioral characteristics.

Given his age, Zack did not yet meet criteria for a psychological diagnosis, though some providers may utilize an adjustment disorder not otherwise specified. The criteria for an adjustment disorder are listed (Table 4.3). In this case, there is not a clearly identifiable stressor beyond Zack having difficulty returning to sleep when not comforted and his history of reflux. His distress to the point of vomiting could be considered to be "in excess of what would be expected from an exposure to the stressor," (Table 4.3 B, point i) though given his age and history of reflux, others may debate that his response might not be excessive. While this diagnosis does not describe Zack's symptoms as accurately as behaviorally based insomnia, practitioners may be able to justify use of the adjustment disorder diagnosis.

Based on the initial information provided by the parents, Zack's sleep difficulties appeared to be related to 2 major aspects of his infancy. First, the colic and underdeveloped diaphragm he had suffered as an infant disrupted his sleep from an early age. Consequently, his parents were more anxious when he cried, due to concerns that he may become upset to the point of vomiting when put to sleep at night. When he was initially referred to the pediatric psychologist, Zack's reflux was reasonably well controlled with omeprazole/sodium bicarbonate, and vomiting occurred only when Zack was extremely upset.

Due to his disrupted sleep during infancy, Zack's parents had been putting him to bed after he was asleep and had been picking him up to comfort him when he cried. Consequently, Zack had developed a learned response such that he was able to return to sleep only when held and comforted by his parents. Rather than an underlying physical response, Zack's sleep difficulties appeared

Table 4.3 DSM-IV diagnostic criteria for adjustment disorder—not otherwise specified

A. The development of emotional or behavioral symptoms in response to an identifiable stressor(s) occurring within 3 months of the onset of the stressor(s).
B. These symptoms or behaviors are clinically significant as evidenced by either:
   i. Marked distress that is in excess of what would be expected from exposure to the stressor.
   ii. Significant impairment in social or occupational functioning.
C. The stress-related disturbance does not meet the criteria for another specific Axis I disorder and is not merely an exacerbation of a pre-existing Axis I or Axis II disorder.
D. The symptoms do not represent bereavement.
E. Once the stressor (or its consequences) has terminated, the symptoms do not persist for more than an additional 6 months.

to be more behavioral in nature, requiring behavioral interventions to assist Zack in learning to sleep independently.

Zack's presentation is quite typical of a child becoming overly tired and stressed. When a child is overly tired, his body initiates a stress response, provoking chemical changes designed to fight fatigue. This then further inhibits the baby's ability to sleep. Research on sleep behaviors of children post-colic suggests that infants between 8 and 12 months and between 14 and18 months of age wake more during the night than their non-colicky peers. Additionally, many babies with colic develop habits that are maintained even after the colic has improved (i.e., being held or rocked until they fall asleep). Children may then demand these rituals, or sleep associations, in order to sleep.

Bibliography

American Psychiatric Association. *Diagnostic and Statistical Manual of Mental Disorders*. 4th ed.-text revision. Washington, DC: American Psychiatric Association; 2000.

Ferber R. *Solve Your Child's Sleep Problems*. New York, NY: Fireside; 2006.

Streisand R, Efron LA. Pediatric sleep disorders. In: Roberts MC, ed. *Handbook of Pediatric Psychology*. 3rd ed. New York, NY: Guilford Press; 2003:578–598.

Weissbluth M. *Healthy Sleep Habits, Happy Child*. New York, NY: Ballantine Books; 2005.

5

45 Days Awake and Counting

MIA ZAHARNA, MD

KUMAR BUDUR, MD, MS

Case History

Simon was a 57-year-old man who came to the sleep center for evaluation of insomnia. He was referred by his psychiatrist after years of sleep related difficulties that were unresponsive to medication or behavioral therapy focusing on sleep hygiene. His chief complaint was, "I never ever sleep. I have not slept in at least 45 days. I may sleep 1 night every few months. I will die if I don't get some sleep." He appeared anxious and upset, and he was desperate to get some relief.

Until 5 years ago, Simon reportedly slept between 8 and 9 hours a night without difficulty. As a child and a young adult, he said, he was a good sleeper. He denied any significant stressors or life events that may have contributed to his difficulty sleeping back then. Gradually he began having difficulty falling asleep, and he stated that within the past 2 years things had worsened to the point where it took 5 to 6 hours to fall asleep. He denied any physical complaints such as urinary frequency/urgency that could be keeping him awake. He also stated that on most nights he did not sleep at all. He lived and slept alone. He recently had been out of town for 3 days at a work-related conference, and he had not been able to sleep. He denied drinking caffeinated beverages or participating in mentally engaging activities past dinner time. He mentioned working on sleep hygiene with his therapist, and he felt he was doing everything right. He felt tired during the day on occasion, but he denied falling asleep even during boring or monotonous activities, such as reading or watching TV. He had stopped driving for the past few months because he was afraid of falling asleep at the wheel, although he never had, nor had he experienced an accident or a near-accident due to sleepiness. He had been voluntarily admitted to an inpatient psychiatric unit 5 times within the past 2 years after reporting to his family suicidal ideations, which he said were solely the result of his inability to sleep. Prior to this, he had never been admitted to a psychiatric unit or experienced suicidal thoughts. During each hospital stay, nursing reports documented, he slept 8 to 9 hours a night without any difficulty falling asleep or maintaining sleep. When he was confronted with the nursing reports, he exclaimed, "That's impossible! I never slept in the hospital, and I never sleep now!"

Simon started drawing on disability insurance 2 years ago for an anxiety disorder that he ultimately ascribed to his sleep problems. His psychiatrist and his primary care doctor had tried him on several hypnotic/sedating medications—including various benzodiazepines, low-dose sedating atypical anti-psychotics, sedative antidepressants, and antiepileptic medications—in an attempt to improve his sleep. These included lithium, valproic acid, zolpidem, zaleplon, eszopiclone, ramelteon, temazepam, clonazepam, lorazepam, trazodone, amitriptyline, quetiapine, olanzapine, and chlorpromazine. He also had tried many anti-anxiety medicines, including the more sedating ones such as mirtazapine and paroxetine, with poor control of his anxiety disorder and not even minimal effect on his insomnia. He felt that he no longer had any problems with anxiety, but he worried about sleep.

There was no history of snoring or witnessed apnea. He did not have any symptoms suggestive of other sleep disorders, such as narcolepsy, restless legs syndrome, periodic limb movement disorders, or parasomnias. The medical history was significant for hypothyroidism, hyperlipidemia, and generalized anxiety disorder. Hypothyroidism was under good control on 100 mcg of levothyroxine in the morning. He had a recent normal TSH. He was taking simvastatin in the morning for hyperlipidemia. He had suffered from anxiety for more than 25 years, and he had been seeing a psychiatrist every 2 months since the diagnosis. He took venlafaxine XR 150 mg daily along with clonazepam 1 mg at night. Further review of systems was unremarkable.

His family history was significant for a sister with depression, a father with hyperlipidemia, and a mother with Type 2 diabetes mellitus. Otherwise, his family was healthy, without any sleep disorders.

Simon was born and raised in Cleveland, Ohio. He had a master's degree in education and taught fourth grade up until 2 years ago, when he went on disability. He was never married and had no children. His 4 siblings and his parents lived near him, and he had a good relationship with his family. He denied any stress related to social- or work-related environments. He denied any alcohol or illicit drug use. He had stopped using caffeinated beverages, hoping that would help him to sleep better at night.

Physical Examination

On examination, Simon was of normal weight with a body mass index of 23.3 kg/m². His oropharyngeal exam showed a Freidman tongue position Grade II. His general and neurological examinations were otherwise unremarkable.

Evaluation

He was advised to wear an actigraph for 2 weeks, complete a sleep log during this period, and obtain a polysomnogram (PSG). The actigraph was requested to get a better idea of sleep-wake schedule, and the PSG was to get objective evidence of sleep. Simon was thrilled that he was to get a PSG at last, as numerous providers in the past felt PSG would not be helpful. Simon was confident that it would prove his point to all.

The PSG showed a sleep latency of 20 minutes and a total sleep time of 7 hours and 30 minutes. The sleep architecture was fairly normal, with wake after sleep onset (WASO) time of less than 10 minutes (Figure 5.1). There was no snoring, and he did not have any apneas or hypopneas. The lowest oxygen saturation during this study was 92%. There were no periodic limb movements or any unusual behavior noted during this sleep study. Interestingly, the morning after PSG he reported not sleeping at all during the study.

On his sleep log, he reported sleeping for only 1 to 2 hours every 2 to 3 days (Figure 5.2), however, actigraphy showed a relatively normal sleep-wake pattern with approximate sleep and wake times of 11 p.m. to midnight and 7 a.m., respectively (Figure 5.3).

Diagnosis

Paradoxical insomnia.

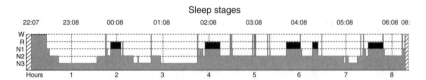

Figure 5.1 A relatively normal sleep architecture showing all stages of sleep and multiple sleep cycles. Note the predominance of deep NREM sleep in the first one-third of the night and the multiple REM periods (black).

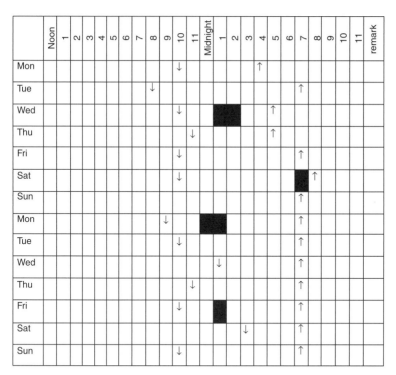

	Noon	1	2	3	4	5	6	7	8	9	10	11	Midnight	1	2	3	4	5	6	7	8	9	10	11	remark
Mon											↓					↑									
Tue							↓												↑						
Wed										↓			■		↑										
Thu											↓				↑										
Fri										↓									↑						
Sat										↓										■ ↑					
Sun																			↑						
Mon								↓			■					↑									
Tue									↓							↑									
Wed												↓				↑									
Thu										↓						↑									
Fri									↓			■				↑									
Sat														↓			↑								
Sun										↓						↑									

Figure 5.2 Sleep log in patient with paradoxical insomnia. Here the patient reports going to bed at around 10 to 11 p.m. on most of the nights and getting out of bed at approximately 7 a.m. However, his reported sleep time during these 2 weeks is just 6 hours all together.

Outcome

Every attempt was made at the initial evaluation to help Simon understand the normal sleep requirements and why it is impossible to continue to function relatively well without sleep for the alleged 45 days. He, however, was adamant that he never sleeps at night, and he got confrontational and at the same time frustrated that no one believed him. Three weeks after the initial visit, Simon returned to the clinic, and this time his brother accompanied him. Simon requested that his brother be present during this visit so that his brother could witness the lack of sleep during the study. The findings on both the actigram and PSG were explained to Simon and his brother. While his brother expressed no surprise, Simon was incredulous of the results and felt they were inaccurate. He chose not to follow up.

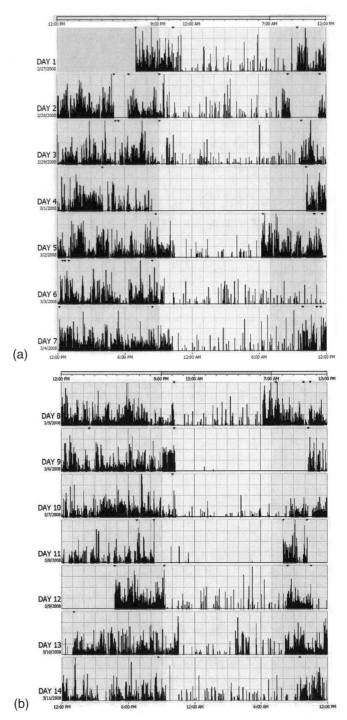

Figure 5.3a and 5.3b Actigraphy showing a relatively normal sleep-wake pattern. The pattern is suggestive of a sleep time at 11 p.m. to mid-night and a wake time of approximately 7 a.m. on most days.

Discussion

This is an extreme case of paradoxical insomnia, which is, surprisingly, not very uncommon in patients who present to a tertiary sleep disorder center.

Paradoxical insomnia was very high in the differential diagnosis because of the nature and severity of insomnia the patient reported at the initial visit, which is not compatible with the normal function of human body. ICSD-2 defines paradoxical insomnia as "a complaint of severe insomnia that occurs without evidence of objective sleep disturbance and without the level of daytime impairment commensurate with the degree of sleep deficits reported" (Table 5.1).

Psychophysiological insomnia should be considered in this patient. Although Simon met the general criteria for insomnia and reported some worries and anxiety associated with his perceived inability to fall asleep, he did not have other features of psychophysiological insomnia, such as ability to sleep better in places other than his bed/home or difficulty falling asleep in bed at desired

---

Table 5.1 ICSD-2 criteria for paradoxical insomnia

A. The patient's symptoms meet the criteria for insomnia.
B. The insomnia is present for at least 1 month.
C. One or more of the following criteria apply:
  i. The patient reports a chronic pattern of little or no sleep most nights with rare nights during which relatively normal amounts of sleep are obtained.
  ii. Sleep-log data during 1 or more weeks of monitoring show an average sleep time well below published age-adjusted normative values, often with no sleep at all indicated for several nights per week; typically, there is absence of daytime naps following such nights.
  iii. The patient shows a consistent, marked mismatch between objective findings from polysomnography or actigraphy and subjective sleep estimates derived either from self-report or a sleep diary.
D. At least 1 of the following is observed:
  i. The patient reports constant or near constant awareness of environmental stimuli throughout most nights.
  ii. The patient reports a pattern of conscious thoughts or rumination throughout most nights while maintaining a recumbent position.
E. The daytime impairment reported is consistent with that reported by other insomnia subtypes, but is much less severe than expected given the extreme level of sleep deprivation reported; there is no report of intrusive daytime sleep episodes, disorientation, or serious mishaps due to marked loss of alertness or vigilance, even following reportedly sleepless nights.
F. The reported sleep disturbance is not better explained by another sleep disorder, medical or neurological disorder, mental disorder, medication use, or substance abuse disorder.

---

bedtime, but no difficulty falling asleep during other monotonous activities when not intending to sleep. Short sleeper is another diagnostic consideration. It is a normal variant wherein people routinely get 5 hours of sleep or less in 24 hours and do not have any daytime impairment. They do not focus on their short sleep period, but rather may express satisfaction with both the quantity and quality of their sleep.

Finally, idiopathic insomnia is another condition that should be ruled out. Idiopathic insomnia is a chronic condition characterized by onset in infancy or childhood with no identifiable precipitant or cause, and the course of this disorder is characterized by lack of sustained remission. Of note, our patient had no difficulty sleeping until 5 years ago, and until then he reportedly slept for 8 to 9 hours every night.

Insomnia is defined as difficulty falling asleep, staying asleep or unrefreshing sleep despite adequate opportunity to sleep, accompanied by some daytime impairment. Patients with paradoxical insomnia, previously termed sleep state misperception, complain of sleeplessness although sleep tests show a normal sleep pattern. Patients will often report spending hours lying awake at night, although bed partners report that the patient appears to be asleep. These patients significantly underestimate their total sleep time and overestimate their sleep latency and wake time after sleep onset. Patients also generally report an unrealistic amount of sleep deprivation, often reporting going several nights without any sleep at all. Daytime effects of the perceived sleep loss varies, but in most cases functional impairment is far less severe than expected given the reported estimated sleep time.

The cause of this disorder is unknown. However it is thought that these patients suffer from an intense awareness of their surroundings throughout the entire night, or a state of hyperarousal consistent with being awake even though all objective measures show the patient is asleep. One study showed that patients with paradoxical insomnia demonstrated significantly increased 24-hour metabolic rate compared with matched normals, suggesting a physiologic hyperarousal state. An overnight sleep study generally shows fairly normal sleep duration and quality. Of note, PSG is not indicated in the diagnosis of insomnia. In our patient, PSG was done to get objective evidence of sleep because of the chronic nature and the patient's perceived severity of the problem.

Although insomnia is a common disorder, affecting from 10%–35% of people in the United States, paradoxical insomnia is relatively rare, affecting fewer than 5% of those with chronic insomnia. Paradoxical insomnia is more common in younger and middle-aged patients. There is no known gender bias, although insomnia in general is more common in women. Patients with paradoxical insomnia are more likely to suffer from depression and anxiety.

There are 2 primary treatment approaches for insomnia in general: pharmacotherapy and cognitive behavioral therapy for insomnia (CBTi). However, paradoxical insomnia is difficult to treat. Studies have shown that benzodiazepines can reduce physiological activation as measured by metabolic rate and body temperature. Studies have also shown that benzodiazepines improve perception of sleep in insomniacs compared to normal subjects. However, the effectiveness of long-term treatment of paradoxical insomnia with benzodiazepines is unknown. The risk of tolerance and abuse, as well as cognitive side effects, must also be considered with benzodiazepine use. CBTi that includes stimulus control, relaxation therapy, and sleep hygiene therapy may also be effective in some patients. In some cases, after patients are shown their normal testing results their sleep perception improves without further treatment. Alas, Simon did not give us that opportunity.

Bibliography

Bonnet MH, Arrand DL. Physiological activation in patients with sleep state misperception. *Psychosomatic Medicine*. 1997;59:533–540.

Mendelson WB. Effects of flurazepam and zolpidem on the perception of sleep in insomniacs. *SLEEP*. 1995;18:92.

6

Alpha Delta: One Sorority You Don't Want to Join!

KAMALA ADURY, MD
KUMAR BUDUR, MD, MS

Clinical History

Joyce, a 50-year-old woman, worked from home as an Internet marketer. She was recently diagnosed with fibromyalgia. During an office visit, she told her rheumatologist about her sleep issues, noting she was able to sleep well until she started having aches and pains a year ago.

Joyce mentioned that when she first started having pain symptoms, she just had difficulty falling asleep. This was mainly because she felt tender and achy, and she frequently changed positions to find a comfortable sleep posture. Over time, she began waking up in the middle of the night with sore, achy arms and legs, "like needles all over my body." She sometimes woke up 3 to 4 times, needing about 30 minutes each time to go back to sleep. She was worried about not being able to sleep through the night and consequently feeling tired or sleepy during the day. However, she soon realized that worrying made her sleep problems worse, and she started listening to a relaxation tape that her husband used for yoga. She found that it distracted her and helped her to relax. Her rheumatologist started her on 20 mg duloxetine, and the dose was gradually increased to 60 mg every morning, whereupon she noted about 50%–60% reduction in pain symptoms. She was tried briefly on an even higher dose but experienced nausea and headaches without further improvement in symptoms. Although the pain symptoms improved, she continued to have difficulty with insomnia and woke up unrefreshed in the morning. At this stage, her rheumatologist decided to seek an opinion from a sleep specialist.

At the sleep center, Joyce reported a typical bedtime of 10 p.m. and almost 60 minutes to sleep onset. During this period she remained in bed, hoping to fall asleep. She denied worrying or thinking about sleep or getting anxious or nervous. She listened to the relaxation tape during this period and denied any other activities such as reading, watching TV, or repeatedly looking at the clock. Once she was asleep, she woke up 2 to 3 times a night, at times spontaneously and sometimes due to pain. Since the pain symptoms had improved on medication, she was able to resume sleep in 10 to 15 minutes. During these awakenings, she simply rested in the bed. She woke up to an alarm at 7 a.m. and felt tired. Joyce felt that her fatigue got worse as the day progressed, and in the afternoon, especially around 2 to 3 p.m., she felt sleepy, too. Since she worked from home, she was able to take a nap lasting for an hour and she felt better, but not necessarily refreshed. She estimated a total sleep time of 6 to 6.5 hours at night. She had a similar schedule during the weekends. Prior to the onset of her symptoms, she reported a total sleep time of about 7.5 to 8 hours every night and felt refreshed in the morning. Joyce had noticed that her sleep deteriorated whenever her fibromyalgia symptoms got worse, especially when the weather changed. She vividly recalled an episode when her family went to vacation in Denver, CO, and she noticed a significant increase in pain symptoms and sleep problems. She attributed this to a sudden change in pressure and humidity. At the time of presentation, she had an Epworth Sleepiness Scale (ESS) score of 11/24 and a markedly elevated Fatigue Severity Scale (FSS) of 56/63.

Joyce had gained about 20 lbs in the past year, mainly because of lack of activity secondary to pain symptoms. Her husband had observed her snoring and sometimes light breathing but no apnea. She denied any episodes of waking up choking or gasping for air. She slept predominantly on her right side, and she woke up with a dry mouth in the morning. She denied symptoms of other sleep disorders, such as restless legs syndrome, periodic leg movement disorder, narcolepsy, and parasomnias.

Except for the diagnosis of fibromyalgia, she did not have any medical problems, and duloxetine was her only medication. She specifically denied acid reflux or symptoms suggestive of thyroid disorder or psychiatric problems. Review of systems was otherwise unremarkable. She denied feeling depressed, lack of interests, and other psychological symptoms of depression, including suicidal ideation. However, she had felt low and depressed for some time after the onset of fibromyalgia and insomnia symptoms. These feelings resolved spontaneously. Her family history was significant for sleep apnea (father and brother) and depression (mother). Joyce had stopped consuming caffeine when she developed insomnia. She did not smoke and drank 1 glass of wine on weekends. She was married for 28 years and had 2 adult children doing well in college. She denied marital and financial problems.

Physical Examination

On examination, Joyce was obese, with a body mass index of 31 kg/m². Her oropharyngeal exam showed Grade I tonsils and a Freidman tongue position

Grade III. Her general and neurological examinations were otherwise unremarkable.

Evaluation

A polysomnogram (PSG) was done to rule out sleep apnea given her history of snoring and recent weight gain. She slept for 348 minutes, resulting in a sleep efficiency of 95%. The sleep latency was 22 minutes, and REM latency was 100 minutes. The overall apnea-hypopnea index (AHI) was 2.3, and the arousal index was 9. The mean oxygen saturation was 95% and the minimum oxygen saturation was 90%. Additional findings on PSG included alpha intrusion during NREM sleep, especially during Stage N3 sleep (Figures 6.1, 6.2).

Diagnoses

Insomnia due to medical condition.
Fibromyalgia.
Primary snoring.

Outcome

Joyce was educated about insomnia and sleep hygiene. Specifically, she was advised not to go to bed unless sleepy and to get out of the bed and do something relaxing if she was unable to sleep within 15 to 20 minutes. She was also advised not to nap during the day to enhance sleep consolidation at night.

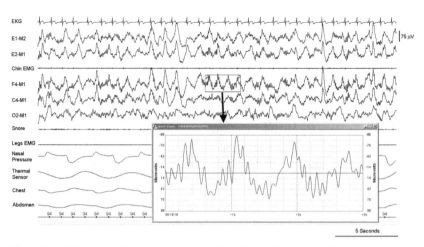

Figure 6.1 Alpha-intrusion on slow-wave sleep. Here alpha waves (frequency of 8–12 Hz) are superimposed over delta waves (frequency of 0.5 to 2 Hz).

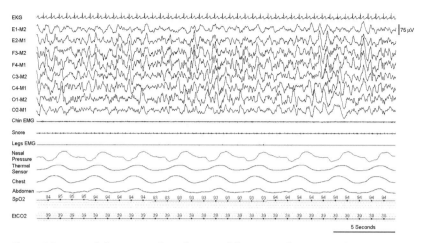

Figure 6.2 Normal slow-wave sleep showing delta waves (frequency of 0.5 to 2 Hz). No superimposed alpha waves are noted (contrast with Figure 6.1).

Pharmacotherapy was also discussed. Since she still had some residual symptoms of fibromyalgia, and she was not able to tolerate a higher dose of duloxetine, she was advised to discuss a trial of pregabalin with her rheumatologist.

At her first follow-up visit, Joyce reported she had been started on pregabalin 50 mg TID 2 weeks prior. She had noticed a remarkable improved in her pain. She was less fatigued during the day and able to avoid napping on all but 2 days per week. She had postponed her bedtime to 10:30 p.m. and found it much easier to fall asleep delaying bedtime until she was sleepy. She now took only 15 minutes to fall asleep. The nighttime awakenings were reduced to 1 or 2 per night, and she was able to reinitiate sleep in 10 minutes. She felt better during the day. She was advised to continue with sleep hygiene, relaxation and pregabalin.

At the second follow-up visit, Joyce was on pregabalin 100 mg TID in addition to duloxetine 60 mg, and she reported doing well. She had stopped taking naps during the day, and she did not report any problems with insomnia. She woke up 1 to 2 times at night spontaneously, but she was able to go back to sleep within a few minutes. She was getting about 7 hours of sleep every night and felt refreshed during the day. She was advised to continue current treatments and return as necessary.

Discussion

Joyce had a typical history of a patient with insomnia due to medical condition (Table 6.1). Joyce met the criteria for insomnia (difficulty falling and staying

Table 6.1 ICSD-2 criteria for insomnia due to medical condition

A. The patient's symptoms meet the criteria for insomnia.
B. The insomnia is present for at least 1 month.
C. The patient has a coexisting medical or physiologic condition known to disrupt sleep.
D. Insomnia is clearly associated with the medical or physiological condition. The insomnia began near the time of onset or with significant progression of the medical or physiologic condition, and it waxes and wanes with fluctuations in the severity of this condition.
E. The sleep disturbance is not better explained by another sleep disorder, mental disorder, medication use, or substance use disorder.

asleep for at least 1 month with daytime impairment). Further, the symptoms of insomnia were not just temporally related to fibromyalgia; they also fluctuated with the pain symptoms. Sleep symptoms are common in patients with fibromyalgia. Another diagnosis that should be considered is psychophysiological insomnia, but Joyce did not have a conditioned difficulty falling asleep. Typically, in such cases, symptoms get better when patients are removed from their usual sleeping environment (e.g., sleeping in a hotel during vacation) but in her case, the symptoms got worse on vacation. Moreover, she denied feeling anxious and tense at night, and she was actually able to relax at night using a relaxation tape. Obstructive sleep apnea syndrome (OSA) should be considered in this case because of the risk factors of perimenopausal status, snoring, awakenings in the middle of the night, unrefreshing sleep, and a crowded posterior airspace. Insomnia due to mental illness is a diagnostic consideration given that Joyce has significant medical problems and insomnia, both of which increase the risk of mental illness. She had some symptoms suggestive of depression after the onset of fibromyalgia and insomnia, but these symptoms resolved spontaneously. During the current assessment, she denied having any problems with depression or anxiety, or any other psychiatric problems. Finally, idiopathic hypersomnia without long sleep time is another diagnostic consideration. Joyce reported feeling sleepy during the day, especially in the afternoon, and she took a nap lasting for 30 minutes on most days. However, the frequency or duration of the naps and the intensity of daytime sleepiness were not typical of that seen in idiopathic hypersomnia, making this diagnosis unlikely.

Insomnia due to medical conditions is a common form of insomnia that can be associated with a host of disorders, including angina, heart failure, asthma, emphysema, Parkinson's disease, gastroesophageal reflux, chronic pain syndromes, and malignancies. In these situations, it is important that the medical condition is optimally treated. Patients should be educated on the implications of the underlying medical condition on sleep and the importance of good sleep hygiene practices. Hypnotic medication may be indicated in some cases. Co-morbid insomnia in patients with medical conditions is associated with higher morbidity and increased health care expenditure.

Joyce's case illustrates the scope of sleep and wake complaints commonly observed in patients with fibromyalgia. These include difficulty falling asleep, recurrent awakenings, unrefreshing sleep, and feelings of daytime tiredness or sleepiness. Patients with fibromyalgia often have alpha intrusion in NREM sleep, particularly in Stage N3 sleep on PSG. This is commonly referred to as "alpha-delta sleep." Alpha delta sleep is seen in patients with a host of disorders, including fibromyalgia, chronic fatigue syndrome, depression, and rheumatoid arthritis. In addition, the PSG of a fibromyalgia patient commonly demonstrates a long sleep latency, a relative increase in Stage NI and a decrease in Stage N3 sleep, increased arousal index, and poor sleep efficiency.

Pregabalin is approved by the FDA for the treatment of fibromyalgia. In clinical trials, patients with fibromyalgia who took pregabalin showed significant improvement in pain, sleep, fatigue, and quality of life compared to patients who took placebo. Duloxetine and milnacipran, both serotonin and norepinephrine re-uptake inhibitors, also are effective in the management of pain-related symptoms associated with fibromyalgia. Both are approved by the FDA for the treatment of pain symptoms in fibromyalgia. Another medication, sodium oxybate, is reported to have shown beneficial effects in fibromyalgia in clinical trials. However, sodium oxybate is not yet approved by the FDA for the treatment of fibromyalgia.

Bibliography

Harding S. Sleep in fibromyalgia patients: Subjective and objective findings. Fibromyalgia Symposium; American Journal of the Medical Sciences. *Fibromyalgia.* 1998;315:367–376.

Tishler M, Barack Y, Paran D, Yaron M. Sleep disturbances, fibromyalgia and primary Sjogren's syndrome. *Clin Exp Rheumatol.* 1997;15:71–74.

7

The Case of the Sleepless Insurance Agent

HARALABOS MERMIGIS, MD

ZAHR ALSHEIKHTAHA, MD, RPSGT

Case History

Stewart was a 52-year-old insurance company executive who presented with insomnia of 5 year's duration. There was no apparent medical, social, or psychological incident precipitating his complaint. His customary time in bed was from 11 p.m. to 7 a.m. on weekdays and until 8 a.m. on weekends. He reported difficulty falling asleep, spending about 45 minutes to an hour awake in bed before sleep onset, but he denied negative thoughts or worries at night. He had multiple awakenings during the night, sometimes associated with shortness of breath, and had difficulty returning back to sleep. He was taking zaleplon or lorazepam twice a week for the last 2 years and was concerned he might get addicted to sleep medication. Stewart endorsed fatigue and daytime sleepiness (Epworth Sleepiness Scale score was 11), which interfered with his productivity at work. He denied depressed mood and scored 9 on the Beck Depression Inventory (BDI). He snored rarely, although his wife observed apneas most nights. He denied hypnagogic hallucinations, sleep paralysis, cataplexy, and symptoms suggestive for restless legs syndrome. He normally consumed 4 caffeinated beverages a day and did not use alcohol or tobacco. He had no significant medical or surgical history and took no regular medications.

Physical Examination

Stewart had a blood pressure of 130/80 mmHg, a heart rate of 70 bpm, a neck circumference of 39 cm, and a body mass index of 24 kg/m². His oropharynx revealed a Mallampati score of 1 with absent tonsils. His cardiac, respiratory, abdominal, neurological, and vascular examinations were unremarkable.

Evaluation

Stewart underwent a polysomnogram (PSG) for suspected sleep apnea. During the night of the study, he slept only 134 minutes, resulting in a sleep efficiency of 43%. The sleep latency was 57 minutes, and he was awake for 117 minutes after sleep onset. He had an apnea-hypopnea index (AHI) of 65, with more than 90% of events being central in nature without Cheyne Stokes breathing pattern (Figure 7.1). There was no snoring. The AHI was normal during REM sleep (Figure 7.2). Respiratory events were associated with mild oxygen desaturation (mean oxygen saturation of 95%, minimum of 90%, desaturation index 24). Significant sleep fragmentation was noted with an arousal index of 38. There were 8 periodic leg movements per sleep hour, only a few resulting in arousal.

Stewart was given the diagnosis of central sleep apnea (CSA). He underwent further testing to assess for the etiology for central apnea. Echocardiogram, chest CT, pulmonary function tests, and brain MRI were normal. His arterial blood gases while awake and breathing room air revealed a PO_2 87, PCO_2 39, and pH 7.43. Consequently, his CSA was thought to be primary in nature, as secondary causes were reasonably excluded.

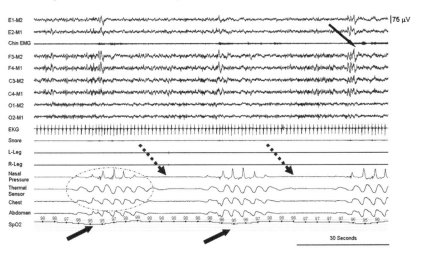

Figure 7.1 Two-minute epoch showing repetitive central apneas during N2 sleep associated with mild oxygen desaturations (bottom arrows) and arousals (top arrow). Central apneas are characterized by a total cessation of airflow in the nasal pressure and thermal sensor channels without evidence of effort in the chest and abdomen (dashed arrows). An abrupt and short ventilation phase without waxing and waning appearance (dotted oval) is observed. The 75 µV bar applies to EOG, EEG, and Chin EMG.

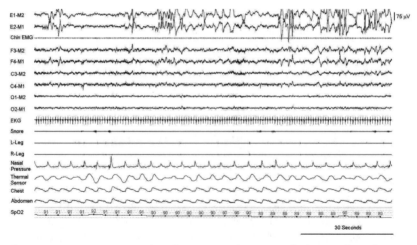

Figure 7.2 Two-minute recording during REM sleep. Note the bursts of rapid eye movements, low EMG in the chin and leg channels, and low-voltage EEG rhythm. Respiratory events are notably absent. The $75\,\mu V$ bar applies to EOG, EEG, and Chin EMG.

Diagnosis

Primary central sleep apnea (Table 7.1).

Outcome

Stewart returned for a positive airway pressure (PAP) titration study. Neither continuous PAP (CPAP) nor bi-level modes with variable pressures adequately reduced central apneas, although he had difficulty acclimating to the device in the laboratory (Figure 7.3). As a result, he underwent a period of habituation on home CPAP at $8\,cmH_2O$ prior to further laboratory testing. Despite his effort

---

Table 7.1 ICSD-2 diagnostic criteria for primary central sleep apnea

Primary central sleep apnea is diagnosed when A, B, and C satisfy these criteria:

A. The patient reports at least one of the following:
   i. Excessive daytime sleepiness.
   ii. Frequent arousals and awakenings during sleep or insomnia complaints.
   iii. Awakenings short of breath.

B. Polysomnographic recording shows 5 or more central apneas per hour of sleep.

C. The disorder is not better explained by another current sleep disorder, medical or neurological disorder, medication use, or substance disorder.

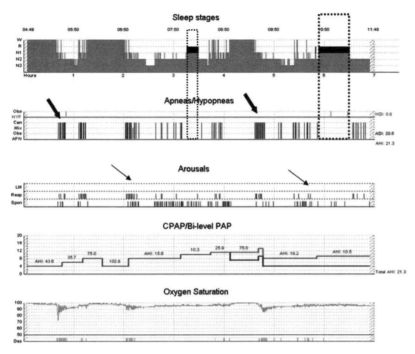

Figure 7.3 Hypnogram of the PAP titration study beginning with CPAP and converting to bilevel PAP. Central apneas (top arrows) became more frequent resulting in multiple arousals (thin arrows) every time the technician tried to increase the pressure. Central events were not present in REM sleep periods (dotted boxed areas) regardless of PAP pressure or mode.

to comply fully with therapy, the data download revealed only 3.4 hours per night of use with a residual AHI of 20. He felt his insomnia was worse with CPAP and had no improvement in his daytime symptoms. A trial of triazolam reduced his sleep latency and night awakenings a bit but did not affect his fatigue and daytime sleepiness. Auto bi-level PAP was no better than CPAP in terms of tolerance, residual apnea, and persistence of daytime sleepiness and fatigue.

Due to Stewart's severe CSA, which persisted despite CPAP and bi-level PAP therapies, a titration with adaptive servo-ventilation (ASV) was recommended. The study began with an expiratory positive airway pressure (EPAP) of $5 \, cmH_2O$, pressure support of 3 to $10 \, cmH_2O$, and a back-up rate of 15 breaths per minute. EPAP was increased every 20 to 30 minutes to abolish respiratory events, desaturations, and arousals. A normal respiratory pattern was achieved at EPAP $8 \, cmH_2O$, pressure support 3 to $10 \, cmH_2O$ and a back-up rate of 15 breaths per minute (Figure 7.4). He returned to the sleep clinic 2 weeks after beginning ASV therapy at home and reported at least 5 hours of use per night, often more. He and his wife described a significant improvement in sleep quality and virtual complete resolution of insomnia, daytime sleepiness, and fatigue.

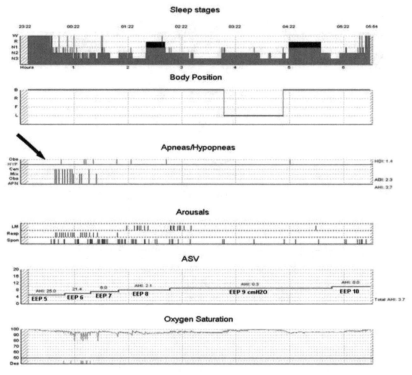

Figure 7.4 Hypnogram of the adaptive servo-ventilation (ASV) titration study
Central apneas persisted at the beginning of the titration (arrow). Respiratory
events were normalized at expiratory positive airway pressure (EPAP) settings of 8,
9, and 10 cmH$_2$O. Minimum pressure support of 3 cmH$_2$O and maximum pressure
support of 10 cmH$_2$O was used with all EPAP settings.

Discussion

Central sleep apnea syndromes are characterized by repeated cessation of airflow during sleep resulting from temporary loss of ventilatory effort (Table 7.2).
CSA typically occurs under circumstances of high altitude or in association
with congestive heart failure (CHF) or stroke. In the latter conditions, Cheyne
Stokes breathing pattern, namely waxing and waning appearance of central
respiratory events alternating with hyperventilation, is observed (Figure 7.5).
CSA rarely occurs at sea level in individuals with no apparent cardiac (systolic
dysfunction), neurologic or pulmonary disease. In such cases, the diagnosis of
primary CSA is made. Primary CSA is an uncommon disorder, representing
fewer than 5% of all cases of sleep apnea in sleep laboratory populations, and by
definition it is a diagnosis of exclusion.

The etiology of primary CSA remains unknown, although it is believed
that the primary mechanism is a genetically based elevated chemosensitivity of

Table 7.2 Classification of central sleep apnea syndromes

Primary (idiopathic) CSA
CSA due to Cheyne Stokes breathing pattern
CSA due to high-altitude periodic breathing
CSA due to medical condition not Cheyne Stokes
CSA due to drug or substance
Primary sleep apnea of infancy (formerly primary sleep apnea of newborn)

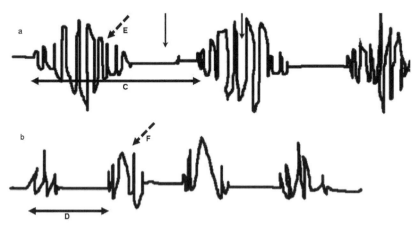

Figure 7.5 Airflow channel signal in a patient with Cheyne Stokes breathing pattern due to CHF (a) and primary CSA (b). The ventilation-apnea cycle is prolonged in Cheyne Stokes breathing pattern (arrow C) compared with CSA (arrow D) and is characterized by a waxing and waning appearance of the ventilation phase (arrow E). An abrupt and short ventilation phase without waxing and waning appearance is seen in primary CSA (arrow F). PCO_2 decreases during the ventilation phase in both cases, reaching the apnea threshold, which results in an apnea. This causes a rise in PCO_2 during the apnea period resulting in hyperventilation, thus perpetuating the cycle.

arterial partial pressure of carbon dioxide (PCO_2). Chemosensitivity refers to the magnitude of ventilatory output to a given change in PCO_2, known as controller gain. In primary CSA, apneas are precipitated by an abrupt increase in tidal volume and minute ventilation, often in association with arousals from sleep, which are accompanied by reductions in PCO_2. In addition, patients with primary CSA, like those with Cheyne Stokes breathing pattern, tend to have hypocapnia during wakefulness. While behavioral influences and neurocompensatory responses strongly oppose apnea even in the presence of marked decreases in PCO_2 during the waking state, this is not the case during sleep. In sleep, primary CSA patients are susceptible to apneic events when the PCO_2 falls below a critical threshold known as the apnea threshold. In primary CSA, the negative feedback system that controls breathing elicits a large ventilatory response when PCO_2 levels rise. The resultant hyperventilatory response drives the PCO_2 below the apneic threshold, producing a central apnea. As a result of the apnea, the PCO_2 rises again, leading to an increase in ventilation, thus perpetuating the cycle.

Primary CSA should be differentiated from Cheyne Stokes breathing pattern. In both conditions, central respiratory events occur primarily during sleep Stages N1 and N2, decrease during stable N3, and disappear in REM sleep because chemosensitivity (controller gain) is reduced during REM sleep and is insufficient to drive the cycling respiration. In primary CSA, the duration of the cycle is shorter (typically 20 to 45 seconds) than in Cheyne Stokes breathing pattern, and more abrupt in onset and offset, lacking a waxing and waning appearance. Oxygen desaturations tend to be less severe, and arousals typically occur at the termination of events. These differences are explained in part by the "recovery phase" in cases of Cheyne Stokes breathing pattern, which is smoother and longer than in primary CSA, reflecting a prolonged arterial circulation time (Figure 7.5).

Stewart represents a typical case of primary CSA due to: (1) compatible symptoms, including sleep onset and maintenance insomnia resulting in poor sleep and daytime sleepiness and fatigue; (2) polysomnographic features, including an AHI of 65 with more than 90% of events being central in nature, cycle length of 35 to 40 seconds with no waxing and waning appearance, and normalization of respiration in REM sleep; and (3) a thorough evaluation that excluded cardiac, pulmonary, and neurologic disorders.

Therapeutic options for primary CSA include pharmacologic therapy, supplemental oxygen during sleep, methods that increase the inspired PCO_2 (inhalation of a CO_2-enriched gas mixture or increase in dead space in PAP devices circuits), and PAP therapy. Some believe that benzodiazepine and nonbenzodiazepine hypnotics not only improve sleep but also decrease apnea frequency, probably by reducing arousals and elevating arterial PCO_2. Triazolam has been the most commonly used benzodiazepine in this setting. Among nonbenzodiazepine agents, zolpidem has been shown to be efficacious in the induction and maintenance of sleep and in the reduction of arousals. The carbonic anhydrase inhibitor acetazolamide may also be effective by producing a metabolic acidosis that shifts the hypercapnic ventilatory response and lowers the apnea threshold.

Several small, short-term trials have shown that oxygen administration reduces respiratory events in patients with primary CSA. However, since this effect has not been confirmed by larger studies, caution is advised, as oxygen may have cardiodepressant effects mediated by O_2 radicals. An increase in inhaled CO_2 sufficient to raise PCO_2 by 1 to 3 mmHg has been shown to eliminate central respiratory events in preliminary studies involving patients with primary CSA. However, this mode of therapy requires further investigation

Nasal CPAP has been shown to be effective in a minority of primary CSA cases. Bi-level PAP therapy is effective in some patients with primary CSA, but deleterious in others by producing hypocapnea. ASV is a more sophisticated method of ventilatory support designed for patients with Chenye Stokes breathing pattern and CHF. Recent studies show promise in primary CSA patients, as illustrated by Stewart's case. Further research is needed to identify the most effective treatments for primary CSA.

Bibliography

Banno K, Okamura K, Kryger, M. Adaptive servo-ventilation in patients with idiopathic Cheyne-Stokes breathing. *J Clin Sleep Med.* 2006;2(2):181–186.

Eckert D, Jordan A, Merchia P and Malhotra A. Central sleep apnea: Pathophysiology and treatment. *Chest.* 2007;131:595–607.

Xie A, Rutherford R, Rankin F, Wong B, Bradley TD. Hypocapnia and increased ventilatory responsiveness in patients with idiopathic central sleep apnea. *Am J Respir Crit Care Med.* 1995;152:1950–1955.

Xie A, Wong B, Phillipson EA, et al. Interaction of hyperventilation and arousal in the pathogenesis of idiopathic central sleep apnea. *Am J Respir Crit Care Med.* 1994; 150:489–495.

8

Out of Sight, Out of Mind

INGA SRIUBIENE, MD
STELLA BACCARAY, RN
NANCY FOLDVARY-SCHAEFER, DO

Case History

Roy was a 49-year-old Caucasian man with ischemic heart failure (HF) who was referred to the sleep disorders center by his cardiologist for evaluation of sleep apnea. He and his wife denied he had any sleep complaints and did not understand why he had been referred. He typically went to bed at 11 p.m. and had no problems falling asleep. He would wake up 5 to 7 times per night, for no apparent reason. However, on occasion, he woke up abruptly feeling short of breath. His usual wake up time was 7 a.m., and he generally felt refreshed in the morning. He estimated a total sleep time of 8 hours. Roy usually slept in the supine position and often woke up in the morning with a dry mouth. On occasion, his wife noted light snoring, which resolved when he rolled onto his stomach. Both he and his wife denied that Roy had any episodes of gasping, choking, or breathing pauses in sleep and daytime sleepiness. He had an Epworth Sleepiness Scale (ESS) score of 6. However, he had experienced fatigue since his myocardial infarction (MI) 1 year prior. He did not take naps. He typically drank three 8-oz cups of coffee per day.

Roy's medical history was remarkable for noninsulin dependent diabetes mellitus (NIDDM), MI complicated by ischemic HF, and recurrent atrial fibrillation (AF) resistant to pharmacotherapy. He had undergone placement of an implantable cardioverter defibrillator (ICD). His medications included aspirin, clopidogrel, atorvastatin, lisinopril, carvedilol, spironolactone, furosemide, and digoxin. A recent echocardiogram (ECHO) revealed a left ventricle ejection fraction (LVEF) of 15% with normal left ventricle (LV) size, severe hypokinesis of mid inferior and mid anterior LV segments, restrictive baseline LV diastolic function, and normal right ventricle size and systolic function. He had a normal HbA1C and thyroid stimulating hormone. A brain natriuretic peptide (BNP) level was 105 pg/ml (normal: 0–99). Roy denied alcohol use and smoked 1 pack of cigarettes per day for 20 years, which he had quit after his MI. He worked as an electrical power plant operator. Due to his recent health issues, he was unable to fully participate in his favorite outdoor activities, golfing and gardening.

Physical Examination

Roy had a blood pressure of 122/88 mmHg, a heart rate of 88 beats per minute and a respiratory rate of 18 breaths per minute. At 140 kg and 186 cm tall, his body mass index was 41 kg/m². His neck circumference was 46 cm. The upper airway examination revealed patent nares and a Grade III Friedman tongue position. His cardiac exam revealed an irregularly irregular rhythm without murmur. The lungs were clear to auscultation, and there were no signs of jugular venous distention or lower extremity edema.

Evaluation

Roy underwent a polysomnogram (PSG) to evaluate for sleep apnea given his history of snoring, fatigue, and obesity. The total sleep time was 439 minutes, resulting in a sleep efficiency of 79%. He fell asleep in 34 minutes and had a REM latency of 74 minutes. He spent 72% of sleep time in the supine position. He spent 17.7% of sleep time in Stage N1, 56.3% in N2, 3.1% in N3, and 22.9% in REM sleep. There were 390 arousals, resulting in an arousal index of 53. Roy snored heavily and had 428 respiratory events comprising 324 apneas (6 obstructive, 185 mixed, and 133 central) and 104 hypopneas (Tables 8.1, 8.2). The apnea-hypopnea index (AHI) was 58. The mean oxygen saturation was 90% with a minimum of 69%. He spent 37% of sleep time with oxygen saturation below 90%. The maximum end-tidal CO_2 (EtCO$_2$) was 47 mmHg, and he spent only 2.6% of sleep time with an EtCO$_2$ above 45 mmHg. Periodic

Table 8.1 Respiratory event summary

	REM Time (min)	REM AHI	NREM Time (min)	NREM AHI	Total sleep time (min)	Overall AHI
Supine	39	57	273	69	312	67
Off-supine	62	29	67	45	128	38
Total	101	40	339	64	440	58

Table 8.2 Apnea-hypopnea index by event type and sleep stage

Apnea index = 44			Total
Obstructive apnea index	1	REM	2
		NREM	1
Mixed apnea index	25	REM	14
		NREM	29
Central apnea index	18	REM	5
		NREM	22
Hypopnea index = 14		REM	20
		NREM	13

breathing consistent with Cheyne Stokes breathing pattern was noted during stages N1 and N2 (Figure 8.1). The average heart rate during sleep was 54 beats per minute, with a range of 50 to 72. There were no periodic limb movements.

Diagnoses

Central sleep apnea (CSA) due to Cheyne Stokes breathing pattern (Table 8.3). Obstructive sleep apnea (OSA).
Ischemic heart failure.

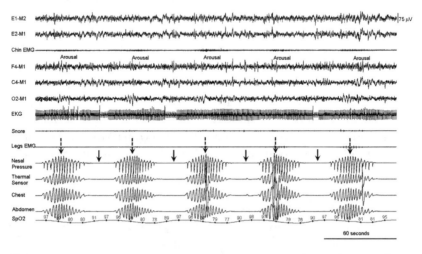

Figure 8.1 Five-minute tracing showing central sleep apnea due to Cheyne Stokes breathing pattern. Note the characteristic crescendo decrescendo pattern of breathing (broken arrows) alternating with central apneas (solid arrows) and arousals, occurring at the peak of respiratory effort.

Table 8.3 ICSD-2 diagnostic criteria for Cheyne Stokes breathing pattern

A. Polysomnography shows at least 10 central apneas and hypopneas per hour of sleep in which the hypopnea has a crescendo-decrescendo pattern of tidal volume accompanied by frequent arousals from sleep and derangements of sleep structure.
   Note: *Although symptoms are not mandatory to make this diagnosis, patients often report excessive daytime sleepiness, frequent arousals and awakenings during sleep, insomnia complaints, or awakenings short of breath.*
B. The breathing disorder occurs in association with a serious medical illness, such as heart failure, stroke, or renal failure.
C. The disorder is not better explained by another current sleep disorder, medication use, or substance use disorder.

Outcome

Since Roy's PSG showed evidence of both OSA and CSA with Cheyne Stokes breathing pattern despite optimization of HF management, a trial of continuous positive airway pressure (CPAP) therapy was recommended. Roy was acclimated to CPAP $5\,cmH_2O$ for 1 week at home before returning to the sleep laboratory for a PAP titration study. CPAP was titrated from $5\,cmH_2O$ to $10\,cmH_2O$, increasing by $2\,cmH_2O$ every 40 minutes to abolish apneas and hypopneas, and by $1\,cmH_2O$ for snoring, oxygen desaturations, and arousals. Since central events and periodic breathing persisted on CPAP $10\,cmH_2O$, bi-level PAP therapy was initiated at an inspiratory positive airway pressure (IPAP) of $8\,cmH_2O$ and an expiratory positive airway pressure (EPAP) of $4\,cmH_2O$ with a back-up rate of 14 breaths per minute (2 to 4 breaths fewer than his respiratory rate in sleep). EPAP was increased by $2\,cmH_2O$ every 40 minutes to abolish apneas; IPAP was increased correspondingly to maximum of $15\,cmH_2O$ to eliminate hypopneas, arousals, snoring, and desaturations. The IPAP-EPAP gradient was maintained at no less than $4\,cmH_2O$. Despite bi-level PAP therapy, the AHI remained unacceptably elevated and higher pressures were poorly tolerated. Consequently, a titration study with adaptive servo-ventilation (ASV) was performed with careful blood pressure and ECG monitoring. ASV was initiated at an EPAP of $5\,cmH_2O$ with a minimum and maximum pressure support of 3 to $10\,cmH_2O$. The EPAP setting was increased by $1\,cmH_2O$ slowly to eliminate respiratory events. At an EPAP setting of $9\,cmH_2O$, respiratory events were completely eliminated and the arousal index and oxygen saturation were normalized.

Roy has used ASV faithfully ever since, wearing it 7 to 8 hours per night, 7 nights per week. He enrolled in a weight-loss program and had lost 8 lbs by his

1-month follow-up visit. His energy level improved, and he and his wife both felt he was better able to perform daily activities. At his most recent follow-up visit, he reported meeting his golf buddies again every Thursday morning for an 8 a.m. tee time. His cardiologist was pleased to find that his LVEF had increased to 30% on his most recent ECHO.

Discussion

Sleep related breathing disorders (SRBD) represent an important, often unrecognized, co-morbidity in patients with HF, affecting 12% to more than 50% of cases. Central sleep apnea, including Cheyne Stokes breathing pattern and OSA, often co-exist. Central sleep apnea is characterized by recurrent episodes of cessation of respiration lasting 10 seconds or longer due to temporary loss of ventilatory drive. Cheyne Stokes breathing pattern, also known as periodic breathing and Cheyne Stokes respiration (CSR), is characterized by recurrent episodes of central apneas and/or hypopneas alternating with prolonged periods of hyperventilation in a crescendo-decrescendo ventilatory pattern. Identifying SRBD in HF patients has important clinical implications, since untreated SRBD can accelerate HF progression by producing a state of increased sympathetic activity due to recurrent oxygen desaturations and arousals. Increased sympathetic activity increases myocardial oxygen demand in the face of reduced oxygen supply. The presence of SRBD is associated with higher levels of BNP (higher BNP correlates with worse outcome in HF patients), longer hospital stays, increased risk of heart transplantation, and death. In addition, SRBD contributes to poorer quality of life in the HF population.

In contrast to patients with OSA, who typically present with snoring, significant daytime sleepiness, and obesity, those with CSA due to CSR (CSA-CSR) tend to experience fatigue, paroxysmal nocturnal dyspnea, and recurrent arousals and awakenings. Risk factors for CSA-CSR in the HF population include male gender, over 60 years of age, presence of AF, and hypocapnia (wake PCO_2 ≤ 38 mmHg). A definitive diagnosis of CSA-CSR is made by PSG.

The old phrase "Out of sight, out of mind"—the idea that something is easily forgotten or dismissed as unimportant if it is not in direct view—applies to breathing disorders in sleep in the HF population. Like the majority of HF patients with SRBD, Roy denied sleep complaints, and his wife did not recognize abnormal breathing patterns in sleep. In fact, he questioned why he was referred to the sleep center. Due to the presence of typical risk factors, his cardiologist maintained a high index of suspicion for SRBD and rightly referred him for sleep testing. Supportive features included intermittent snoring and frequent night awakenings, at times associated with shortness of breath. Pertinent findings on physical examination included obesity, large neck girth, and a crowded upper airway. Despite the relative paucity of sleep complaints, Roy's PSG demonstrated severe sleep apnea having both central and obstructive components and periodic breathing. His presentation and sleep evaluation illustrate the importance of maintaining a high clinical suspicion for SRBD in HF patients, even in the absence of notable sleep complaints, as untreated sleep disorders can have detrimental effects on cardiac function and quality of life.

The differential diagnoses in patients with central events on PSG include:

(1) Primary CSA. This rare form of SRBD was ruled out in Roy's case by the presence of HF. In addition, Roy's PSG was characterized by a crescendo-decrescendo pattern of breathing lasting almost invariably longer than 45 seconds, a feature of CSA-CSR. In contrast, central apneas are terminated more abruptly, and the length of the cycle is shorter in patients with primary CSA.

(2) Sleep related hypoventilation/hypoxemic syndrome can be distinguished from CSA-CSR by the presence of hypercapnic respiratory failure (wake $PCO_2 > 45$ mmHg) and more pronounced oxygen desaturations in sleep. Even though Roy had significant oxygen desaturations, the $EtCO_2$ consistently remained below 45 mmHg.

(3) CSA due to drug or substance abuse is typically characterized by a history of opioid use for at least 2 months or a history of substance abuse. Neither of these applied to Roy.

The treatment of CSA due to CSR includes optimization of HF medical therapy, which may improve or even abolish respiratory events. In patients with persistent apnea despite optimal medical therapy, especially if accompanied by severe oxygen desaturations and refractory HF, ventilatory support during sleep should be administered. Nocturnal oxygen supplementation, noninvasive positive pressure ventilation (NPPV) with CPAP, bi-level PAP, and ASV have been used in this setting. Blood pressure monitoring should be performed when PAP is introduced, before, during and on the morning after titration, as treatment can increase intrathoracic pressure and decrease cardiac output, resulting in hypotension and decreased coronary blood flow.

Early studies found that CPAP significantly reduced or eliminated respiratory events and improved LVEF in patients with CSA-CSR and systolic HF, in some cases improving survival. The Canadian Continuous Positive Airway Pressure for Patients with Central Sleep Apnea and Heart Failure Trial (CANPAP) showed that CPAP therapy reduced CSA, improved nocturnal oxygen saturation, decreased sympathetic activity, and increased LVEF. However, it failed to demonstrate improvement on the primary outcomes of transplantation-free survival and death. In fact, the early divergence in the event rates initially favored the control group but after 18 months favored the CPAP group. As a result of the CANPAP trial, CPAP therapy for treatment of predominantly CSA in HF patients in order to prolong survival is no longer recommended, but it remains the treatment of choice for OSA. A subsequent post-hoc analysis of the CANPAP database suggested that reduction of the AHI (< 15) by CPAP in patients with CSA might improve both LVEF and transplant-free survival, indicating that CPAP therapy could be beneficial in select patients with HF. However, further investigation is required to determine the efficacy and safety of CPAP therapy in this setting.

Limited data are available on other forms of PAP therapy for treatment of CSA in HF patients. Recent studies indicate that bi-level PAP therapy could be an effective alternative for HF patients with CSA-CSR who do not respond to CPAP. Bi-level PAP may not only reduce central respiratory events and normalize breathing patterns, it may also improve LVEF in HF patients. ASV is a novel therapy used to treat all forms of CSA and periodic breathing. It provides a small, continuous EPAP to eliminate obstructive events and a variable IPAP to eliminate central events when required. ASV was found to be more effective than CPAP in treating CSA, increasing LVEF, and improving quality of life in a small series of HF patients. Larger trials are needed to assess the beneficial effects of ASV on cardiovascular outcomes.

Bibliography

Arzt M, Floras JS, Logan AG, Kimoff RJ, Series F, Morrison D, Ferguson K, Belenkie I, Pfeifer M, Fleetham J, Hanly P, Smilovitch M, Ryan C, Tomlinson G, Bradley TD. Suppression of central sleep apnea by continuous positive airway pressure and transplant-free survival in heart failure: A post hoc analysis of the Canadian Continuous Positive Airway Pressure for Patients with Central Sleep Apnea and Heart Failure Trial (CANPAP). *Circulation.* 2007;(115):3173–3180.

Garcia-Touchard A, Somers VK, Olson LJ, Caples SM. Central sleep apnea: Implications for congestive heart failure. *Chest.* 2008;133(6):1495–1504.

Hastings PC, Vazir A, Meadows GE, Dayer M, Poole-Wilson PA, McIntyre HF, Morrell MJ, Cowie MR et al. Adaptive servo-ventilation in heart failure patients with sleep apnea: A real world study. *Int J Cardiol.* 2008;139:17–24.

Pepin JL, Couri-Pontarollo N, Tamisier R, Levy P. Cheyne Stokes respiration with central sleep apnoea in chronic heart failure: Proposals for a diagnostic and therapeutic strategy. *Sleep Med Rev.* 2006;10(1):33–47. Epub 2005 Dec 22.

9

Can't Breathe or Won't Breathe: How Would I Know if I Am Asleep?

BRUCE COHEN, MD

JYOTI KRISHNA, MD

Case History

By the age of 13, Shirley had been through it all. In 1998, when Shirley was 4 years old, she was found to have neurofibromatosis Type 1 (NF1) and a visual pathway glioma. The visual pathway glioma was treated with 6 months of intravenous chemotherapy (carboplatin and vincristine), which resulted in shrinkage and subsequent long-term stabilization of the tumor. When Shirley was 7 years old, she developed headaches and vomiting. The MRI scan showed a diffuse intrinsic brainstem mass, which was presumed to be a glioma (Figure 9.1). Based on the location, it was decided not to perform a diagnostic biopsy. She was treated empirically with temozolomide. The mass continued to grow and it was decided to perform a biopsy of the mass, which determined the tumor to be, in fact, a low-grade infiltrating astrocytoma. Since it had enlarged while Shirley was on chemotherapy, there had been discussion to try a different chemotherapeutic approach, but it was decided to treat with a standard course of external beam radiotherapy. The treatment resulted in an improvement in symptoms and shrinkage of the mass, and she had been in clinical and radiographic remission since that time. In 2007, at age 12, she developed a sixth cranial nerve palsy and was found to have papilledema. Coupled with a history of long-standing ventriculomegaly, she underwent a third ventriculostomy. During surgery, her CSF pressure was found to be elevated, and the procedure resulted in effectively treating the increased intracranial pressure.

On routine follow-up with her neuro-oncologist for tumor surveillance in 2008, Shirley complained of feeling tired all the time. Her parents noted mood

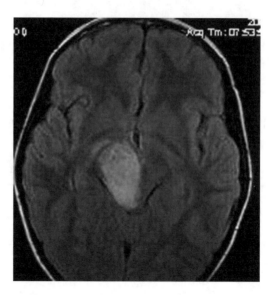

Figure 9.1 The brain MRI shows an axial FLAIR sequence demonstrating a right sided intrinsic infiltrating glioma (bright white area) involving the mid pons and midbrain.

changes and a decline in her school performance. Further history determined that she had poor sleep habits. She stayed awake until very late in the night and she would then sleep until 2 p.m. Her weight was steady at the 50th percentile, and despite having a history of 2 different brain tumors, her neurological examination was normal. The MRI was stable and there was no evidence of a change in the ventricular size or recurrence of the tumors. Due to the new history of excessive daytime fatigue, school failure and poor sleep patterns, Shirley was referred for a consult with a sleep specialist.

In the sleep clinic, Shirley was noted to be comfortable but very quiet. Historical details were thus obtained after Shirley's mother, Mrs. Hastings, asked her husband to wait in the lobby with Shirley. In hushed tones, Mrs. Hastings told us that this is how she preferred Shirley's medical discussions to proceed. She felt that repeated references to neurological issues of the past were best avoided in front of Shirley. She was tearful as she described her fears for her daughter's welfare. With the tumor under control, Shirley's sleep had become the focus of her attention. She noted that her daughter felt increasingly tired during the day with difficulty in falling asleep, daytime sleepiness, and delayed rise times. If allowed to awaken spontaneously, Shirley seemed to feel more rested and would not nap. Typically, Shirley would be on her computer "chatting" until 2 a.m. and usually awoke only after 11 a.m. Once asleep, she generally slept through the night without complaining of any symptoms suggestive of restless legs, bruxism, enuresis, or parasomnias. She did not snore, but she seemed to choke on her saliva at times. The erratic rhythm of her breathing, punctuated with long pauses and restlessness, really worried her mother, who began co-sleeping with her daughter "to keep an eye on her."

Review of systems was unremarkable. Specifically, there were no headaches, nausea, or seizure-like symptoms. Shirley was being home schooled both because of her sleep cycles and complex medical affairs as well as her inability to handle a full day's curriculum without breaks. She had only a few friends and generally remained sedentary ever since her treatment for the brainstem tumor.

Physical Examination

Shirley was noted to be quiet and withdrawn. The physical exam was unchanged since she had seen the neuro-oncologist. Specifically, her BMI was 25 kg/m^2, BP was $122/77 \text{ mmHg}$, and SpO_2 in room air was 99%. Her tonsils were surgically absent. She had mild retrognathia and tongue position was Friedman Grade II. The nasal septum was midline, and the turbinates appeared normal. Her neurological exam was normal as well.

Evaluation

A polysomnogram (PSG) was ordered with plans to do a multiple sleep latency test (MSLT) in case of a normal PSG. A delayed sleep protocol was used for the PSG, and lights were turned out at 1:32 a.m. The total record time was 554 minutes with a sleep efficiency of 66.8%. The sleep latency was 11.5 minutes and REM latency was 198 minutes. Of the total sleep time (TST), 91.5% was spent in supine position, and sleep stage distribution included 6.1% N1, 42.5% N2, 20.2% N3, and 31.2% REM.

The arousal index was 25.3 with 86 stage shifts. The apnea-hypopnea index (AHI) was 21.4 (39 hypopneas and 93 apneas). Of the apneas, there were 1 obstructive, 2 mixed, and 90 central events (Figure 9.2). The REM AHI was 56.6; NREM AHI was 5.4.

Oximetry showed mean SpO_2 of 96.0% with a nadir of 83.0%. Time below 90% was 1.8% of TST. $EtCO_2$ data showed time above 45 mmHg was 1.9% of TST.

Leg movements were not significantly elevated, with a PLM index 5.3 and PLM arousal index 1.3. Of note, the MSLT was cancelled due to severely abnormal PSG findings.

Diagnoses

Central sleep apnea (CSA) due to medical condition (brainstem glioma) not Cheyne Stokes.
Delayed sleep phase syndrome (DSPS).

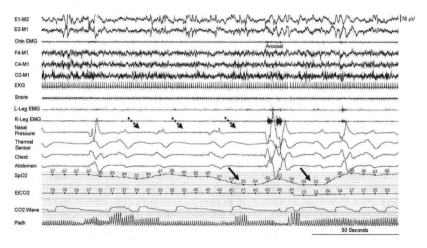

Figure 9.2 Baseline polysomnogram showing a 2-minute epoch in stage REM. Note multiple central apneas with no respiratory effort or airflow (broken arrows) and accompanying "see-saw" desaturations (solid arrows). The CO_2 waveform shows a distinct plateau signifying that end-tidal gases are truly being sampled. The regularity of the plethysmogram similarly is reassuring for reliable SpO_2 readings.

Outcome

At the return visit, the sleep study results were discussed with mother. As before, she preferred not have Shirley be part of the discussion. However, after explaining to her that treatment options included a nasal mask and a positive airway pressure (PAP) machine every night for the foreseeable future, mom agreed to have the child be part of the discussion. Shirley listened to her complicated sleep related diagnoses patiently. She remained quiet and accepting of our advice and her mother's decision to go ahead with a management plan. We respected the mother's request to minimize reference to the past medical issues in future discussions.

It was decided to treat sleep related breathing disorder characterized predominately by central apneas with bi-level PAP with a back-up rate. Nasal mask fitting was done as an outpatient in the sleep clinic, during which the child and parent had an education session involving PAP therapy, mask care, and familiarization with the PAP delivery system. Education included discussion of circadian rhythms and phase delay as well as sleep hygiene. Based on her quiet demeanor, the parents were encouraged to consider referral to clinical psychology to help evaluate her for possible depression as well as provide her the mental tools to accept and adhere to the planned sleep related therapy. She was to continue her usual follow-up with neuro-oncology.

The plan was to be executed beginning with a period of PAP for habituation in the hospital setting on empirically chosen low starting-pressure settings with plans for a subsequent full-night study in the hospital using a mobile PSG unit to assure acceptable control of respiration. Thus, Shirley was admitted to the Cleveland Clinic Children's Hospital to be observed for a few nights while on bi-level PAP at pressures of $8/4\,cmH_2O$ and a back-up rate of 10 per minute. Cardiology referral was obtained, due to the longstanding sleep apnea, and pulmonary hypertension was ruled out. Her acceptance of the mask was adequate. After 2 days of habituation, blood gases, drawn just prior to awakening, were reassuring. She was discharged home on these pressures after a bedside PSG on current pressures confirmed acceptable respiratory status. A few weeks later, a formal titration in the sleep laboratory was done and an optimal pressure of 9/4 cmH_2O with back-up rate of 12 breaths per minute was prescribed (Figure 9.3). This corrected her bradypnea and alleviated central apnea quite well.

Over the next few months, Shirley reported more energy in the waking period since the start of PAP therapy which she used for 6 to 7 hours nightly. She became more interactive, though still laconic. The family felt more relaxed knowing that the machine would back up Shirley's breathing should it falter in the night. A battery back-up in case of power interruption was arranged. This was a very reassuring scenario for them. Her mother's own sleep improved as a result.

DSPS with contribution from poor sleep hygiene continued to be a problem, however. Mrs. Hastings admitted that the child's medical issues had resulted in laxity in bedtime rules and limits. She was willing to gradually work towards bedtime limit setting. Other interventions for circadian shift were deferred for future by her request. The possibility of depression was discussed. While Shirley's mother did not deny this, she did say the child was now much more open and interactive at home and disagreed with the need for a referral. NF1, optic, and brainstem gliomas remained stable, according to her neuro-oncologist.

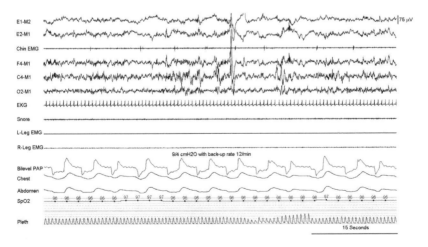

Figure 9.3 A 1-minute epoch in stage REM showing successful bi-level positive airway pressure titration at $9/4\,cmH_2O$ and a back-up rate of 12 per minute.

Discussion

NF1 is a genetic disorder that occurs in about 1 in 3500 people. The NF1 gene is located on the long arm of chromosome 17, near the centromere. It is a large gene, comprising 279,347 base pairs located within 60 exons. The gene product is neurofibromin, a protein comprising 2818 amino acids. Neurofibromin functions as GTPase-activating protein (GAP), which serves in the normal (nonmutated) state as a regulatory switch to prevent tumor formation. NF1 is an autosomal dominant disorder, meaning that the heterozygote state (1 normal or wild gene copy and 1 abnormal or mutant gene copy) can cause the disease. When a second mutation occurs in a cell, which can be triggered by an environmental event, for example, the wild allele can "mutate," an event referred to as loss of heterozygosity, resulting in tumor formation. Further, there are other functions of neurofibromin that are not known, and there are an enormous number of different mutations and deletions with the NF1 gene that can cause neurofibromatosis. Therefore, at this time there is no clear genotype-phenotype correlation. Mutations in the NF1 gene express themselves in an autosomal dominant fashion and have a very high spontaneous mutation rate, with about half of cases having neither parent affected with the condition.

The clinical features of NF1 include multiple cafe-au-lait macules, freckling in the axilla and groin, cutaneous and subcutaneous neurofibromas, plexiform neurofibromas, characteristic bony abnormalities that include, but are not limited to, sphenoid wing dysplasia and thinning of the tibia and Lisch nodules of the iris. There is an increased risk of visual pathway gliomas, which are about 4600 times more common in those with NF1 than those without the disorder. There are no specific therapies at this time that can be used to treat the cutaneous manifestations of the disease. Because of the frequency of visual pathway tumors in this disease, treatment has been well-studied in controlled clinical trials. Usually at presentation, chemotherapy is the preferred method of treatment, reserving radiotherapy for consideration when trials of different chemotherapy agents have failed or if tumor relapse occurs. Though not as common as visual pathway tumors, the occurrence of a brainstem tumor in NF1 is not infrequent. These tumors may present with hydrocephalus that leads to increased intracranical pressure and focal cranial nerve deficits, as what happened with Shirley, as well as ataxia and long tract signs. The histology can be either low-grade or high-grade glioma.

This case illustrates several issues. Children with chronic illnesses, especially those who have undergone traumatic and painful procedures in the past, need a lot of encouragement and loving handling to enlist their cooperation for future care. Medically fragile children may unknowingly be victims of the so-called "vulnerable child syndrome," with parental overprotection and tendency to shield the child from any chance of further negative experience. This may result in interference with care or even erroneous diagnoses. This may also bias medical caregivers to dismiss observations from such parents, especially if they do not seem part of the expected. This child was astutely investigated by the neuro-oncology team, and due attention was paid to the mother's concern for night-time breathing and sleep related issues.

In Shirley's case, sleep related breathing disorder with predominant central apneas and bradypnea was most likely caused by her prior brainstem tumor, or it was a possible effect of radiotherapy on brainstem integrity. Other causes of central sleep apnea (CSA), such as primary CSA, Cheyne Stokes respiration, or CSA secondary to drug or substance use, were not considerations. Other well-classified hypoxemia-hypoventilation syndromes were not likely, due to the lack of evidence of hypercarbia and the pattern of hypoxia fluctuating in a "see-saw" pattern with the changing airflow. The pattern in hypoxia-hypoventilation syndromes involves more sustained alterations in gas exchange lasting several minutes or longer.

The decision to initiate the PAP therapy in the hospital was a personal physician choice reflecting the high parental anxiety, need for patient encouragement, and the potential for inducing acid-base disequilibrium with unsupervised empiric ventilation. Blood gas analysis provided further reassurance to all concerned that the therapy was acceptably instituted.

There are numerous reports of sleep related manifestations of intracranial neoplasms. Many such cases have associated excessive daytime sleepiness or secondary narcolepsy. MSLT testing may be beneficial. Sleep related breathing disorders may be responsible for daytime sleepiness, however. This was true in Shirley's case, with circadian delay and inadequate sleep hygiene as co-morbid features. Depression was considered to be playing a role additionally, but the parents refused further workup in this context. In the end, treatment of CSA resulted in substantial improvement to daytime function, and gradual progress continues with regard to the DSPS and sleep hygiene by means of behavioral modifications alone.

Bibliography

Boitano, LJ. Equipment options for cough augmentation, ventilation, and non-invasive interfaces in neuromuscular respiratory management. *Pediatrics*. 2009;123:S226–S230.

Ito K, Murofushi T, Mizuno M, Semba T. Pediatric brain stem gliomas with the predominant symptom of sleep apnea. *Int J Pediatr Otorhinolaryngol*. 1996;37:53–64.

Neurofibromatosis: A Handbook for Patients, Families and Health Care Professionals. Allen Rubinstein, Bruce Korf, eds. Thieme Publishers New York; 2005.

Rosen GM, Bendel AE, Neglia JP, Moertel CL, Mahowald M. Sleep in children with neoplasms of the central nervous system: case review of 14 children. *Pediatrics*. 2003;112:e46–54.

10

Three's a Charm

HARALABOS MERMIGIS, MD

ZAHR ALSHEIKHTAHA, MD, RPSGT

Case History

Thomas was a 72-year-old man who presented to the sleep center complaining of excessive daytime sleepiness (EDS), loud snoring, witnessed apneas, frequent awakenings during sleep, and unrefreshing sleep. He and his wife were concerned about how his progressively worsening EDS interfered with social activities and driving. He often cancelled on his friends in favor of a nap and was unable to stay awake during movies with his family. He had 2 near-accidents in the last year due to dozing behind the wheel. His Epworth Sleepiness Scale (ESS) score was 14. He slept in the guest room for the last 5 years due to the disruptive nature of his snoring and reported a 50- to 60-lb weight gain over the same time frame. Thomas's typical bedtime and rise time were 10 p.m. and 6 a.m., respectively. He denied insomnia, hypnagogic hallucinations, sleep paralysis, cataplexy, and symptoms of restless legs syndrome.

His past medical history was significant for gastroesophageal reflex, coronary arterial disease status post angioplasty and stent placement 4 years prior, atrial fibrillation, hypertension, hyperlipidemia, and depression. He drank 3 cups of coffee daily but denied alcohol use, and he was a nonsmoker. His medications included sertraline, amlodipine, metoprolol, warfarin, and esomeprazol.

Physical Examination

Thomas had a blood pressure of 140/80 mmHg, a heart rate of 71 beats per minute and a respiratory rate of 14 breaths per minute. His body mass index was 37kg/m^2 and his neck circumference was 43 cm. The upper airway examination revealed a Mallampati score of 3 with Grade 0 tonsils. The remainder of his physical examination was unremarkable.

Evaluation

Thomas was referred for a polysomnogram (PSG) to rule out obstructive sleep apnea (OSA) given his history of snoring, witnessed apneas, EDS, and recent weight gain. During the study, 266 minutes of total sleep time was recorded, resulting in a sleep efficiency of 66%. There were 338 respiratory events comprising 132 apneas (99 obstructive, 20 mixed, and 13 central) and 206 hypopneas (Figure 10.1). The apnea-hypopnea index (AHI) was 76 (supine 81; off-supine 61; REM 60; NREM 78). The mean oxygen saturation during the study was 85%, with a minimum oxygen saturation of 61%. The arousal index was 42. No periodic limb movements were observed (Figure 10.2).

Thomas was diagnosed with severe OSA and a continuous positive airway pressure (CPAP) titration study was scheduled. Prior to the titration study, he was acclimated at home to CPAP set at $5 \text{cmH}_2\text{O}$ pressure. During CPAP titration, obstructive events were eliminated at a pressure of $10 \text{cmH}_2\text{O}$. However, frequent central apneas and arousals appeared resulting in a central apnea index ranging from 18 to 51 (Figure 10.3). None of the tested pressures eliminated central events (Figure 10.4). As a result, a bilevel titration was initiated, but central events continued at all tested pressures. In addition to the PSG, he

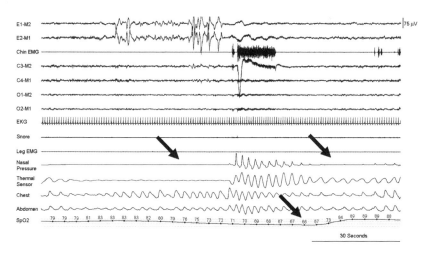

Figure 10.1 Two-minute PSG tracing showing repetitive obstructive apneas during REM sleep (upper arrows). Note that respiratory events are associated with severe oxygen desaturations (lower arrow) and arousals. The $75\,\mu\text{V}$ bar applies to EOG, EEG, and Chin EMG.

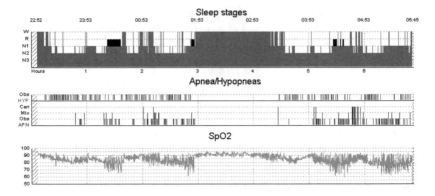

Figure 10.2 Hypnogram of the diagnostic PSG. Note the presence of frequent respiratory events, the majority of which are obstructive in nature, associated with arousals and desaturations.

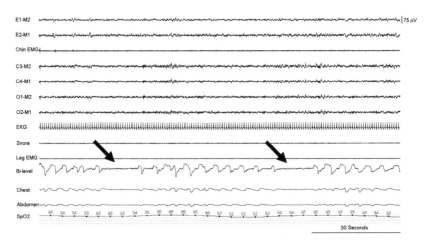

Figure 10.3 Emergence of central apneas without Cheyne Stokes respiration (arrows) during bi-level titration at IPAP 16 cmH$_2$O/EPAP 10 cmH$_2$O. The chest and abdominal channels show no evidence of effort during events. Ventilation phases between the central apneas have no waxing and waning pattern. The 75 μV bar applies to EOG, EEG, and Chin EMG.

underwent a chest CT scan that was normal and an echocardiogram revealing an ejection fraction of 60% with no abnormalities noted.

Diagnosis

Complex sleep apnea.

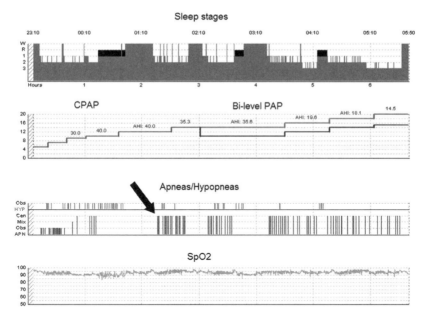

Figure 10.4 Hypnogram of the titration study using CPAP and bilevel PAP. A marked reduction in obstructive apneas and hypopneas is seen, however, frequent central events (arrow) emerged on CPAP and bilevel PAP suggesting the diagnosis of complex sleep apnea. Note the absence of central events during REM sleep.

Outcome

Thomas was prescribed CPAP 8 cmH$_2$O at home for acclimatization for a 2-week period prior to further testing. The data download revealed he used CPAP about 5 nights per week for an average of 4.5 hours per night and registered a residual AHI of 29. He reported no improvement in his daytime sleepiness while using CPAP, and his ESS was unchanged. As a result, a titration study with adaptive servo-ventilation (ASV) was performed. The study was initiated at an expiratory positive airway pressure (EPAP) of 6 cmH$_2$O, pressure support (difference between inspiratory positive airway pressure [IPAP] and EPAP) from 3 to 10 cmH$_2$O, and a back-up rate of 15 breaths per minute. EPAP level pressures were increased by 1 cmH$_2$O every 20 to 30 minutes to abolish obstructive respiratory events while aiming to avoid the appearance of central events. A normal respiratory pattern without arousals and desaturations was achieved at EPAP 8 cmH$_2$O, pressure support from 3 to 10 cmH$_2$O and back-up rate of 15 breaths per minute (Figure 10.5). Within days of use at home, Thomas and his wife noted a marked improvement in daytime symptoms and complete cessation of snoring, apneas, and night awakenings. At his 3- and 6-month follow-up visits, he reported an average nightly use of 6 hours, 6 nights per week. His ESS score

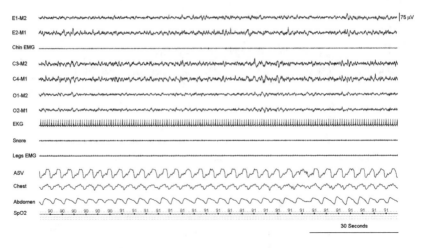

E1-M2	75 μV
E2-M1	
Chin EMG	
C3-M2	
C4-M1	
O1-M2	
O2-M1	
EKG	
Snore	
Legs EMG	
ASV	
Chest	
Abdomen	
SpO2	90 90 90 90 90 90 91 91 91 91 91 91 91 91 91 91 91 91 91 91 91 91 91 91 91 91 91 91

30 Seconds

Figure 10.5 Two-minute epoch during the adaptive servo-ventilation (ASV) titration study. Normalization of breathing pattern without respiratory events, arousals, or desaturations is observed at EPAP 8 cmH$_2$O, pressure support from 3 to 10 cmH$_2$O and back-up rate 15 breaths per minute. The 75 μV bar applies to EOG, EEG, and Chin EMG.

was 7, and his wife joked that she got her "old Thomas" back. Thomas described his satisfaction with his ASV device as "Three's a charm," noting the number of PAP machines he tried before his sleep problem finally resolved.

Discussion

Complex sleep apnea is a form of central sleep apnea (CSA) characterized by the persistence or emergence of central respiratory events during CPAP titration or during bi-level PAP therapy without a back-up rate once obstructive events have disappeared. Patients with complex sleep apnea have predominately obstructive or mixed apneas during the diagnostic study. With use of a PAP device, a pattern of respiratory events meeting the criteria for CSA emerges.

Thomas represents a typical case of complex sleep apnea. Severe OSA was observed on the diagnostic PSG, and both CPAP and bi-level PAP titrations failed to adequately reduce the AHI, due to the appearance of central events. Titration was then performed with ASV, resulting in normalization of the AHI and improvement in sleep quality and daytime symptoms. Treatment was deemed appropriate due to the severity of OSA, co-morbid disorders (coronary artery disease and atrial fibrillation) and clinical features (EDS leading to impaired quality of life and drowsy driving).

The prevalence of complex sleep apnea is estimated to be as high as 13%–15% in U.S. and Australian populations, although smaller percentages (around 5%)

have been reported in Japanese series. The male sex is more predominant than in other forms of sleep related breathing disorders. No distinct clinical features are predictive of complex sleep apnea.

While the pathophysiology of complex sleep apnea is poorly understood, affected individuals are believed to have anatomic and physiologic vulnerability to OSA in addition to central breathing control instability leading to chemoreflex dysfunction. High loop gain, defined as the ratio of a corrective response (i.e., hyperpnea) to a disturbance (i.e., apnea), is required. If the corrective response is greater than the disturbance (loop gain > 1), small disturbances can lead to a self-sustaining oscillatory pattern. Complex sleep apnea is characterized by central apneas followed by hyperventilation indicative of a high loop gain (Figure 10.6). In patients with OSA and high loop gain, application of PAP in the form of proportional assist ventilation can produce ventilatory instability leading to periodic breathing.

It has long been noted that some patients with predominately obstructive events during diagnostic PSG develop central events after successful elimination of obstructive events with CPAP or even tracheostomy. One important consideration in determining the optimal treatment modality is whether the central events during PAP titration are transient in nature. Complex sleep apnea has been classified as CPAP-emergent and CPAP-persistent cases. The first group refers to those cases in which central events emerge during CPAP titration but disappear with continued CPAP use. The second group describes those patients in whom central events persist despite continued treatment with CPAP or bi-level PAP therapy. Some experts believe that the majority of complex sleep

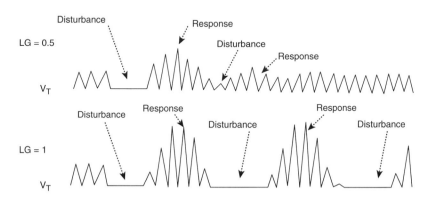

Figure 10.6 Comparative ventilatory responses to apnea (the first disturbance) in 2 individuals with different loop gain (LG). In the upper tracing, a LG of 0.5 produces a regular ventilatory pattern. In the lower tracing, a heightened LG (LG =1) results in an exaggerated response with subsequent oscillation. V_T = tidal volume. From White DP: Pathogenesis of obstructive and central sleep apnea. *Am J Respir Crit Care Med.* 2005;172:1363–1370. © ResMed 2009. Used with permission.

apnea belongs to the CPAP-emergent group and represents either an instability of the respiratory drive at sleep-wake transitions or prominent "post hyperpnea pause" with such a frequency to meet the criteria for CSA.

Complex sleep apnea results in significant sleep fragmentation as a result of repetitive arousals and awakenings. When left with markedly fragmented sleep, CPAP is not an adequate treatment modality unless one speculates that central events will abate with time. At this time, while no simple solution can be proposed for what is, by definition, a complex problem, patients with features of complex sleep apnea require careful laboratory assessment and follow-up. And when it comes to pressure settings, more is not better. The goal is to find a pressure that minimizes obstructive events without precipitating central ones. When central events emerge on CPAP, they often become more frequent with higher CPAP pressures. When this occurs after first trying higher pressures, the technologist should down-titrate to find the optimal pressure overall. In such cases, ASV should be considered.

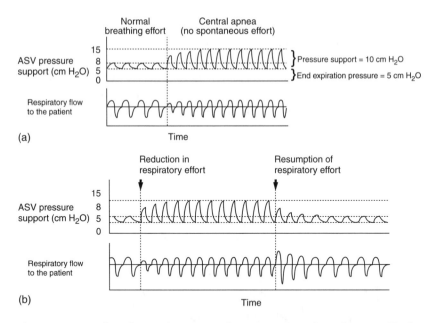

Figure 10.7 ASV algorithms. When a central event occurs and ventilation suddenly drops below the target (a), pressure support rapidly increases over a few breaths to keep ventilation at the target. As breathing resumes and total ventilation exceeds the target (b), pressure support is rapidly reduced back toward the minimum setting used. This reduces the likelihood of overventilation and hypocapnia, which can lead to vocal cord closure and further apneas. With permission from ResMed VPAP Adapt SV and Adaptive Servo-Ventilation, Technology Fact sheet, www.resmed.com

ASV is a sophisticated method of ventilatory support designed to treat Cheyne Stokes breathing pattern in heart failure patients. Recent studies demonstrate promising results in the treatment of complex sleep apnea. The ASV device adapts to the patient's ventilatory needs on a breath-by-breath basis and automatically provides target ventilation (90% of the patient's recent average ventilation). The settings vary by manufacturer and include a range of choices for EPAP, variable pressure support, and variable back-up rate if needed. When central respiratory effort ceases, machine support (i.e., pressure swing amplitude) increases from the minimum pressure support setting used to the level required to maintain ventilation at 90% of the long-term average calculated continuously by the device. When normal spontaneous effort resumes, support decreases to the minimum setting used, over a similar time period. Using this algorithm, respiration is gradually normalized and associated arousals and desaturations eliminated (Figure 10.7).

Does every complex sleep apnea patient need ASV? Should CPAP acclimatization be performed in all complex sleep apnea suspects first? Is there a way to reliably recognize whether central events are transient or not? Presently, these questions remain unanswered. Further investigation of this challenging subset of sleep apnea is required.

Bibliography

Allam JS, Olson EJ, Gay PC, Morgenthaler TI. Efficacy of adaptive servo-ventilation in treatment of complex and central sleep apnea syndromes. *Chest.* 2007;132:1839–1846.

Gilmartin GS, Daly RW, Thomas RJ. Recognition and management of complex sleep-disordered breathing. *Curr Opin Pulm Med.* 2005;11:485–493.

Lehman S, Antic NA, Thompson C, Catcheside PG, Mercer J, McEvoy RD. Central sleep apnea on commencement of continuous positive airway pressure in patients with a primary diagnosis of obstructive sleep apnea-hypopnea. *J Clin Sleep Med.* 2007;3:462–466.

Morgenthaler TI, Kagramanov V, Hanak V, Decker PA. Complex sleep apnea syndrome: Is it a unique clinical syndrome? *Sleep.* 2006;29:1203–1209.

Morgenthaler TI, Gay PC, Gordon N, Brown LK. Adaptive servoventilation versus noninvasive positive pressure ventilation for central, mixed, and complex sleep apnea syndromes. *SLEEP.* 2007;30:468–475.

11

Ahhh… The Comforts of Home

STELLA BACCARAY, RN

NOAH ANDREWS, RPSGT

NANCY FOLDVARY-SCHAEFER, DO

Case History

Will was a 50-year-old man who accepted the notion that being sleepy was simply a fact of life. In denial, he presented to the sleep clinic accompanied by his wife after she made an appointment, unbeknownst to him. She was certain he had obstructive sleep apnea (OSA) and was concerned about potential complications. He had a history of "horrific snoring" that was first noted when he had gotten married 24 years prior. He reported daytime sleepiness and had an Epworth Sleepiness Scale (ESS) score of 18. When reading the newspaper, he would be asleep in minutes. He could never finish watching a movie with his 2 daughters, which became the standing joke of the household. He worked as a financial manager for a large material handling dealership and would doze at work during meetings unless he was actively participating. He reported typically sleeping 7 hours at night, and he rarely felt refreshed on awakening. He would take a 15-minute nap most days that rejuvenated him for no more than 1 or 2 hours. He drank five to six 8-oz cups of coffee a day as a temporary fix. He preferred to sleep on his side but occasionally would awaken from sleep in the morning and find himself on his back with a dry mouth. While he admitted to only occasionally gasping or choking in sleep, his wife witnessed apneas almost nightly.

Will's medical history was notable for obesity and hyperlipidemia. Over the past year, he had gained 25 lbs; his wife noticed more apneas and he noticed a worsening of his daytime sleepiness. He had 3 cousins with OSA. Of these, 2 had prescribed continuous positive airway pressure (CPAP) therapy, and the third underwent uvulopalatopharyngoplasty. For years, his father snored and gasped during sleep, but to his mother's chagrin, the father refused to be evaluated.

Physical Examination

On physical examination, Will had oropharyngeal crowding with a Friedman tongue position Grade III but no craniofacial abnormalities. His blood pressure was 146/84mmHg. His height was 5'10" and he weighed 280 lbs. His body mass index (BMI) was 36kg/m^2 and neck circumference was 47 cm (18.5 inches). The examination was otherwise normal.

Evaluation

Based on Will's history and exam, a polysomnogram (PSG) was recommended to screen for OSA. Due to the presence of excessive daytime sleepiness (EDS), he was invited to participate in a clinical trial comparing laboratory PSG and portable monitoring (PM) in patients with a high probability of OSA. Wary of spending the night in the sleep laboratory, he decided to participate and was relieved to be assigned to sleep testing in the comfort of his own home. He was instructed on how to hook himself up and start the study on his own (Figure 11.1). He was encouraged to abstain from caffeine and napping that day and to try and sleep on his back that night. He was asked to note the time he went to bed, the time he fell asleep, and the time he woke up, and instructed to return the device the next day.

Will's home PSG revealed recurrent obstructive apneas and hypopneas producing oxygen desaturations as low as 76% and bradytachyarrhythmias (Figure 11.2). The apnea-hypopnea index (AHI) was 73, indicating severe OSA. The AHI was higher in the supine position, but it was severely abnormal off-supine as well (Table 11.1).

Diagnosis

Obstructive sleep apnea syndrome (OSAS).

Outcome

Will was instructed on the importance of weight loss and the avoidance of sleep deprivation and driving when drowsy. Based of the severity of OSA and lack of

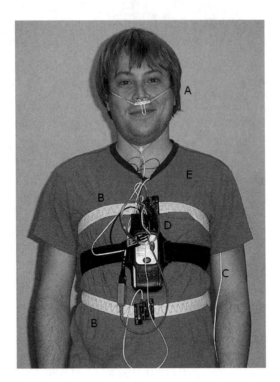

Figure 11.1 Portable PSG hook-up. Illustration of a portable recording unit. The device includes nasal transducer and thermistor to measure airflow (A), chest and abdominal respiratory inductance plethysmography to monitor effort (B), pulse oximetry placed on the fingertip to monitor oxygen saturation (C), the recorder itself placed around the torso (D), and ECG placed directly on the chest wall (E).

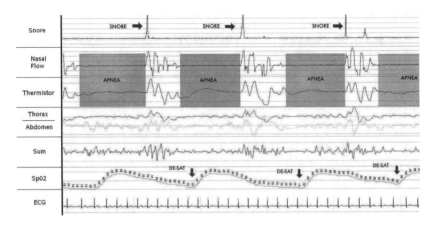

Figure 11.2 Portable PSG tracing of obstructive sleep apnea. Two-minute tracing showing recurrent snore artifact (upper, horizontal arrows) followed by cessation in nasal pressure and airflow signals (shaded boxes) and persistent, though reduced, respiratory effort, followed by oxygen desaturation (lower, vertical arrows) in the supine position.

Table 11.1 Portable monitoring data summary

Analyzed Time: 7 hours 50 minutes (470.9 minutes)
Analysis Start Time: 14.6.2008 at 0:39 a.m.
Analysis Stop Time: 14.6.2008 at 8:30 a.m.

Apnea/hypopnea (A/H)

Recording time min	455.3
A + H count (events/h)	553 (73)
Supine A + H count (events/h)	401 (82)
Off-supine A + H count(events/h)	152 (56)

Position Time min

Supine	298.6
Off-supine	165.4
Upright	6.9

Oxygen saturation

Average oxygen saturation %	93
Lowest oxygen saturation %	76
Oxygen desaturation (4%) events (events/h)	550 (73)

ECG bpm

Mean heart rate	72
Minimum heart rate	39
Maximum heart rate	117

Apnea/hypopnea statistics

Type	Number	Supine	Off-supine	AHI	Mean sec	Longest sec
Apnea	460	350	110	61	25.4	59.3
Obstructive	459	349	110	61	25.4	59.3
Central	1	1	0	0.1	15.4	15.4
Hypopnea	93	51	42	12	21.0	39.3
Total	553	401	152	73	24.6	59.3

a significant positional component, an oral appliance or positional therapy would not have been adequate. Will underwent a home auto CPAP titration study over 6 nights. The study recorded snoring, apneas and hypopneas, and flow limitation while the device automatically adjusted pressures based upon its programmed algorithm. It increased pressure as needed to maintain airway patency and decreased pressure if no events were detected over a predetermined period of time. He used the auto CPAP device for 6 hours and 4 minutes, on average, per night. Normalization of the AHI occurred at a pressure of 12 cmH$_2$O, which corresponded to the 90th percentile pressure, the level of pressure that was exceeded only 10% of the time. In other words, Will spent 90% of total titration time at a pressure of 12 cmH$_2$O or less (Figure 11.3).

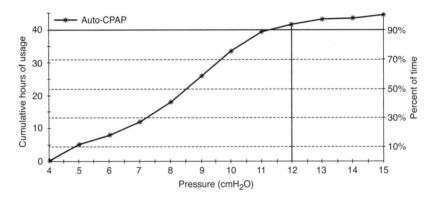

Figure 11.3 Auto CPAP Time at Pressure. The 90th percentile pressure of 12 cmH$_2$O is the level of pressure exceeded only 10% of the time.

One month after starting treatment with therapeutic CPAP, Will began to awaken from sleep in the middle of the night gasping for air. He also reported mouth dryness when using the nasal mask and nasal pillows, and his compliance data showed a significant mask leak. A chin strap resolved these issues. His ESS score was reduced to 6, and he and his family were pleased with his progress. At his next follow-up visit, 2 months later, his ESS score was 4. He was tolerating CPAP and using it nightly. The machine became an essential part of his airline carry-on items during out-of-town business trips. His wife no longer reported snoring or apneas. Now he is able to stay awake during meetings and watch late-night movies with his daughters. He no longer naps. He still drinks coffee, but not to stay awake. He simply likes the taste.

Discussion

Will demonstrated the clinical and polysomnographic criteria of OSA, including snoring, witnessed apneas, EDS, and recurrent respiratory events associated with oxygen desaturation, arousal, and bradytachyarrhythmias (Table 11.2). Predisposing factors include oropharyngeal crowding, large neck circumference, obesity, male gender, and a family history of OSA. He denied having irritable, unusual sensations in his legs, or leg jerks at night. He also denied cataplexy, sleep paralysis, and vivid dreams. He did not sleep walk, sleep talk, or act out his dreams. Thus, based on his evaluation, a sleep related movement disorder, narcolepsy, and parasomnia were unlikely culprits.

A variety of screening tools are available to help identify OSA in the clinical setting. Two of the more common ones are the ESS and the STOP Questionnaire. The ESS is a self-administered survey that measures one's likelihood of dozing

Table 11.2 ICSD-2 adult obstructive sleep apnea diagnostic criteria

A, B, and D or C and D satisfy the criteria:

A. At least 1 of the following applies:
   i. The patient complains of unintentional sleep episodes during wakefulness, daytime sleepiness, unrefreshing sleep, fatigue, or insomnia.
   ii. The patient wakes with breath holding, gasping, or choking.
   iii. The bed partner reports loud snoring, breathing interruptions, or both during the patient's sleep.

B. Polysomnographic recording shows:
   i. Five or more scoreable respiratory events (i.e., apneas, hypopneas, or RERAs) per hour of sleep.
   ii. Evidence of respiratory effort during all or a portion of each respiratory event. (In the case of a RERA, this is best seen with the use of esophageal manometry.)

or

C. Polysomnographic recording shows:
   i. Fifteen or more scoreable respiratory events (i.e., apneas, hypopneas, or RERAs) per hour of sleep.
   ii. Evidence of respiratory effort during all or a portion of each respiratory event. (In the case of a RERA, this is best seen with the use of esophageal manometry.)

D. The disorder is not better explained by another current sleep disorder, medical or neurological disorder, medication use, or substance use disorder.

off during 8 everyday situations (Appendix 1). The total score ranges from 0 to 24; a score of 10 or more is considered abnormal and signifies EDS.

The STOP questionnaire comprises 4 questions (1) Do you *snore* loudly? (S), (2) Do you often feel *tired*, fatigued or sleepy during daytime? (T), (3) Has anyone *observed* you stop breathing during sleep? (O), and (4) Do you have or are you being treated for high blood *pressure?* (P).

Responders who answer "yes" to 2 or more questions are considered at high risk for OSA. The sensitivity for predicting OSA is greater when combined with other known risk factors, such as a high BMI, age over 50, large neck circumference, and male gender.

In recent years, there has been a growing awareness among health care professionals and the general public of OSA and its associated morbidity and mortality. Estimates are that more than 80% of affected individuals are undiagnosed. Consequently, the demand for sleep related services has increased, and the availability of laboratory PSG is thought to be insufficient to meet these demands. Laboratory PSG requires the attendance of a sleep technologist for an 8-hour recording period, rendering it labor intensive, and therefore costly. While laboratory PSG remains the gold standard, PM offers an alternative for some patients. In March 2008, the Centers for Medicare & Medicaid Services (CMS) issued a decision allowing for coverage of CPAP therapy based upon a diagnosis of OSA by home sleep testing, subject to the stated requirements.

Sleep monitoring devices are classified into 4 types. The most comprehensive is a Type I device, which is an attended in-laboratory PSG. Type II devices record the same variables as Type I devices but can be used outside of the laboratory without the attendance of a technologist. Type III devices do not record variables needed to stage sleep (EEG, EOG, and submental EMG). Four physiologic variables are measured, including 2 respiratory variables (respiratory effort and airflow), 1 cardiac variable (heart rate or ECG), and arterial oxyhemoglobin saturation. Some Type III devices detect additional signals such as body position, snoring, and actigraphy. Type III devices can be used unattended. Type IV devices, as defined AASM, record 1 or 2 variables and can also be used unattended. For instance, these could include arterial oxyhemoglobin saturation and airflow. However, CMS requires that Type IV devices measure at least 3 variables. The 2008 CMS decision provides coverage for CPAP in adults diagnosed with OSA by clinical evaluation and a positive study using a Type I, Type II, Type III, or Type IV device measuring at least 3 variables.

In 2007, the Portable Monitoring Task Force of the American Academy of Sleep Medicine published clinical guidelines for the utility of PM (Table 11.3). In brief, PM may be considered as an alternative to in-laboratory PSG in patients with a high probability of moderate to severe OSA in the absence of co-morbid sleep disorders and medical conditions that might compromise the test's accuracy.

These clinical guidelines also state that:

(1) At a minimum, PM must record airflow, respiratory effort, and blood oxygenation,
(2) PM testing should be performed under the auspices of an AASM-accredited comprehensive sleep medicine program with written policies and procedures,
(3) An experienced sleep technologist must apply the sensors or directly educate patients in sensor application,
(4) PM device must allow for display of raw data with the capability of manual scoring or editing of automated scoring by a qualified sleep technologist,
(5) A board certified sleep specialist or an individual who fulfills the eligibility criteria for the sleep medicine certification examination must review the raw data from PM using scoring criteria consistent with current published AASM standards,
(6) Under the conditions specified above, PM may be used for unattended studies in the patient's home,
(7) A follow-up visit to review test results should be performed for all patients undergoing PM, and
(8) Negative or technically inadequate PM tests in patients with high pretest probability of moderate to severe OSA should prompt in-laboratory PSG.

Table 11.3 Indications for portable monitoring

1. PM for the diagnosis of OSA should be performed only in conjunction with a comprehensive sleep evaluation that must be supervised by a practitioner with board certification in sleep medicine or one who fulfills the eligibility criteria for the sleep medicine certification examination. In the absence of a comprehensive sleep evaluation, there is no indication for the use of PM.
2. Provided that the above recommendations have been satisfied, PM may be used as an alternative to PSG for the diagnosis of OSA in adult patients with a high pretest probability of moderate to severe OSA. PM use in older patients (> 65 years of age) who are more likely to have both co-morbid conditions and co-morbid sleep disorders should be approached cautiously.
   2.1. PM is not appropriate for the diagnosis of OSA in patients with significant co-morbid medical conditions that may degrade the accuracy of PM, including, but not limited to, moderate to severe pulmonary disease, neuromuscular disease, or heart failure.
   2.2. PM is not appropriate for the diagnostic evaluation of OSA in patients suspected of having other sleep disorders, including central sleep apnea, periodic limb movement disorder, insomnia, parasomnias, circadian rhythm disorders, or narcolepsy.
   2.3. PM is not appropriate for general screening of asymptomatic populations, including high risk populations such as patients with heart failure, hypertension or bariatric surgery candidates.
3. PM may be indicated for the diagnosis of OSA in patients from whom in-laboratory PSG is not possible by virtue of immobility, safety, or critical illness.
4. PM may be indicated to monitor the response to non-CPAP treatments for OSA, including oral appliances, upper airway surgery, and weight loss.

OSA is a potentially serious health problem associated with significant morbidity. Patients with moderate to severe OSA are at increased risk of hypertension, cardiac arrhythmias, diabetes, and stroke. They are also more likely to experience motor vehicle accidents, impaired work performance, and reduced quality of life. PM represents a reasonable alternative to in-laboratory PSG for patients suspected to be at high risk for OSA. Regardless of the diagnostic technique employed, the importance of early diagnosis and treatment of OSA cannot be overemphasized.

Bibliography

Berry R, Parish J, Hartse K. The use of auto-titrating continuous positive airway pressure for treatment of adult obstructive sleep apnea. An American Academy of Sleep Medicine Review. *SLEEP*. 2002;25:148–173.

Centers for Medicare & Medicaid Services. Continuous Positive Airway Pressure (CPAP) Therapy for Obstructive Sleep Apnea (OSA). 2008. Available at: http://www.cms.hhs.gov/MLNMattersArticles/downloads/MM6048.pdf. Accessed on August 15, 2009.

Chung F, Yegneswaran B, Liao P, Chung SA, Vairavanathan S, Islam S, Khajehdehi A, Shapiro CM. STOP questionnaire: A tool to screen patients for obstructive sleep apnea. *Anesthesiology.* 2008;108:812–821.

Portable Monitoring Task Force of the American Academy of Sleep Medicine. Clinical guidelines for the use of unattended portable monitors in the diagnosis of obstructive sleep apnea in adult patients. *J Clin Sleep Med.* 2007;3:737–747.

12

Teaching Tommy How to Breathe

WILLIAM NOVAK, MD
JULIANNE SLIWINSKI, RPSGT

Clinical History

Tommy, a 71-year-old grandfather and entrepreneur, presented to the sleep disorders center for evaluation of sleep apnea during an out-of-town visit. He had
recently been diagnosed with atrial fibrillation and complained of snoring and
shortness of breath during the night. His usual sleep duration was 10 hours,
but he woke in the morning feeling unrefreshed. He had trouble staying alert
during the day and scored 17 on the Epworth Sleepiness Scale (ESS).

Physical Examination

Tommy's physical exam showed him to be a well-built gentleman (he indicated
that he exercised daily). His body mass index was $25.9 \, \text{kg/m}^2$ and neck size was
15.5 inches. The oral examination revealed a small tongue with a Friedman
tongue position Grade II and a Mallampati score of I. He had a slight nasal septal
deviation on anterior examination. The rest of his exam was unremarkable.

Evaluation

Tommy underwent an overnight polysomnogram (PSG) and was found to have
severe obstructive sleep apnea syndrome (OSA) with an apnea-hypopnea index
of 30. Respiratory events were more frequent and prolonged in REM sleep, where
oxygen desaturations plummeted to 56%. Due the severity of OSA, positive

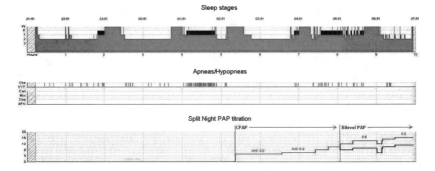

Figure 12.1 Hypnogram from the split-night polysomnogram showing frequent hypopneas during the diagnostic portion of the PSG, with increased frequency in REM sleep. During the second half of the night, titration with CPAP was performed followed by bi-level PAP due to CPAP intolerance. The patient had frequent arousals and awakenings and complained of pressure intolerance using both modalities.

airway pressure (PAP) therapy was administered during the second half of the study (Figure 12.1). Despite the use of continuous PAP (CPAP) and bi-level PAP, respiratory events persisted and Tommy complained of mask discomfort and difficulties tolerating higher PAP settings.

Since it was thought that some of Tommy's PAP difficulties would resolve over time, a period of acclimation with CPAP 5 cmH₂O was recommended before returning for further titration 1 month later. During the full-night titration study (Figure 12.2), he was started on bi-level PAP due to persistent complaints of CPAP intolerance at home. However, he felt it was still difficult to breathe, stating that it "forced me to breathe a way I didn't want to." He requested to

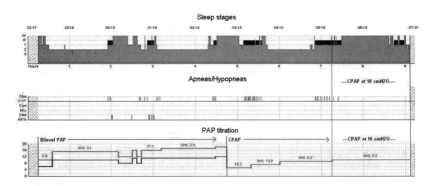

Figure 12.2 Hypnogram of full-night titration study beginning with bi-level PAP with conversion to CPAP due to persistent pressure complaints. The AHI was normalized and oxygen desaturations abolished on CPAP 10 cmH₂O, although sleep time at this pressure was of brief duration.

terminate the titration but was persuaded to try CPAP 1 more time. The AHI in both REM and NREM sleep normalized, and oxygen desaturations resolved on a CPAP pressure of $10\,cmH_2O$. However, in the morning, he refused to use CPAP, as he felt as if he were being suffocated.

Once home, Tommy tried CPAP, bi-level PAP, and an auto-titrating device, but he continued to report mask leaks, mask discomfort, and feelings of suffocation. Whenever he thought there might be a leak, his wife would tighten the nasal mask to the point where the skin over the bridge of his nose would be reddened and irritated in the morning. He tried other types of interfaces, but these problems persisted. Despite heroic efforts, he felt the bi-level PAP was forcing him to breathe, and he could not exhale with CPAP. He was unable to use any of the devices for more than 2 hours per night. He continued to find sleep unrefreshing, and his daytime sleepiness persisted, though his wife reported some reduction in snoring with use of PAP therapy.

On another business trip to Cleveland, 2 months later, Tommy returned to the sleep center desperate for a new solution. Other OSA treatment options, including surgery and an oral appliance, were felt not to be good options based on his upper airway examination. Instead, he was offered a session on diaphragmatic breathing (Figure 12.3). The technologist asked Tommy to breathe deeply into his lungs using his diaphragm. As the diaphragm descends, it pushes the stomach out of the way, causing a slight bulge. She demonstrated how this could be performed while standing, sitting, or lying supine. While supine on the bed, it was easy for him to monitor his performance by feeling his abdominal movements with his hand as the lower lungs expanded and contracted. The technologist suspected that Tommy had been breathing shallowly into the upper chest and that the weaker accessory expiratory muscles were unable to push air out against the CPAP pressure, leading to a sense of suffocation. This intervention taught him to use his abdominal muscles instead.

Diagnoses

Obstructive sleep apnea syndrome.
Positive airway pressure therapy intolerance.

Outcome

Since his lesson in diaphragmatic breathing nearly 1 year prior, Tommy continues to use CPAP on a nightly basis. While he still does not use the device the entire night (he often wakes up due to nocturia, takes the mask off, and forgets to replace it), he sleeps an average of 6 hours per night using CPAP. He no longer experiences mask leaks and feels that he's in control of the machine, not the

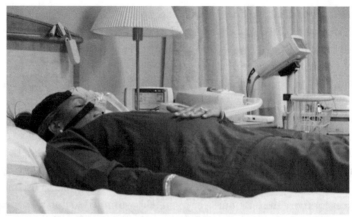

(a)

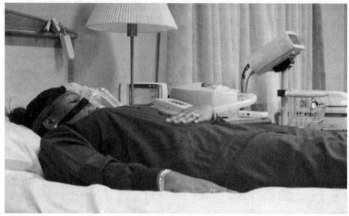

(b)

Figures 12.3a and 12.3b Demonstration of diaphragmatic breathing for PAP intolerance. During inspiration (a), diaphragmatic breathing brings in more air than thoracic breathing and draws it deep into the lungs, causing the stomach to move slightly out of the way. The subject can feel this by placing a hand on the abdomen. Note the protrusion of the abdomen with an outward movement of the left hand. During expiration (b), the subject uses the abdominal muscles to push air out of the lungs, exhaling enough air to make room for plenty of fresh air. In this way, she avoids the feeling of suffocation. Note the compression of the abdomen and the inward movement of the left hand.

other way around. His snoring has resolved, and daytime sleepiness has markedly improved. He scored a 9 on the ESS at his most recent visit.

Discussion

Comfortable PAP use necessitates the patient exhale against positive pressure. When this does not occur, complaints of pressure intolerance and mask leaks arise.

This can be corrected by breathing diaphragmatically. At birth, we use the diaphragm to breathe. As children, we're told to stand up straight and pull in the abdomen, resulting in shallow thoracic breathing using muscles of the neck, shoulders, and upper chest—the respiratory accessory muscles. Singers and athletes—swimmers in particular—breathe diaphragmatically on a routine basis, but during exercise or a performance, they use the accessory muscles for extra inspiration. Before and after exertion, they allow these muscles to rest. Most of the rest of us can get by in spite of shallow thoracic breathing, although at the end of the day we may need a shoulder massage to get rid of the tension. For some of us, this tension is great enough to interfere with sleep at night.

Sleep apnea patients using PAP therapy are challenged to breathe correctly in order to optimize the treatment modality and minimize issues that contribute to poor compliance. When first placed on CPAP even at low pressure settings, many patients either become startled by the constant rush of air or feel they are not getting enough air. Many describe this as Tommy did - a sense of suffocation, sometimes so intense they request to abort the titration study. Bi-level PAP may be an alternative therapy to CPAP in this setting, providing a lower positive pressure during expiration.

Respiratory biofeedback can help teach patients how to breathe diaphragmatically (Figure 12.4). In this technique, a belt placed around the patient's abdomen generates a signal as the abdomen expands and contracts with respiration. The patient observes the signal on a computer screen rising as the

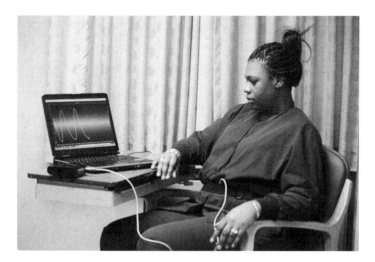

Figure 12.4 Use of biofeedback for diaphragmatic breathing. The subject is demonstrating biofeedback to monitor diaphragmatic breathing. When she breathes deeply into the lungs, the diaphragm moves downward, causing the abdomen to move forward, and the waveform on the computer screen rises. When she contracts her abdominal muscles to exhale, the waveform falls.

abdomen protrudes and falling as it contracts. When breathing is shallow, the magnitude of the signal declines, providing the patient with immediate feedback about his breathing technique.

In Tommy's case, bi-level PAP was equally challenging to CPAP because he felt the change in pressure from inspiration to expiration and back was controlling his natural respiratory drive. A 15-minute training session in diaphragmatic breathing helped him relax and focus on proper breathing techniques. Once he learned diaphragmatic breathing, he was able to tolerate CPAP and his sleep complaints resolved.

Bibliography

Bourne, EJ. *The Anxiety and Phobia Workbook*. 3rd ed. Oakland, Calif: New Harbinger Publications;2000.

Rakel D. Breathing exercises. In Rakel D., ed. *Integrative Medicine*. Philadelphia, Pa: WB Saunders; 2003: 693–696.

13

When Weight Loss Is Not Enough

ROOP KAW, MD

CHARLES BAE, MD

Case History

TJ was a 31-year-old man who was always tired. He was told by family and friends for years that he snored loudly and stopped breathing during sleep, but he did not believe this. However, over the past 10 years he had gained 130 lbs, and at 358 lbs he was the heaviest he had ever been. During the past year, he woke up many times with a sensation that he was choking and feared he would die in his sleep. He had tried countless diets and most recently lost 100 lbs, only to gain it all back, plus 40 lbs more. He finally decided to see his primary care physician, who referred him for a bariatric surgery evaluation.

TJ reported extreme tiredness and easy fatigability even after 7 to 9 hours of sleep. He went to bed by midnight and usually fell asleep within minutes, but he woke up 3 to 4 times per night, sometimes to go to the bathroom and more recently due to coughing and choking sensations. He usually slept on his back, and he woke up with a dry mouth most mornings. He woke up at 8 a.m., never feeling rested and with a headache at least a few times per week. He scored 12 on the Epworth Sleepiness Scale (ESS) and 55 on the Fatigue Severity Scale (FSS). Despite his complaints, TJ did not take naps and denied falling asleep when driving.

TJ's medical history was notable for asthma and hypertension. He took hydrochlorothiazide with potassium and omega-3 fish oil daily. He was a supervisor at a chemical distribution warehouse and was not very active at work. He did not exercise. He drank 1 or 2 pots of coffee and smoked a pack or 2 of cigarettes a day. He denied alcohol and recreational drug use.

Physical Examination

TJ was 6'5" tall and weighed 358 lbs. His body mass index (BMI) was 42.4 kg/m²
and his neck circumference was 22 inches. He had a crowded oropharyngeal
cavity with a low lying palate and a Grade IV Friedman tongue position. The
lungs were clear to auscultation bilaterally. The cardiac exam revealed normal
heart sounds with no murmur. The rest of the examination was unremarkable.

Evaluation

A polysomnogram (PSG) was performed as part of TJ's bariatric surgery evaluation given his history of snoring, witnessed apneas, and fatigue. The diagnostic
portion of the study revealed severe obstructive sleep apnea (OSA) with an
apnea-hypopnea index (AHI) of 108. Obstructive apneas and hypopneas were
associated with oxygen desaturations reaching a nadir of 68%, arousals, and
recurrent bradytachycardiaarrhythmia. After 2 hours of recording, continuous positive airway pressure (CPAP) therapy was initiated and a pressure of
12 cmH$_2$O normalized the AHI, abolished snoring and maintained oxygen saturation above 90% (Figure 13.1).

Diagnoses

Obstructive sleep apnea syndrome.
Morbid obesity.

Outcome

TJ was started on CPAP 12 cmH$_2$O. He used the device 5 to 6 hours per night and
reported a 60% improvement in sleep symptoms. He was not waking up as
many times during the night and no longer woke up feeling like he was choking.
As his tiredness resolved, he started walking 1 to 2 miles per day and lost over
25 lbs in 3 months. Five months after starting CPAP, he underwent a laparoscopic Roux-en-Y gastric bypass (RYGB) surgery. He resumed CPAP immediately
postoperatively and continued use for another 6 months, by which point he had
lost 65 lbs. He felt that the CPAP pressure was too high, so stopped using it.
Off CPAP, his sleep remained more consolidated and he woke up in the morning
feeling rested, so he retired the machine to his closet.

One year after surgery, TJ's weight plateaued at 245 lbs. He underwent a
second PSG that demonstrated an AHI of 22 with oxygen desaturations no
lower than 90%, a marked improved over his initial study. TJ opted to remain off

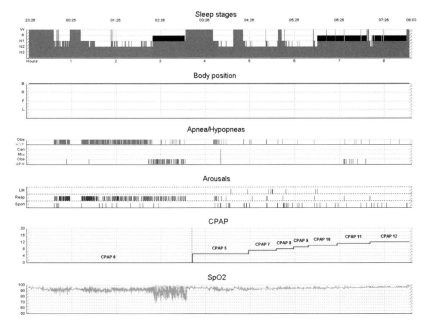

Figure 13.1 Split-night study before bariatric surgery. Note the presence of frequent respiratory events associated with arousals and severe REM-related oxygen desaturations in the initial (baseline) portion of the study. In the second part of the study, CPAP produced a marked reduction in apneas, hypopneas and arousals, normalized oxygen saturation, and improved sleep consolidation.

CPAP, as he and his wife felt that his OSA had completely resolved. He scored 4 on the ESS and 22 on the FSS at the time of his last follow-up visit.

Discussion

Bariatric surgery helps morbidly obese individuals (BMI > 40 kg/m²) lose weight after traditional weight loss methods fail. The 2 most common types of surgeries are the RYGB (restrictive and malabsorptive) and gastric banding (restrictive), both of which can be performed laparoscopically (Figure 13.2). People lose less weight with gastric banding, but there are fewer complications. It is not known whether a particular type of bariatric surgery has the advantage in reducing the AHI in OSA patients.

Untreated OSA is associated with perioperative complications that can be prevented with proper assessment and planning. Altered respiratory mechanics, pulmonary hypertension, and postoperative pulmonary embolism are major contributors to poor outcomes in obese patients who undergo bariatric surgery.

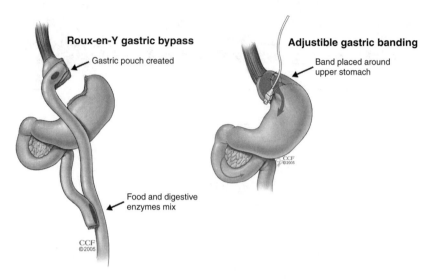

Figure 13.2 Bariatric surgery procedures. Weight loss with gastric banding is achieved through a restrictive mechanism. Weight loss with the Roux-en-Y bypass is achieved through a combination of restrictive and malabsorptive mechanisms. From Brethauer et al. *Cleve Clin J Med.* 2006;73(11):993–1007. Reprinted with permission, Cleveland Clinic Center for Art and Photography © 2005–2009. All rights reserved.

In patients undergoing surgeries including gastric bypass procedures, arrhythmias and conduction abnormalities due to sleep apnea-related hypoxemia have been reported. In a review of more than 3000 patients undergoing bariatric surgery at a single institution, sleep apnea was found to be a positive predictive factor for anastomotic leaks. In another study of patients undergoing bariatric surgery, OSA was associated with a longer length of hospital stay (odds ratio 5:5).

Preoperative Assessment

The prevalence of OSA in patients undergoing bariatric surgery ranges from 58%–91%. Polysomnography remains the gold standard for the diagnosis of OSA. In one of the largest studies, only 19% of 249 patients presenting for bariatric surgery had a clinical history suggestive of OSA, while the diagnosis was confirmed by PSG in 91%. In another study, mandatory screening using PSG reduced respiratory complication-related ICU stay from 34% to 9%. As a result, preoperative PSG and treatment of OSA when detected has been advocated in all bariatric surgery candidates.

Perioperative Airway Management

Airway management in bariatric surgery patients can pose unique challenges. Areas of concern include intubation, maintaining adequate oxygenation while intubated, and extubation.

Intubation challenges vary in awake and sedated patients. Mask ventilation may require that 2 anesthesia providers use a 2- or 3-handed bilateral jaw thrust and mask seal. In addition, oropharyngeal and/or nasopharyngeal airways may be needed in situ with airway pressure relief valve and a mask seal set to deliver CPAP 5 to 15 cmH$_2$O. If difficulty with either mask ventilation or tracheal intubation is expected, the American Society of Anesthesiology Difficult Airway Algorithm recommends that intubation and extubation be performed while the patient is awake. This requires judicious administration of sedative and analgesic medications that can compromise the airway of OSA patients. If intubation is performed with the patient asleep, it is important to fully preoxygenate the obese patient given the smaller functional residual capacity (FRC) contributing to a greater tendency to desaturate during apneic episodes compared with the normal-weight patient. The use of benzodiazepines should be avoided due to their depressant effects on the central nervous system and upper airway musculature.

In morbidly obese patients undergoing laparoscopic bariatric surgery, recurrent oxygen desaturations can occur despite supplemental oxygen. The following methods are suggested to improve ventilation and increase oxygenation in obese patients.

(1) Reverse Tredelenburg position: The Reverse Tredelenburg position (RTP) improves oxygenation in anesthetized obese patients and enables better exposure of the subdiaphragmatic region, allowing mechanical ventilation with safe levels of airway pressure. It also decreases the push of abdominal contents on the diaphragm thereby increasing FRC. With the patient positioned head-up, oxygen desaturations due to obstructive events are less severe and shorter in duration. However, any advantage with regard to lung function, atelectasis, and shunting in the 25° head-up position is lost when positive pressure ventilation is commenced.

(2) Pre-induction and maintenance positive end-expiratory pressure (PEEP): Preoxygenation with 100% oxygen (FIO$_2$= 1.0) and 10 cm PEEP for 5 minutes before the induction of general anesthesia and PEEP administration during mask ventilation and after intubation reduces immediate post-intubation atelectasis and improves immediate post-intubation arterial oxygenation. In obese patients, the improvement in oxygenation achieved with PEEP is significant and increases the time to desaturation. In contrast, in normal-weight patients, PEEP does not

appear to increase PaO$_2$ or decrease the alveolar-arterial (A-a) O$_2$ gradient.

(3) Perioperative CPAP: Prophylactic use of CPAP in the first 24 hours after surgery significantly reduces the risk of pulmonary restrictive syndrome that occurs in morbidly obese patients after gastroplasty. In one study, a 16% (95% CI: 2.9–29.3) absolute risk reduction in the rate of respiratory failure was reported with use of noninvasive ventilation during the first 48 hours post-extubation. However, postoperative CPAP carries a theoretical risk of anastomotic leak resulting from the increase in pressurized air into the stomach and proximal anastomosis. RYGB comprises 2 anastomoses: a proximal gastrojejunostomy and a distal jejuno-jejunostomy. In one study, among 1067 patients who underwent RYGB—including 420 with OSA, 159 of whom used CPAP—no relationship was found between CPAP use and anatomic disruption of RYGB. It was recently suggested that CPAP/Bi-level PAP may not be required in OSA patients after a laparoscopic RYGB provided they are closely monitored and pulmonary status is optimized by aggressive incentive spirometry and early ambulation. Further studies are required to validate this approach.

In patients with known or suspected OSA, care must be taken to ensure that neuromuscular blockade is fully reversed and the patient is arousable prior to extubation. Full recovery from neuromuscular blockade should be demonstrated by a neuromuscular blockade monitor, sustained head lift for more than 5 seconds, and confirmation of an adequate vital capacity and peak inspiratory pressure. This should be performed with an oral or nasopharyngeal airway in place. Extubation should be attempted in the semi-upright or lateral position. CPAP should be immediately available after extubation. In the early postoperative period, oxygen should be administered by face mask. However, oxygen used to treat desaturations does not prevent carbon dioxide retention secondary to obstructive episodes. In patients with known OSA, CPAP therapy should be resumed soon after extubation to allow for the safe use of analgesic and anesthetic medications. Oxygen supplementation (2 to 4 liters/min) via a sideport on the CPAP mask can generate a moderately high inspired oxygen concentration. To reduce the tendency of upper airway obstruction postoperatively, the patient should be maintained in the lateral position if possible.

Perioperative Pain Management

The use of narcotics should be limited in patients with OSA in favor of alternative forms of analgesia, such as nonsteroidal antiinflammatory medications, nerve blocks, or local analgesics. If narcotics are required for pain control, patient-controlled analgesia with restricted dosing and no basal rate should be considered. In obese patients, larger fat stores provide an increased volume of distribution for lipid-soluble drugs, such as benzodiazepines and narcotics. Since this leads to decreased clearance, maintenance doses should be administered less frequently. In contrast, water-soluble drugs, such as neuromuscular blocking agents, have a much more limited volume of distribution, and maintenance doses should be based on ideal body weight to avoid overdosing. Whether epidural agents have an advantage in this setting is unknown. Respiratory arrest has been reported in patients with OSA administered epidural opioids 2 to 3 days postoperatively. Patients with suspected OSA requiring IV narcotics should be monitored closely, with naloxone readily available.

Postoperative PAP Management

Bariatric surgery patients with OSA should be informed in advance of the need to continue PAP in the postoperative period, since it can take months to over a year to achieve an optimal body weight. As weight loss occurs, PAP requirements likely will decrease. Pressure intolerance may lead to noncompliance in the postoperative period. Auto-titrating PAP devices may be more tolerable when pressure changes are expected over time. Once the weight loss has plateaued or the goal weight is achieved, a PSG should be repeated, as significant OSA persists in some patients even after significant weight loss in the absence of daytime symptoms as in TJ's case. A recent meta-analysis showed that even though there was a 71% decrease in the AHI after bariatric surgery, nearly two-thirds of OSA patients had a mean residual AHI that was greater than 15. Careful follow-up is therefore needed, since some patients may need to be treated for residual sleep apnea. In addition, sleep apnea can recur if weight loss is not sustained.

Bibliography

Brethauer SA, Chand B, Schauer PR. Risks and benefits of bariatric surgery: Current evidence. *Cleve Clin J Med.* 2006;73(11):993–1007.

El Solh A, Aquilina A Pineda L, et al. Noninvasive ventilation for prevention of post-extubation respiratory failure in obese patients. *Eur Respir J.* 2006;28:588–595.

Greenburg DL, Lettieri CJ, Sliasson AH. Effects of surgical weight loss on measures of obstructive sleep apnea: A meta-analysis. *Am J Med.* 2009;122(3):535–542.

Hallowell PT, Stellato TA, Schuster M, Graf K, Robinson A, Crouse C, Jasper JJ. Potentially life-threatening sleep apnea is unrecognized without aggressive evaluation. *Am J Surg.* 2007;193:364–367.

Halowell PT, Stellato TA, Petrozzi MC, et al. Eliminating respiratory intensive care until stay after gastric bypass surgery. *Surgery.* 2007;142(4):608–612.

Sergio H, Scott D, Robert S, Zhaoping L, Carson L, Mark S, James A, Edward E. Safety and efficacy of postoperative continuous positive airway pressure to prevent pulmonary complications after Roux-en–Y gastric bypass. *J Gastrointest Surg.* 2002;6(3):354–358.

Shenkman Z, Shir Y, Brodsky JB. Perioperative management of the obese patient. *Br J Anaesth.* 1993;70:349–359.

14

"Advancing" the Treatment of Obstructive Sleep Apnea

SALLY IBRAHIM, MD
ROBERT ARMSTRONG, DMD

Case History

Michael was a 54-year-old man with history of obstructive sleep apnea (OSA) and difficulty breathing through the nose for many years. He tried continuous positive airway pressure (CPAP) therapy on multiple occasions, but he could not tolerate the pressure. Michael had worsening nasal congestion despite the use of a nasal corticosteroid and a variety of different PAP interfaces. He underwent a series of surgeries, including tonsillectomy in childhood and rhinoplasty, septoplasty with bilateral turbinate reduction, and open revision of septorhinoplasty for repair of nasal vestibular stenosis as an adult. His nasal breathing during the day improved and snoring was reduced, but he continued to report nonrestorative sleep and excessive daytime sleepiness (EDS). He scored 11 on the Epworth Sleepiness Scale (ESS). He felt sleepy driving into work most mornings and had difficulty with concentration during business transactions, often missing key points during meetings. He woke up in the morning with a dull bifrontal headache. He presented to the sleep disorders center hoping for a more definitive surgical option.

Michael had no significant medical history. He underwent a chin implant for cosmetic reasons. He took no regular medications and did not smoke or use alcohol.

Physical Examination

On examination, Michael had a Grade II Friedman tongue position. Anterior rhinoscopy examination revealed a slight nasal septum deviation toward the right with external valve collapse, right greater than left. Flexible laryngoscopy examination showed a large tongue base with a retroverted epiglottis. The Mueller maneuver produced a mild collapse at the palatal level, but moderate collapse at the levels of the hypopharynx and tongue base. His side profile suggested mild hypoplasia of both jaws with a blunted throat angle. The remaining examination was normal.

Evaluation

Since it had been several years since Michael underwent sleep testing and his sleep symptoms had progressed with time, a polysomnogram (PSG) was performed. The study revealed an apnea-hypopnea index (AHI) of 50 with frequent arousals and severe oxygen desaturations. Cephalometric analysis with lateral radiograph (Figure 14.1) showed evidence of maxillary and mandibular hypoplasia. The SNA (angle from the sella to nasion to a point A just anterior to the superior portion of the maxilla) measured at 78 degrees (normal 82 ± 2 degrees). The SNB (angle from the sella to nasion to a point B just anterior to the inferior portion of the mandibular) measured at 73 degrees (normal 80 ± 2 degrees). See Chapter 20 for an illustration of cephalometric angles.

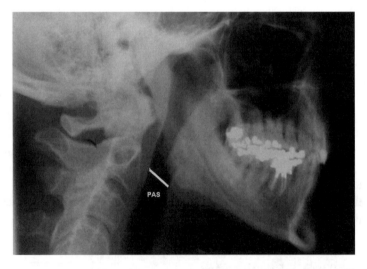

Figure 14.1 Preoperative lateral cephalogram illustrating mild hypoplasia of both jaws with a blunted throat angle. The line denotes the width of the posterior airway space (PAS).

Diagnoses

Severe obstructive sleep apnea.
Maxillary and mandibular hypoplasia.

Outcome

Michael was categorized as having a Fujita Class II airway obstruction (see discussion) with minimal improvement after multiple nasal surgeries. He was deemed a good candidate for maxillomandibular advancement (MMA). He underwent a Le Fort I maxillary osteotomy and bilateral sagittal split mandibular ramus osteotomies with a bi-maxillary advancement of 8 mm (Figure 14.2 A–C). He spent 3 days in the intensive care unit and was discharged to home on the fourth postoperative day. He maintained 2 weeks of wire maxillomandibular fixation and an additional 4 weeks of elastic fixation along with strict compliance to a no-chew diet. He returned for weekly postoperative follow-up appointments for weight, pain, incision, and occlusion checks. A postoperative lateral cephalogram revealed an improvement of the posterior airway space (PAS; Figure 14.3). Repeat PSG several months postoperatively showed a marked reduction in AHI (from 50 to 6) and arousals and normalization of oxygen saturation in sleep (Table 14.1). He reported more refreshing sleep and improvement in daytime function. His ESS was reduced from 11 to 4 (now normal) and his work performance improved.

Discussion

MMA surgery is an option for select patients with OSA. The surgery involves a series of osteotomies through the maxilla and mandible to allow for the bony segments to be repositioned in such a way that there is adequate bone-to-bone contact for stable healing. The maxilla is cut from the malar buttress to the piriform rim and along the nasal septum. This is followed by separation from the cranial base through osteotomies through the pterygoid plates. Once completed, the maxilla is advanced into the new position and maintained with several titanium microplates and screws. The mandibular osteotomies are placed medially along the ramus, above the lingula of the mandible where the inferior alveolar nerve enters the mandible. A second osteotomy is placed along the anterolateral aspect of the ramus and external oblique ridge of the mandible, and a third vertical osteotomy is completed from the inferior border of the mandible to join up with the second osteotomy. The 2 segments of the mandible are separated using osteotomies, which allows for the mandible to fracture along the inferior border.

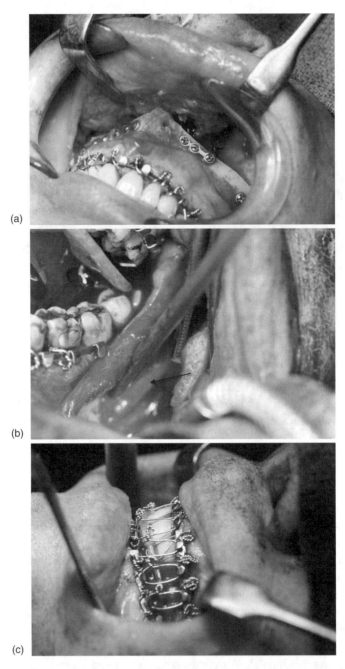

Figure 14.2 Intraoperative photos of MMA. First, a Le Fort I osteotomy is completed and fixated using titanium microplates in the new advanced position (a). Following the mandibular sagital split osteotomy, the bone segments are separated exposing the inferior alveolar neurovascular bundle (arrow) (b). Finally, wire maxillomandibular fixation of the dental arches within an acrylic splint to assure proper dental occlusion is maintained in the new skeletal position after advancement (c).

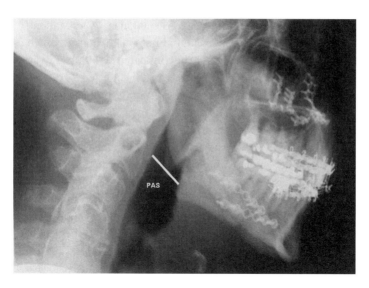

Figure 14.3 Postoperative lateral cephalogram following maxillomandibular advancement. The line denotes the width of the posterior airway space (PAS). Note the increase in PAS compared to the preoperative image (Figure 14.1).

Table 14.1 Polysomnographic data before and after maxillomandibular Advancement

	AHI	Arousal index	Mean SpO$_2$ (%)	Min SpO$_2$ (%)	% TST with SpO$_2$<90%
Pre-MMA	50	50	92	77	27
Post-MMA	6	14	95	90	0

Once completed, the inferior alveolar nerve will be contained entirely within the distal segment, and the condyle of the joint is maintained with the proximal piece. The mandible can then be advanced upon itself so that it is lengthened but maintains bony contact between both pieces. The pieces are then secured in the new position using microplates and/or microscrews. Wire maxillomandibular fixation may or may not be performed postoperatively depending upon the method of fixation (Figure 14.2). The entire procedure is carried out through the oral cavity to avoid facial scarring.

Though the surgery is invasive, it is highly effective in carefully chosen patients. Good candidates for MMA are those with maxillomandibular insufficiency who typically have obstruction at the hypopharyngeal level with or without velopharyngeal obstruction, such as in Michael's case. Airway obstruction is evaluated using the Fujita classification. A Type I obstruction reflects retropalatal/velopharyngeal narrowing (posterior to the soft palate). A Type III obstruction indicates compromise at the retrolingual/hypopharygneal level (posterior to the tongue base). A Type II obstruction is a combination of Type 1 and III, both retropalatal and retrolingual narrowing. Patients with a Fujita Type III airway obstruction are ideal to be considered for MMA. Airway narrowing can be measured using cephalometric analysis. A cephalogram uses lateral plain films to make skeletal measurements to estimate the PAS. Typically, patients with mandibular insufficiency will have stenotic hypopharyngeal airway space shadows when compared to those patients with normally positioned mandibles. A PAS less than 9 mm can be associated with hypopharyngeal obstruction. Measurements of key angles can be made from the cephalogram in order to quantitate skeletal discrepancies. This allows for determining optimal positioning of the maxilla and mandible in relation to the other skeletal landmarks (Figure 14.1). Angles below normal suggest maxillary and/or mandibular deficiency. After advancement, these angles change, with the net effect being expansion of the PAS (Figure 14.3).

The exact mechanism of improvement of OSA after MMA is unclear, but it is likely due to the anterior advancement of the pharyngeal tissues attached to the jaws, soft palate, and tongue, causing an enlargement of the velohypopharyngeal airspace. Current practices have suggested an average advancement of 8 to 10 mm to produce meaningful improvement. Additionally, the lateral pharyngeal wall collapsibility improves after MMA. Response rates are variable, depending on one's interpretation of success. Published success rates range from 96%–100%, when success is defined as at least 50% reduction in the AHI and/or AHI less than 20.

The complications associated with MMA surgery include neurosensory deficits, especially of the inferior alveolar nerve, causing parasthesias and sensory deficits in the chin and lip, bony nonunion, bleeding, malocclusion, and surgical site infection. With alterations of the facial skeleton and external soft tissue drape, there will be a change in facial appearance. In patients with significant bi-maxillary hypoplasia, these changes may be seen as an aesthetic plus. However, patients should be prepared for a noticeable change and made aware that this surgery is not a cosmetic-based treatment. The majority of patients report an improvement in sleep quality and reduction in OSA symptoms, as in Michael's case. Objective improvement has been shown by postoperative PSG, with most studies reporting improvement in AHI, oxygen saturation, and sleep architecture, including increased REM sleep time.

Bibliography

George LT, Barber D, Smith BM. Maxillomandibular advancement surgery: an alternative treatment option for obstructive sleep apnea. *Atlas Oral Maxillofac Surg Clin North Am.* 2007;15(2):163–177.

Li KK, Guilleminault C, Riley RW, Powell, NB. Obstructive sleep apnea and maxillomandibular advancement: An assessment of airway changes using radiographic and nasopharyngoscopic examinations. *J Oral Maxillofacial Surgery*. 2002;60:526–530.

Prinsell J. Maxillomandibular advancement surgery for obstructive sleep apnea syndrome. *JADA*. 2002;133:1489–1497.

Riley R, Guilleminault C, Herran J, Powell N. Cephalometric analyses and flow-volume loops in obstructive sleep apnea patients. *SLEEP*. 1983;6(4):303–311.

15

The Case of the Windblown Bus Driver

ALAN KOMINSKY, MD, FACS

Clinical History

Jerry was a 46-year-old bus driver for the municipal transit service in Cleveland who presented to the sleep disorders clinic for upper airway surgical consideration. He had been diagnosed at another sleep center with obstructive sleep apnea (OSA) and had had failed a continuous positive airway pressure (CPAP) trial due to pressure intolerance on his prescribed pressure of 15 cmH$_2$O. He had a history of nasal fracture, which made breathing through his nose very difficult. Following his CPAP experience, he had had nasal surgery to improve his airway.

Jerry reported typically sleeping 8 to 9 hours per night. He worked the second shift and went to bed by 1 a.m. While he denied nighttime awakenings, he usually felt unrefreshed on awakening. He denied daytime sleepiness and had an Epworth Sleepiness Scale (ESS) score of 3. Falling asleep while driving was never a problem, and he denied accidents or near-accidents due to sleepiness or fatigue. He had been a snorer as long as he could remember, and his wife had become quite irritated with it, resulting in marital friction. She noted that over the past 5 years he had begun to have pauses in breathing while asleep. Jerry denied cataplexy, hypnagogic hallucinations, sleep paralysis, and symptoms of restless legs. He was otherwise healthy, with no chronic illnesses.

Sleep Evaluation

A split-night polysomnogram (PSG) was performed as Jerry felt his breathing had improved considerably since nasal surgery. In the diagnostic portion, he had an apnea-hypopnea index (AHI) of 50 with a minimum oxygen saturation of 91% and an arousal index of 40. The titration was initiated at CPAP 6 cmH$_2$O with a full face mask and titrated to abolish respiratory events. Due to persistent apneas, at higher pressures, therapy was switched to bi-level PAP. At a pressure of 17/12 cmH$_2$O, the AHI was normalized (2.7), although his arousal index remained elevated and mild snoring persisted.

Jerry subsequently underwent a head and neck examination by an otolaryngologist. This revealed a midline nasal septum, but his turbinates were markedly hypertrophic. He had Grade II tonsils and a Friedman tongue position of Grade III. He was minimally overweight, with a BMI of 28 kg/m². There was no retrognathia. In order to assess the airway anatomy and visualize the dynamics of the airway, flexible fiberoptic laryngoscopy was performed. A moderate-sized adenoid was observed. There was narrowing of his airway at the level of the soft palate. The Mueller maneuver was performed, and Jerry had collapse at the palatal and tonsillar levels and narrowing of the posterolateral hypopharyngeal walls (see videos 1 and 2).

Diagnoses

Obstructive sleep apnea syndrome.
Adenoid, turbinate and tonsillar hypertrophy.

Outcome

Problems arose when Jerry tried to use his new bi-level therapy at home. He liked it better than CPAP, but he still felt the pressure was too high. He felt abdominal bloating in the mornings and complained of persistent nighttime awakenings. He felt "windblown."

Based on Jerry's upper airway physical findings, he was deemed a candidate for surgery. He was informed of his anatomic findings and how they related to OSA. The discussion focused around his nasal obstruction due to enlarged turbinates and adenoid hypertrophy. Based on the fiberoptic exam showing collapse at the tonsillar and palatal levels, tonsillectomy with uvulopalatopharyngoplasty (UPPP) was recommended. He was informed that this strategy would improve his nasal airway and likely decrease his optimal CPAP pressure making the therapy more tolerable. Furthermore, he was estimated to have a 40%–50% chance of a surgical "cure," meaning that PAP therapy would no longer be required. After discussing the options, a staged surgical approach was decided upon. He underwent an adenoidectomy and submucous resection of the turbinates without fracture (lateralization of the turbinates) as the first stage. Six weeks later, expanded sphincter pharyngoplasty type UPPP was performed.

Jerry healed nicely after surgery and 3 months later another PSG was performed. His AHI was 33. CPAP at 8 cmH$_2$O normalized the apnea-hypopnea and arousal indices. Further surgery to improve the hypopharyngeal airway—including tongue base reduction or advancement, hyoid suspension, and maxillomandibular advancement—were discussed. He was thrilled to be able to tolerate CPAP and chose not to pursue further surgery, since his OSA symptoms had resolved.

Discussion

Jerry's case exemplifies a common problem with PAP treatment in patients with OSA: pressure intolerance. Finding an appropriate treatment required a routine examination of his head and neck as well as flexible fiberoptic laryngoscopy. Nasal obstruction is frequently an impediment to CPAP use. While Jerry had a history of nasal fracture and septoplasty to reconstruct his deviated septum, his turbinates were enlarged to the point where nasal breathing was compromised. Further restricting the nasal airway was an enlarged adenoid pad. The combination of these findings precluded PAP therapy.

Jerry's oral examination showed a large tongue and small- to medium-sized tonsils and was staged based on a scale described by Friedman. The tonsils are scaled from 0 to IV based on size and relationship to other oropharyngeal structures (Figure 15.1): (1) Grade 0: surgically removed or completely atrophied, (2) Grade I: within the tonsillar fossae, (3) Grade II: to the edge of the tonsillar pillars, (4) Grade III: Extend beyond the tonsillar pillars, but are not touching, and (5) Grade IV: "kissing" or nearly touching.

Tongue position is graded based on visualization of the intraoral structures with the mouth open and tongue relaxed and not protruded (Figure 15.2): (1) Grade I: can visualize the entire uvula and tonsils (or pillars), (2) Grade II: can visualize some of the uvula, but not tonsils, (3) Grade III: Can visualize soft palate, but no uvula, and (4) Grade IV: can visualize only hard palate.

Staging is based on the following combinations of tongue and tonsil size (assuming a BMI < 40 kg/m^2 since weight reduction is generally recommended in patients with higher BMI prior to considering upper airway surgery):

Stage	Tongue position	Tonsil size
Stage I:	I or II	III or IV
Stage II:	I or II	I or II
	III or IV	III or IV
Stage III:	III or IV	0, I, or II

Jerry was a Stage III. Friedman's published data suggest that Stage III cases have a low likelihood of cure (defined as reduction of the AHI by 50% and an

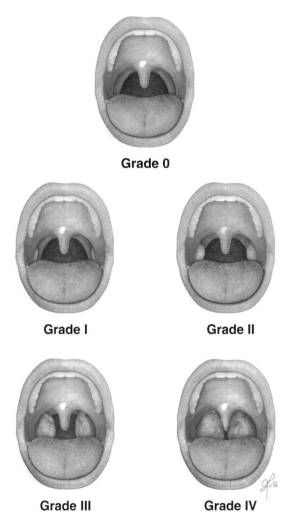

Grade 0

Grade I   **Grade II**

Grade III   **Grade IV**

Figure 15.1 Tonsil size. See text for grading scale. Reprinted with permission, Cleveland Clinic Center for Art and Photography © 2005–2009. All rights reserved.

AHI < 20 OR a reduction of the apnea index [AI] by 50% and an AI < 10) with palate surgery alone. Consideration of surgery was further complicated by concerns that some post-UPPP patients are less tolerant of CPAP because of air leak from the mouth.

As a result, a staged approach was recommended to improve Jerry's nasal airway with turbinate reduction, removal of the adenoids, and tissue-sparing UPPP. Current trends in palate surgery are leaning toward more conservative techniques. Pang and Woodson described a technique that spares palate mucosa and advances the palate forward by reorienting the palatopharyngeus

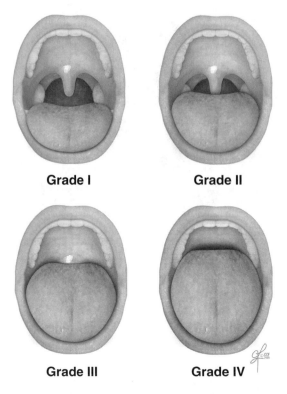

Grade I   Grade II

Grade III   Grade IV

Figure 15.2 Tongue position. See text for grading scale. Reprinted with permission, Cleveland Clinic Center for Art and Photography © 2005–2009. All rights reserved.

muscle after tonsillectomy. The uvula may or may not be shortened or removed using this technique. This type of procedure is in contrast to the traditional UPPP, in which a significant portion of the soft palate, tonsils, and anterior tonsillar pillars is removed. This newer technique decreases the chance of postoperative complaints of dysphagia and globus, and the lack of tissue removal may decrease mouth leak with subsequent CPAP therapy.

The literature on outcome of surgical intervention for OSA is conflicting, due to the number of different types of procedures employed, lack of standardization in pre- and postoperative sleep testing, and variation in definitions of what constitutes a success. Historically, success rates (as defined above) for UPPP have been reported in the range of 40%–50%. This is based on a landmark meta-analysis of OSA patients who underwent surgery regardless of the site of obstruction. In fact, the success rate exceeded 83% in patients with retropalatal obstruction. This meta-analysis pointed out additional limitations of the surgical literature. For example, the probable site of obstruction was determined in fewer than 50% of cases. In addition, surgical studies tend to have small sample sizes and short follow-up periods. In a more recent study, survival rates of nearly 21, 000 veterans with OSA treated with CPAP therapy and UPPP were compared. Surgery conferred a survival advantage over CPAP with CPAP patients being 31% more likely to have died at any point in time. This study underscores the role of surgery in the treatment of OSA in patients who will not or cannot use PAP therapy.

With few exceptions, such as obvious airway obstruction from severely hypertrophied tonsils, surgery for OSA in adults should be reserved as a salvage procedure for patients who fail PAP therapy. While Jerry had severe OSA, milder cases of apnea can be equally challenging, in terms of both PAP tolerance and upper airway anatomic obstruction. Recommending a UPPP in a patient with mild OSA should be done with caution. Traditional UPPP has long-term side effects and can even worsen OSA. Patients with mild OSA are frequently seeking relief from snoring—not the apnea. In such cases, a minimally invasive procedure such as palatal implants may be considered.

The primary goal of the surgeon in treating OSA patients is to improve upper airway obstruction to the point at which PAP therapy is no longer required. When this may not be possible, improving PAP tolerance, and compliance, in turn, also constitutes a success. Jerry's case illustrates how CPAP tolerance can improve and pressure requirements lessen after upper airway surgery. Surgery helped convert this windblown bus driver from a bi-level PAP failure to a CPAP success.

Bibliography

Friedman M, Ibrahim H, Lee G, Joseph NJ. Combined uvulopalatopharyngoplasty and radiofrequency tongue base reduction for treatment of obstructive sleep apnea/hypopnea syndrome. *Otolaryngol Head Neck Surg.* 2003;129(6):611–621.

Mortimore IL, Bradley PA, Murray JA, Douglas NJ. Uvulopalatopharyngoplasty may compromise nasal CPAP therapy in sleep apnea syndrome. *Am J Respir Crit Care Med.* 1996;154(6 Pt 1):1759–1762.

Pang KP, Woodson BT. Expansion sphincter pharyngoplasty: A new technique for the treatment of obstructive sleep apnea. *Otolaryngol Head Neck Surg.* 2007;137(1):110–114.

Sher AE, Schechtman KB, Piccirillo JF. The efficacy of surgical modifications of upper airway in adults with obstructive sleep apnea syndrome. *SLEEP.* 1996;19(2):156–177.

Weaver EM, Maynard C, Yueh B. Survival of veterans with sleep apnea: Continuous positive airway pressure versus surgery. *Otolaryngol Head Neck Surg.* 2004;130:659–665.

16

No Sleep for the Squeaky Infant

RAHUL SETH, MD
JYOTI KRISHNA, MD
PAUL KRAKOVITZ, MD

Clinical History

Cole was a boy born at 7 lbs, 1 oz at a gestational age of 36 weeks. The pregnancy was complicated only by the late delivery of prenatal care. APGAR scores were 8 and 9, at 1 and 5 minutes respectively, after an uncomplicated vaginal birth. The patient was born with an imperforate anus and anal atresia requiring an anoplasty and diverting colostomy on his first day of life. He was kept intubated with an appropriately sized endotracheal tube for 2 days and was subsequently extubated. He was discharged home at 2 weeks of age in stable condition without any significant breathing difficulties while in the hospital.

His mother reported that his breathing problems began at that time with mild audible inspiratory stridor. Cole's stridor worsened over the next several weeks to the degree that his mother felt he was "struggling to breathe." When re-evaluated at age 2 months, his breathing difficulties were characterized as being present most of the time, with high-pitched inspiratory noise that was not dependent on position. His stridor was not associated with an increase in work of breathing, apneic episodes, or cyanosis.

Additionally, his stridor did not interfere with his ability to feed, as he was able to drink a bottle in 5 minutes without choking or coughing. Cole was started on famotidine, and a modified barium swallow showed no evidence of aspiration. His weight was consistently stable at the fifth percentile. A pediatric neurology evaluation was reassuring for absence of neurological or motor delays.

His stridor continued to improve over time but remained noticeably worse at night. He then underwent reversal of his colostomy at age 4 months, with intubation only for the duration of the procedure. After this surgery, Cole's mother noted a significant worsening of his stridor. This was accompanied with mild tachypnea and suprasternal retractions with exertion and after feeds. He was placed on oral steroids for a suspected upper airway swelling following the recent intubation, but this did not help. His oral intake decreased to 2 ozs of feeds by bottle prior to having to cease feeding to take rest. By 5 months, Cole had stopped gaining weight and his growth began to falter. He was noted to have significant snoring and excessive movements during sleep that had both been worsening. His grandmother described him as "sounding like a grown man snoring." His breathing compromise continued to be significant without any improvement as he aged.

Examination

In clinic his weight was below the fifth centile. His vital signs were normal. The neurological examination was unremarkable. No cranio-facial dysmorphology was apparent. The abdomen had well-healed scars from his prior surgeries. Mild retractions of his chest wall were noted, and inspiratory stridor was apparent when he cried for a feed. His lung sounds were, however, normal.

Evaluation

Cole was sent for an evaluation by otolaryngology, where flexible fiberoptic laryngoscopy (FFL) revealed evidence of the suspected diagnosis of laryngomalacia (see video 1). At 7 months of age, Cole underwent pediatric polysomnography, revealing severe obstructive sleep apnea (OSA) with an apnea-hypopnea index (AHI) of 32.0 (Table 16.1).

Diagnosis

Obstructive sleep apnea secondary to laryngomalacia.

Outcome

Given this degree OSA and failure to thrive in the setting of laryngomalacia, Cole was taken to the operating room for a direct laryngoscopy, bronchoscopy, and evaluation of the airway. His epiglottis was found to be floppy, along with

Table 16.1 Polysomnography Data

	Age (months)	Respiratory events	Hypopneas	Apneas	Obstructive apneas	Central apneas	Mixed apneas	Oxygen nadir (%)	% TST with SpO$_2$ <90%	Supine sleep (% TST)	Supine AHI	Total AHI
Pre-Surgeries	7	240	202	38	23	10	5	79	3.6	96.8	29.5	32.0
Post-Surgeries	9	123	122	1	0	1	0	78	0.5	91.0	12.6	14.4
Supplemental Oxygen	10	33	24	9	3	6	0	86	0.0	49.1	2.2	3.6

Of note, due to oxygen therapy during the supplemental oxygen test, the AHI, a priori, is not accurately represented due to masking of desaturations. TST = Total sleep time.

the aryepiglottic folds foreshortened with redundant mucosal tissue. The subglottis was closely examined for stenosis given his previous intubations, but no abnormalities were found. Given the severity of OSA as a consequence of laryngomalacia, he underwent aryepiglottoplasty of the left side of the larynx. This was performed through a rigid suspended operating laryngoscope and under high-power microscopic visualization. The left aryepiglottic fold was divided along with the trimming of redundant tissue along the left arytenoid adjacent to the aryepiglottic fold. The procedure was staged, with the right side aryepiglottoplasty performed 1 month later.

After the bilateral staged procedures, Cole's breathing improved significantly with resolution of inspiratory stridor. Despite this, his mother described continued mild nightly snoring, which was much reduced from the past. A repeat sleep study was obtained with the baby now 9 months old. This study revealed an AHI of 14.4 (reduced from preoperative AHI of 32.0). He spent only 0.5% of his sleep time with an oxygen saturation below 90% (Table 16.1).

Due to the continued sleep apnea, a trial of continuous positive airway pressure (CPAP) therapy via nasal mask was attempted as an inpatient on the pediatric floor. Appropriate education, mask fitting, and desensitization were attempted. Cole did not tolerate the mask, however, and the family did not wish to pursue this further. The baby was therefore started on low-flow oxygen therapy via nasal cannula during sleep at a rate of 0.5 L/minute. Another sleep study was obtained to titrate the oxygen with care to monitor for hypercarbia. The study revealed an AHI of 3.6 (Table 16.1). It was understood, however, that due to oxygen therapy, the AHI from this study was not an accurate representation of the respiratory flow reductions that would otherwise have qualified as hypopneas or apneas were there to be associated desaturations. Hypnograms from presurgeries, postsurgeries, and supplemental oxygen titration studies pictorially reflect these findings (Figure 16.1). Improvement was noted with each successive intervention performed. Along with significant improvement of sleep apnea, Cole had resolution of both stridor and work of breathing postsurgically.

Discussion

Laryngomalacia is the most common cause of stridor in infants, accounting for 65%–75% of all cases of evaluated stridor, and it is the most common congenital laryngeal anomaly. The onset of stridor associated with laryngomalacia is usually shortly after birth. There is a slight male predominance. The stridor and respiratory symptoms of laryngomalacia worsen until age 4 to 6 months. Fortunately, laryngomalacia is a condition that is usually self-limited, with improvement and resolution of symptoms without therapy at about 12 to 18 months of life in most infants.

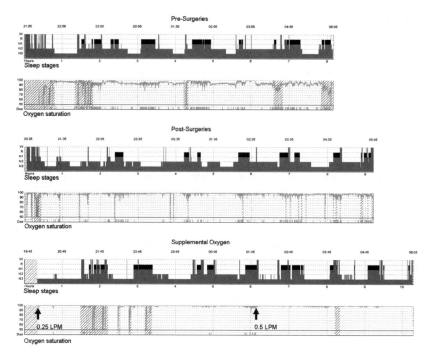

Figure 16.1 Abbreviated hypnograms obtained from sleep studies done presurgeries, postsurgeries, and then with administration of supplemental oxygen. Note the improvement in the oxygenation tracings with each successive intervention. See text and Table 16.1 for details.

The etiology of laryngomalacia is unknown, and histological examination of excised laryngeal tissue from laryngomalacia reveals submucosal edema and lymphatic dilation. Interestingly, gastroesophageal reflux is thought to be an important cofactor in the disease process, as it occurs in up to 80% of infants with laryngomalacia, and usually resolves after treatment or resolution of symptoms. There is a high incidence of neuromuscular problems in affected infants; therefore, some investigators believe the disorder represents a state of hypotonia creating a lack of coordinated muscular laryngeal inlet dilation. Others propose that the laryngeal cartilages lack structural strength creating a state of supraglottic collapse. Regardless of the proposed etiology, there is a loss of gross normal architecture of the laryngeal anatomy (Figure 16.2).

Laryngomalacia symptomatically is characterized by inspiratory stridor. In general, airway obstructions that are extrathoracic produce an inspiratory stridor, while intrathoracic obstructions (for example, tracheal stenosis) produce an expiratory stridor. The inspiratory stridor of laryngomalacia is attributable to the inward collapse of the supraglottic laryngeal structures during inspiration. Most notably, shortened aryepiglottic folds can prolapse medially,

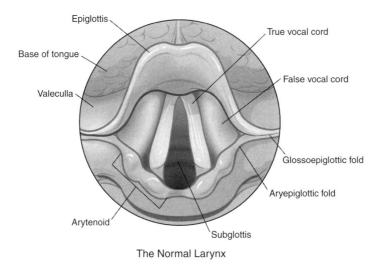

Epiglottis

Base of tongue

Valecula

Arytenoid

True vocal cord

False vocal cord

Glossoepiglottic fold

Aryepiglottic fold

Subglottis

The Normal Larynx

Figure 16.2 The anatomy of a normal larynx. Compare this to the typical findings in laryngomalacia shown in Figure 16.3. Reprinted with permission, Cleveland Clinic Center for Art and Photography © 2005–2009. All rights reserved.

redundant arytenoid mucosa can prolapse anteriorly, a posteriorly displaced epiglottis can prolapse posteriorly, or any combination of these may occur during inspiration to produce the problematic airway obstruction and stridor (Figure 16.3).

Although most children with laryngomalacia will have resolution of stridor associated with laryngomalacia by 12 to 18 months of age, an estimated 5%–15% of children with laryngomalacia have a severe form of the disease. They present with chronic dyspnea, failure to thrive, pulmonary hypertension, weight loss, and/or OSA. These infants may require surgical intervention. The decision to perform a supraglottoplasty is tailored for each individual infant and the severity of disease. In general, the accepted indications for supraglottoplasty are: (1) presence of resting dyspnea or intense respiratory effort; (2) obstructive sleep apnea syndrome (OSAS); (3) hypoxia, hypercapnia, cyanotic episodes, apneas, or apparent life-threatening events; (4) pulmonary hypertension or cor pulmonale; (5) inability to feed; (6) failure to thrive; and (7) weight loss.

The differential diagnosis of laryngomalacia primarily includes other airway lesions, such as laryngeal cyst or cleft, subglottic stenosis, tracheomalacia, and vocal cord paralysis. In-office FFL is used to assist in determining the etiology of respiratory findings. Operating room examination of the airway with direct laryngoscopy and bronchoscopy is advocated in those children with respiratory findings consistent with severe laryngomalacia, suspicion of a synchronous lesion of the larynx, and in infants who will likely require surgical intervention for the laryngomalacia.

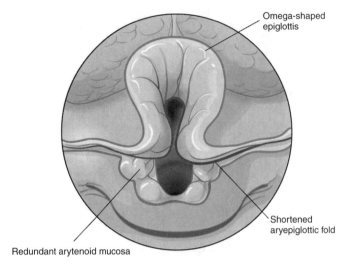

Omega-shaped
epiglottis

Shortened
aryepiglottic fold

Redundant arytenoid mucosa

Larynx of Laryngomalacia

Figure 16.3 Characteristic findings of laryngomalacia during inspiration. The epiglottis is omega shaped and posteriorly displaced. The arytenoids have redundant mucosa that can enter the airway opening, and the aryepiglottic folds are shortened. All of these effects cause narrowing of the airway, as depicted. Reprinted with permission, Cleveland Clinic Center for Art and Photography © 2005–2009. All rights reserved.

Surgical intervention for severe laryngomalacia aims at addressing the anatomical site of supraglottic obstruction by any combination of 3 procedures: (1) redundant mucosal tissue of the arytenoid cartilages is trimmed if this is excessive and prolapsing into the airway, (2) shortened aryepiglottic folds reducing the laryngeal inlet are divided to decrease tethering of the anterior and posterior supraglottis, and, (3) a posteriorly displaced epiglottis is sutured anteriorly to a denuded area of the base of tongue (rarely performed). The first 2 procedures are called aryepiglottoplasty; the third is named epiglottopexy. These procedures collectively are termed supraglottoplasty and are performed in the operating room under direct laryngoscopy with the aid of microscopic visualization. Microsurgical instruments are used to perform the operation. Tissue resection is done using either cold instrumentation or CO_2 laser. The established potential complications of supraglottoplasty include persistent airway obstruction requiring further surgery, supraglottic stenosis, granuloma, synechia formation, dysphagia, aspiration, and, rarely, even death. Of these, the most common is aspiration, which appears to have a higher likelihood of occurrence if present preoperatively. The aspiration generally is initially managed conservatively, with feeding tube or gastrostomy tube necessitated in cases of failed medical management or continued failure to thrive.

Supraglottoplasty has been shown to have a nearly 90% success rate in improving the respiratory compromise associated with severe laryngomalacia. Specifically, supraglottoplasty is associated with a significant improvement of OSAS in infants. Generally, a unilateral procedure is carried out initially. Unilateral procedures have been associated with a 90% success rate; if unsuccessful, however, aryepiglottoplasty is performed on the contralateral side in a staged fashion. Staging the procedure may help prevent supraglottic stenosis, an uncommon complication of bilateral aryepiglottoplasty. In rare cases where these interventions do not ameliorate the symptoms, revision aryepiglottoplasty or tracheostomy may be needed.

Combined with surgery, appropriate medical evaluation and treatment must be performed in a child with severe laryngomalacia. Given the high rate of gastroesophageal reflux disease in infants with laryngomalacia, medical treatment with anti-reflux agents is necessary. The reflux generally resolves as the laryngomalacia improves or after supraglottoplasty. Additionally, evaluation for neuromotor development is needed if there is any suspicion of delay. Snoring, restless sleep, or witnessed apneic pauses during sleep should prompt a sleep study evaluation.

In the present case, Cole displayed severe laryngomalacia with worsening stridor and significant sleep apnea. This eventually led to failure to thrive, weight loss, and progressive respiratory compromise. Surgical management with staged bilateral aryepiglottoplasty was able to nearly eliminate the infant's stridor and significantly decreased the AHI. Although CPAP was not tolerated, supplemental oxygen delivery augmented therapy and further improved the patient's respiratory status. As demonstrated, a team approach to severe laryngomalacia is necessary to achieve optimal patient outcomes.

Bibliography

Olney DR, Greinwald JH, Smith RFH, Bauman NM. Laryngomalacia and its treatment. *Laryngoscope*. 1999;109:1770–1775.

Valera FC, Tamashiro E, de Araujo MM, Sander HH, Kupper DS. Evaluation of the efficacy of supraglottoplasty in obstructive sleep apnea syndrome associated with severe laryngomalacia. *Arch Otolaryngol Head Neck Surg*. 2006;132:489–493.

Zoumalan R, Maddalozzo J, Holinger LD. Etiology of stridor in infants. *Ann Otol Rhinol Laryngol*. 2007;116:329–334.

17

For this Teen, Life Begins after OSA!

JENNIFER SCIUVA, MSN, PNP
JYOTI KRISHNA, MD

Case History

Joe's only source of enjoyment was his artwork. Crayons and paint brushes were his best friends, and paintings adorned his small bedroom. At 14, he was a reserved and laconic African-American boy who stayed away from other kids. His grandparents had custody of him since he was an infant because his mother abused alcohol and drugs during pregnancy. For many a sleepless night, his grandfather had watched over the infant's jittery wakefulness and restless sleep as he recovered from the effects of his antenatal drug exposure. As he grew up, his grandparents noted he had some problems with learning and behavior, though not severe enough to be in special classes at school. His friends would make fun of him because of his small head, odd face, and speech. He found comfort in staying at home after school, content to be with his grandparents. Their nurturing care brought him through all that. One problem seemed to remain; Joe struggled to breathe during sleep. While breathing pauses were of some concern during early infancy, Joe quickly got over that issue, and everyone was glad to see the last of the apnea monitor when Joe turned 1 year old. This new concern was different, and it was getting worse.

In the sleep center, Mr. Harris appeared quite concerned about his grandson. He told us about his frequent trips to Joe's bedroom to reassure himself the child was still breathing. Loud snoring, snorting sounds, and pauses in his breathing during sleep had been worsening for the last 5 to 7 years. Further, Joe began to complain of sleepiness at school and cringed with embarrassment when his grandfather added a comment on his frequent episodes of bedwetting. He slept an adequate 10 hours per night, and napped 2 times per week for 1 hour, yet Joe fell asleep at school daily. Bedwetting occurred 3 or 4 times per week since age 6 years. This was surprising in a child who had been dry at night since he was 4. His past medical history included a diagnosis of fetal alcohol syndrome, sinusitis, and seasonal allergies. Joe did not have any other systemic disorders. Specifically, he denied cardiopulmonary complaints. He was not on any daily medications. Family history was negative for sleep disorders.

Physical Examination

The physical exam showed weight of 120 lbs (54.5 kg, 60th percentile); height of 4'10" (147.3 cm, <5th percentile); body mass index (BMI) of 25.2 kg/m^2 (> 90th percentile). The head circumference was on the smaller side (49 cm). He had mid-facial hypoplasia, small palpebral fissures, crowded oropharynx, and dental malocclusion consistent with physical characteristics of in-utero alcohol exposure. He also had inferior turbinate hypertrophy and hyponasal speech. His tonsillar size was Grade III and Friedman tongue position was Grade IV. The neurological exam showed a slight left pronator drift but was otherwise unremarkable. The back did not reveal any midline cutaneous stigmata.

Evaluation

A working diagnosis of obstructive sleep apnea (OSA) was made with hypersomnia very likely secondary to this. Due to daytime sleepiness, enuresis, and lack of energy despite adequate sleep time, several investigations were ordered, including a polysomnogram (PSG) followed by a multiple sleep latency test (MSLT). Specifically, the plan was not to proceed with MSLT if the PSG showed evidence of significant OSA. Other labs included metabolic profile and complete blood count (CBC) as well as urinalysis to screen for renal and urinary pathology on account of enuresis.

Joe and his guardians were scheduled to return 1 week after the testing to discuss the results, but they were called in urgently the very next day because the sleep study was severely abnormal (Figures 17.1 and 17.2). The apnea-hypopnea index (AHI) was close to 93 events per hour with a mean O_2 saturation of 83% and a nadir in the 50s. The end-tidal CO_2 (EtCO$_2$) data was not reliable due to severe airflow limitation and multiple arousals. No cardiac rhythm disturbance was noted, aside from a much exaggerated sinus arrhythmia. His waking O_2 saturations were normal at 97%. The CBC, metabolic profile, and urinalysis were within normal limits. The MSLT was not done once the AHI was noted to be severely elevated.

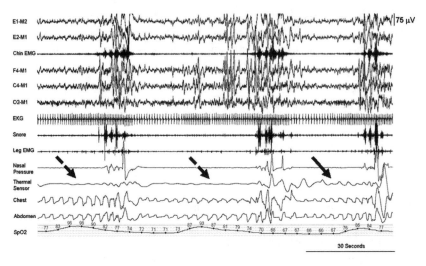

Figure 17.1 A 2-minute epoch from the baseline preoperative polysomnogram showing severe desaturations with apnea (broken arrows) and hypopnea (solid arrow) events. The EtCO$_2$ channel was not reliable.

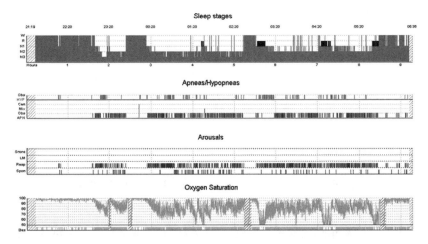

Figure 17.2 Hypnogram summarizing findings of the baseline preoperative polysomnogram. Note the fragmented sleep architecture with multiple periods of stage Wake interrupting sleep. There are numerous respiratory events marked as apneas and hypopneas as well as repetitive arousals and accompanying desaturations.

Diagnoses

Obstructive sleep apnea syndrome, pediatric (Table 17.1).
Sleep enuresis.
Fetal alcohol syndrome.

Outcome

During his follow-up office visit, Joe dozed off in the exam room, and this time he gave us the opportunity to witness the severity of his disease first-hand. While asleep in a sitting position in a hard-backed chair, Joe suffered several frank apneic episodes with 30–45 second pauses. Based upon this, he was sent immediately to the hospital for direct admission in the cardiopulmonary monitoring

---

Table 17.1 ICSD-2 diagnostic criteria for Pediatric Obstructive Sleep Apnea

A. The caregiver reports snoring, labored or obstructed breathing, or both snoring and labored or obstructed breathing during the child's sleep.
B. The caregiver reports observing at least one of the following:
   i.   Paradoxical inward rib-cage motion during inspiration.
   ii. Movement arousals.
   iii. Diaphoresis.
   iv. Neck hyperextension during sleep.
   v.   Excessive daytime sleepiness, hyperactivity, or aggressive behavior.
   vi. A slow rate of growth.
   vii. Morning headaches.
   viii. Secondary enuresis.
C. Polysomnographic recording demonstrates 1 or more scorable respiratory events per hour (i.e., apnea or hypopnea of at least 2 respiratory cycles in duration).
D. Polysomnogram demonstrates either i or ii:
   i.   At least 1 of the following is observed:
      a) Frequent arousals from sleep associated with increased respiratory effort.
      b) Arterial oxygen desaturation in association with the apneic episodes.
      c) Hypercapnia during sleep.
      d) Markedly negative esophageal pressure swings.
   ii. Periods of hypercanpnia, desaturation, or hypercapnia and desaturation during sleep associated with snoring, paradoxical inward rib-cage motion during inspiration, and at least one of the following:
      a) Frequent arousals from sleep.
      b) Markedly negative esophageal pressure swings.
E. The disorder is not better explained by another current sleep disorder, medical or neurological disorder, medication use, or substance abuse disorder.

---

unit and an urgent cardiac and ENT evaluation was ordered. An EKG was done which showed normal sinus rhythm. Also, an echocardiogram was done which showed normal cardiac anatomy and no evidence of right ventricular hypertrophy or pulmonary hypertension. He underwent surgery, which included adenotonsillectomy and somnoplasty of the inferior turbinates. His postsurgical course included need for oxygen and bi-level positive airway pressure (PAP) therapy in the hospital intensive care unit setting. He was discharged home after 3 days on empiric bi-level PAP of $12/6\,cmH_2O$ with supplemental O_2 at 2 liters per minute. Over the following 2 months, he was weaned off his oxygen. The bi-level PAP support remained, but a follow-up PSG was ordered to evaluate the improvement after surgery and need for continuing PAP support. In preparation for this study, Joe was asked to discontinue the PAP use for a week prior to the PSG in order that the new data be reflective of his true postoperative baseline.

The 3-month postoperative PSG showed the AHI was still in severe range, albeit much improved at 42/h (Figure 17.3). Oxygenation during sleep improved with a mean O_2 saturation of 95% and most desaturations now in the 80s. What was most striking about Joe was the change in his personality. The withdrawn, laconic Joe had morphed into a teen who was much more confident in himself. He was very talkative and assertive. He felt more rested and alert during the day. He denied falling asleep during school any more and naps were now rare. He grinned as he informed us he no longer had nocturnal enuresis. He stated that he had resumed wearing the bi-level PAP every night for most of the

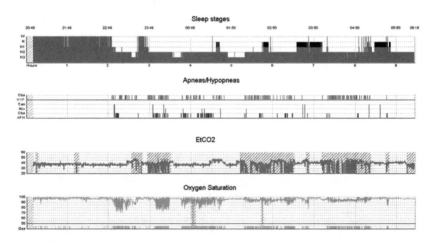

Figure 17.3 Hypnogram summarizing findings of the postoperative polysomnogram. Note the significant improvement over the baseline study. The sleep architecture is more consolidated. The desaturations are less severe than before surgery. The $EtCO_2$ signal is shown here since it was more reliable and significant sleep related hypoventilation (defined as more than 25% of total sleep time with $EtCO_2 > 50\,mmHg$) was not noted. However, severe OSA persists, calling for further therapy.

time he was asleep. This made him feel better. While there were no pressure effects on his facial skin from this, he did complain of nasal congestion.

A PAP titration study was recommended to optimize prescribed pressures. In the meantime, he was encouraged to continue using the PAP device. Fluticasone was prescribed for upper airway congestion problems. His grandfather was encouraged to have Joe evaluated by an orthodontist with the hope that this treatment might additionally help with residual OSA. His grandparents were very happy and grateful for the visible benefit they had observed. Just before departing, Joe asked for a few minutes alone with the sleep physician and confided that he had body image issues due to small head size and he wondered what the girls thought of him? He asked a referral be made to pediatric "head specialist" for a formal opinion on this issue. Indeed, laconic Joe had come along way!

Unfortunately, this was the last we saw of him. He was contacted multiple times by phone and encouraged to return. He always said he felt much better and his quality of life was improved after visiting us and that he would come soon to follow up when he had the time. Life, we guess, was looking good after OSA! We wonder how much better it would be if he only allowed us another chance to optimize his prescription PAP settings.

Discussion

Several issues bear reflection in this case. While African-American descent appears to be associated with higher prevalence of OSA, in this teen the primary risk was related to cranio-facial factors stemming from fetal alcohol exposure, as well as large adenoids and tonsils. Further, due to his significant dental malocclusion, an orthodontic evaluation was suggested to the family.

The implications of severe OSA in children are important since OSA is unlikely to regress spontaneously. If untreated or treated late, pediatric OSA may lead to significant morbidity affecting multiple organ systems. For instance, severe OSA may lead to pulmonary hypertension and cor pulmonale, systemic hypertension, failure to thrive, developmental delay, school failure, and, in rare cases, death.

Adenotonsillectomy is the first-line treatment for pediatric OSA. The surgical management should not be taken lightly, as children with severe OSA are more likely to need extended cardiopulmonary monitoring postoperatively. They have been known to exhibit greater likelihood of postoperative pulmonary edema and may require respiratory support. Based on this, it is recommended that severe OSA be managed with a multidisciplinary approach with adequate in-hospital care to avert any potential for perioperative morbidity. The family should be advised of the increased potential for complications in such cases. Unfortunately, a high initial AHI and presence of anatomical risk factors predict the patient who is less likely to revert to a normal AHI after surgery. Such patients need postsurgical evaluations and close follow-up for residual OSA.

Sleep enuresis has been associated with OSA and may revert with treatment of sleep related breathing disorders. Other consequences of OSA include problems with behavior, learning, attention, memory, poor school performance, and lower quality of life. This was explained to the family in the hope that they would continue to work with us in effectively treating Joe's residual OSA and return to us in the future for ongoing surveillance.

Bibliography

American Academy of Pediatrics. Clinical Practice Guideline: Diagnosis and management of childhood obstructive sleep apnea syndrome. *Pediatrics*. 2002;109: 704–712.

Crabtree VM, Varni JW, Gozal D. Health-related quality of life and depressive symptoms in children with suspected sleep-disordered breathing. *SLEEP*. 2004;27:1131–1138.

Gozal D, Kheirandish-Gozal L. Sleep apnea in children—treatment considerations. *Paediatr Respir Rev*. 2006;7 Supp l1:S58-61. Epub 2006:Jun 5.

Walker P, Whitehead B, Rowley M. Criteria for elective admission to the pediatric intensive care unit following adenotonsillectomy for severe obstructive sleep apnea. *Anaesth Intensive Care*. 2004;32:43–46.

18

This Thing Is Impossible!

LOUTFI ABOUSSOUAN, MD
ZAKK ZAHAND, RPSGT
PETRA PODMORE, REEGT, RPSGT

Case History

John was an 82-year-old, semi-retired gentleman who presented to the sleep center for further management of obstructive sleep apnea (OSA). His apnea was diagnosed at age 70, and he was started on continuous positive airway pressure (CPAP) therapy. He discontinued CPAP after just 1 month. He described it as annoying, causing more sleep disruption for both him and his wife than the OSA itself, and he decided he was just not going to use that "impossible thing."

Over the 12 years since his last sleep study, John had gained 30 lbs, and his list of medical problems and prescription medications had grown. He had had a stroke 3 years prior, and his wife was concerned after reading about sleep apnea and its relation to strokes in Reader's Digest. Though she was initially disturbed by John's loud snoring, it was now the sheer silence during the night that most alarmed her. She would often wake up to find him with his mouth wide open, not breathing at all, and she would shake him awake, fearing he might be dead. His breathing would then start back again after a big snort.

John himself had little appreciation for the poor quality sleep and excessive daytime sleepiness (EDS), although his wife felt it interfered with his ability to function at work and at home. He downplayed his symptoms, though he admitted taking catnaps and had an Epworth Sleepiness Scale (ESS) score of 13. Business associates privately told him he frequently fell asleep in meetings. On weekends, he slept most of the day in front of the television or at the kitchen table. He averaged about 7 hours of sleep per night. He was not aware of his loud snoring and denied difficulty falling asleep, though he woke up 4 to 5 times per night to urinate. He preferred to initiate sleep on his side, but his stroke made it uncomfortable to sleep on his right. He would wake up most mornings on his back with a dry mouth and a dull headache.

John's medical history included a left hemispheric lacunar infarction, Type II diabetes mellitus, hyperlipidemia, spinal stenosis, and venous insufficiency. His medications included insulin, sitagliptin, simvastatin, metoprolol, esomeprazole, and celecoxib. He had a 30 pack-year smoking history but quit after his stroke. He had been married for 45 years and had 2 grown children. He was starting to think about complete retirement, but he felt a responsibility to his lifelong real estate business. He still served as the director of a large real estate investment trust.

Physical Examination

On examination, John was 5' 10" tall and weighed 244 lbs (body mass index of 35 kg/m²). He had a blood pressure of 110/55 mmHg, a heart rate of 65 bpm, and a respiratory rate of 12. His neck circumference was 43.5 cm. The upper airway exam was notable for a Grade IV Friedman tongue position. There was lateral crowding of the oropharynx with a narrow velopharyngeal space. The cardiac and lung examinations were normal. He had a right hemiparesis most notably affecting his right (dominant) hand, right sided hyperreflexia, and reduced vibration in his feet with absent ankle jerks bilaterally. His mental status, language, and cranial nerves were normal, save for a subtle right facial droop.

Evaluation

John was referred for an overnight polysomnogram (PSG) with an order to perform a CPAP titration if his apnea-hypopnea index (AHI) was 15 or higher. During the diagnostic portion of the study, the AHI was 72, with a supine index of 83 and an off-supine index of 61 (Table 18.1). CPAP was titrated from 5 cmH$_2$O to 12 cmH$_2$O. None of the pressures normalized the AHI in the supine position, and an overall residual AHI of 9 at the highest pressure of 12 cmH$_2$O was noted. Central apneas emerged at higher CPAP pressures (Figure 18.1). A CPAP pressure of 12 cmH$_2$O with heated humidification and positional therapy (side sleeping) was recommended as well as a repeat titration with bi-level PAP if symptoms were to persist since CPAP did not abolish events in the supine position.

Table 18.1 Apnea-hypopnea statistics during the split-night polysomnogram

CPAP (cm H$_2$O)	Sleep Time (min)	% Supine	Obstructive (n)	Mixed (n)	Central (n)	Hypo- pneas (n)	AHI	Supine AHI	Off-supine AHI
None	126.5	49	92	0	0	59	72	83	61
5	69.5	0	0	0	0	0	0	0	0
6	61.5	0.5	0	0	0	1	1	0	1
7	19.5	100	4	1	4	8	52	52	0
8	25.0	100	2	0	10	9	50	50	0
10	25.0	100	7	2	31	4	106	106	0
12	72.0	7.6	1	0	9	1	9	98	2

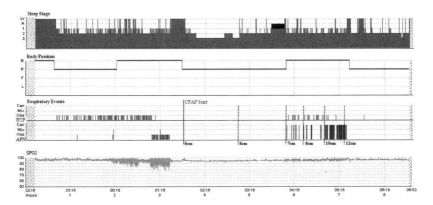

Figure 18.1 Hypnogram of a split-night study. Note the emergence of central apneas at higher PAP pressures.

Start of CPAP and Development of Air Leaks

Due to the challenges John had had tolerating PAP therapy in the past, a detailed education session and mask fitting was performed in the presence of his wife. He felt most comfortable with a full face mask, but his dominant hand weakness made it difficult to apply it on his own. The physician encouraged persistence with CPAP therapy and emphasized its immediate benefits on sleep quality, daytime symptoms, and mood, as well as its long-term cardiovascular benefits, particularly given his medical history.

John started CPAP therapy and took it with him to Florida for the winter. He returned to the sleep clinic 4 months later, appearing sleepy, with dark circles under his eyes and a host of PAP complaints. He continued to wake up 3 to 4 times per night to urinate and found it difficult to remove and reapply the mask on his own. His prior stroke and low back pain prevented him from sleeping comfortably in any one position for extended periods of time, and the frequent position changes led to mask leaks disrupting sleep for himself and his wife. He was refitted with a nasal mask that that could be applied with one hand. Additional education was provided on proper mask fit and technique of hose disconnection without removing the head gear for trips to the bathroom. To be sure, John and his wife provided a return demonstration of mask application and removal and knowledge of the machine features and equipment.

Pressure Problems Prompt a Switch to an Auto-adjusting Device

One month later, John returned to the sleep clinic, continuing to report problems with his CPAP unit. Out of sheer frustration, he had stopped using it altogether shortly after his last visit. While the mask no longer seemed to be the problem, the pressure was. With the 20-minute ramp feature, he was able to fall asleep at the starting pressure on the side, but the pressure was not enough when he was on his back. Yet he felt that the pressure was too high during the night, causing him to wake up repeatedly. To address the positional variability of his OSA, an auto-adjusting CPAP unit was prescribed with a range of $5\,cmH_2O$ to $16\,cmH_2O$. The device was able to detect the degree of obstruction and adjust the pressure over time.

Still no Joy Despite Adherence

On his follow-up visit 1 month later, John remained frustrated because he continued to be sleepy and fatigued (ESS of 12) despite what he thought was excellent compliance with Auto PAP. In fact, he liked the new machine. He was able to sleep better, could shift positions without disrupting the fit of the mask, and was not awakening from pressure changes. A data download revealed that he had used the device for more than 4 hours 78% of nights with a mean nightly usage of 6 hours (Figure 18.2, Table 18.2). His residual AHI was 41.

Switch to Adaptive Servo-ventilation

John's physician was concerned that the emergence of central events on the initial sleep study and the persistence of events on the auto-titrating device represented complex sleep apnea. A repeat titration study performed with bi-level PAP again showed poor control of respiratory events due to central apneas, confirming his suspicion. An adaptive servo-ventilation (ASV) device was prescribed with an EPAP of $5\,cmH_2O$, a pressure support range of 4 to $15\,cmH_2O$ above EPAP, and a back-up rate of 10 breaths per minute (see Chapter 10 for more on complex sleep apnea and ASV).

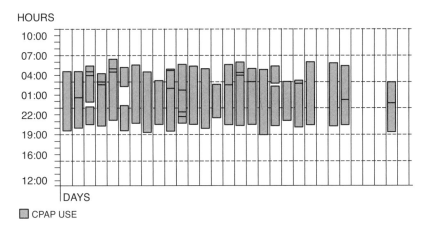

HOURS

DAYS

☐ CPAP USE

Figure 18.2 Adherence data on an auto-titrating device over 30 days. Consecutive days are shown on the X axis. Hours of the day are shown on the Y axis, with shaded areas representing actual hours of device use.

Table 18.2 PAP tracking downloads

	Auto-titrating device	Adaptive servo-ventilation
Days in download	19	8
Pressure cmH$_2$0	Median 11.4	Average peak pressure 13
Days without device usage	2	0
Percent of days used > 4 hours	78	100
Average nightly usage	6 hours 10 min	6 hours 12 min
Mean AHI	41	1

Diagnoses

Complex sleep apnea.
Left hemispheric stroke with residual right hemiparesis.

Outcome

Two weeks later, John returned for follow-up. He appeared much more alert and was quite satisfied, as he felt he finally had made a breakthrough. He reported much more consolidated sleep, fewer nocturnal trips to the bathroom, and improved daytime sleepiness (ESS was 5). A data download of the first 8 days of use showed excellent compliance with a residual AHI of 1 (Table 18.2). John felt much more positive about the therapy. His wife was sleeping more soundly as well.

Discussion

PAP therapy is the treatment of choice for most adult patients with moderate to severe OSA. Short- and long-term benefits of successful PAP include improvements in EDS, cardiovascular outcomes, cognitive function, and psychological testing, and reduction in motor vehicle and occupational accidents, to say nothing of improved quality of life for the spouse. However, the use of CPAP is challenging for many patients, with objective measurements indicating that only 40%–60% adhere to treatment, defined as at least 4 hours of use for 70% of nights. Some programs have shown objective adherence rates as high as 80%. Adaptation to CPAP is usually established within the first 3 months of treatment, but John's case illustrates the importance of persistence and patience, as PAP adherence can take much longer.

Efforts to enhance the PAP experience should be made expeditiously, in order to optimize adherence. Mask fitting, nasal issues, and sleep position should be assessed before the titration study. Physical limitations, as in John's case, should be taken into account. Other factors include spousal considerations (concern for the bed partner's sleep); lifestyle issues, such as traveling with PAP; and being able to use it watching TV or reading. Educational interventions, persistence, and follow-up are critical for success. Patients should be instructed on the pathophysiology of OSA and its long-term consequences, expectations of treatment, and use and care for the machine, interface and tubing. Involvement of the bed partner is an important aspect of the education process.

Dissatisfaction with the PAP interface is a leading barrier to the use the device. This can be due to difficulties with poor fit and dislodgement due to position changes, leaks, skin abrasion, and claustrophobia. PAP interface technology is constantly improving and masks in various shapes, styles, materials, and sizes are available (Figure 18.3). Nasal (anatomic obstruction, nasal congestion, dryness, epistaxis) and pressure (difficulty exhaling, aerophagia) issues can also compromise compliance. Many of these issues can be addressed successfully by a knowledgeable health care provider (Table 18.3).

Third party payers are increasingly requiring documentation of use and benefit in order to continue coverage. The educational component of CPAP therapy is particularly important in the context of the new Medicare Certificate of Medical Necessity (CMN) policy for coverage of CPAP devices. Specifically, in addition to a Medicare-covered sleep study, the requirements for initial (first 12 weeks) device certification include: (1) a face-to-face clinical evaluation by the treating physician prior to the sleep test to assess for OSA, and (2) patient and/or caregiver instruction from the supplier of the CPAP device and accessories in the proper use and care of the equipment.

Continued coverage beyond the first 3 months requires that, no sooner than the 31st day but no later than the 91st day of treatment, there is demonstration of clinical benefit by: (1) a face-to-face clinical re-evaluation by the treating

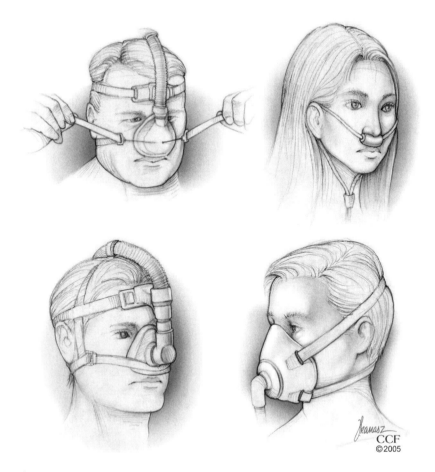

Figure 18.3 Examples of PAP mask interfaces. Reprinted with permission from Cleveland Clinic Journal Press.

physician with documentation that OSA symptoms are improved, and (2) objective evidence of PAP adherence reviewed by the treating physician, defined as use of CPAP than 4 or more hours per night on 70% of nights during 30 consecutive days anytime during the first 3 months of use.

John's case also demonstrates the importance of changing the mode of PAP delivery in patients intolerant of fixed CPAP. Some studies have shown that auto-titrating devices improve adherence, though the difference between the mean pressure on the auto-titrating device and the fixed CPAP pressure tends to be small. Nevertheless, the use of an auto-titrating device may be justified when there are marked changes in AHI with positional variation, across sleep stages and with progressive weight loss after bariatric surgery. Bi-level PAP should also be considered in patients with pressure intolerance, as it reduces the average delivered pressure.

Table 18.3 PAP complications and management strategies

Problem	Potential intervention
Interface related	
Mask leak or discomfort	Alternative interfaces, mask fitting and education
Mouth leaks	Full face mask, chin straps, lower pressure with positional therapy, change interface, bi-level pressure or auto-titrating device
Dry eyes/conjuctivitis/ bloodshot eyes	Alternative interfaces, correct mask leaks
Pressure sores/skin breakdown	Alternative interfaces, avoid over-tightening, tape or foam barrier
Claustrophobia	Nasal interface, desensitization (mask without headgear or pressure then add headgear, tubing, then pressure as anxiety decreases), behavioral therapy
Impairment in dexterity	Use masks that can be placed with 1 hand
Unknowing removal of mask during sleep	Assess for comfort with interface and pressure
Difficulty placing the mask after removal	Keep the mask on and disconnect hose
Nasal related	
Nasal obstruction	Otolaryngology assessment, nasal strip
Nasal congestion	Nasal saline sprays or gels, heated humidification, full face masks, oral interface, nasal strip
Nasal rhinitis	Heated humidifier, nasal steroid or ipratropium
Nasal dryness	Heated humidifier
Epistaxis (nose bleeds)	Nasal saline sprays or gels, heated humidification
Pressure related	
Gastric bloating	Gas relief medication, nocturnal oral patency device, behavior modification
Pressure intolerance	Ramp feature, bi-level pressure or auto-titrating devices, lower pressure with positional therapy
Machine related	
Noise from machine	Check that filters are clean and free from obstruction, assess machine for repair
Persistent symptoms despite adherence	Download PAP tracking data to assess adherence, review for leaks, assess adequacy of prescribed pressure, evaluate for alternative diagnoses such as complex sleep apnea

Residual obstructive events or the emergence of central events may also contribute to poor PAP adherence. In John's case, PAP therapy itself resulted in the development of central apneas, fulfilling the diagnosis of complex sleep apnea. While selection of lower pressures with continued PAP use may result in resolution of complex sleep apnea over time, this was not the case here. Complex sleep apnea was probably a contributing factor to John's poor adherence after mask and pressure issues were resolved, since ASV normalized the AHI and improved his symptoms.

John's presentation also highlights the use of PAP tracking features in confirming adherence and treatment adequacy. While the use of PAP tracking has yet to be shown to improve adherence, it does provide a means of monitoring compliance and can be used to guide therapy.

As general awareness of OSA increases, so too will the use of PAP therapy and the challenges of adherence. John's case highlights the importance of a program of active support, encompassing communication between healthcare providers and home care professionals, individualized education including the patient and family, frequent follow-up in the office or by phone, and the use of PAP tracking devices to confirm adherence and guide therapy. Access to a health care provider in the first weeks of PAP treatment is critical in ensuring long-term success. While intensive monitoring is costly and labor intensive, the incentive to ensure successful outcomes is greater than ever.

Bibliography

Berry RB. Improving CPAP compliance, man more than machine. *Sleep Med.* 2000;1:175–178.

Kakkar RK, Berry RB. Positive airway pressure treatment for obstructive sleep apnea. *Chest.* 2007;132:1057–1072.

Kribbs NB, Pack AI, Kline LR, et al. Objective measurement of patterns of nasal CPAP use by patients with obstructive sleep apnea. *Am Rev Respir Crit Care Dis.* 1993;147:887–95.

Morgenthaler TI, Kagramanov V, Hanak V, et al. Complex sleep apnea syndrome: Is it a unique clinical syndrome? *SLEEP.* 2006;29:1203–1209.

Pépin JL, Krieger J, Rodenstein D, Cornette A, Sforza E, Delguste P, Deschaux C, Grillier V, Lévy P. Effective compliance during the first 3 months of continuous positive airway pressure. A European prospective study of 121 patients. *Am J Respir Crit Care Med.* 1999;160:1124–1129.

Reeves-Hoche MK, Meck R, Zwillich CW. Nasal CPAP: An objective evaluation of patient compliance. *Am J Respir Crit Care Dis.* 1994;149:149–154.

Waldhorn RE, Herrick TW, Nguyen MC, O'Donnell AE, Sodero J, Potolicchio SJ. Long-term compliance with nasal CPAP therapy of obstructive sleep apnea. *Chest.* 1990;97:33–38.

19

Of Broken Homes, Chocolate, and Apnea

JENNIFER SCIUVA, MSN, PNP
JYOTI KRISHNA, MD

Case History

Annie presented to the sleep clinic at age 11 with snoring and apneas witnessed by her mother when co-sleeping. There was no history of nocturnal sweats, morning headaches, limb jerks, or unusual nocturnal behavior during sleep. Sleep history further confirmed sufficient sleep for age amounting to 9 hours on weeknights, with weekend oversleep of 2 hours. She was generally in bed by 9 p.m. and denied symptoms of restless legs or insomnia. Annie also denied sleepiness at school but did nap for 1 hour after school. Aside from weight gain, she had a history of allergic rhinitis, asthma, and polycystic ovarian disease as well as Type-2 diabetes. She had undergone adenoidectomy a year ago for recurrent ear infections. Her current medications included desloratidine, metformin, and montelukast by mouth, and budesonide, fluticasone-salmeterol, and albuterol by inhaler.

Born into a large Italian family, Annie adored all of the pastry her grandmother "made from scratch." When Annie was 9, her parents separated due to many problems in their marriage. With her brother in the custody of their father, it was just Annie and her mother left living together. She thus began co-sleeping with her mother for security. This was also the start of Annie's weight problem, as she turned to food, especially chocolate, for comfort. It was obvious this was the one aspect of her life she was able to control, even as she dreamed of the time when the family would be together again.

Physical Examination

On examination, Annie had inferior turbinate hypertrophy, Grade II-III tonsillar size, a Grade III Friedman tongue position, and acanthosis nigricans on the neck. Her body mass index was $41.25 \, \text{kg/m}^2$. The remainder of the physical examination was unremarkable.

Evaluation

A polysomnogram (PSG) was ordered which showed moderate to severe obstructive sleep apnea (OSA) with a positional component. The overall apnea-hypopnea index (AHI) was 20.9, the REM index 23.7, supine index 50.0, and non-supine index was 13.1. The mean SpO_2 was 92% with a nadir of 73%, and saturations were below 90% for 13.4% of total sleep time. No hypercapnia was noted (Figure 19.1).

Diagnoses

Obstructive sleep apnea, pediatric.
Morbid obesity.
Co-morbid Type 2 diabetes and polycystic ovarian disease.

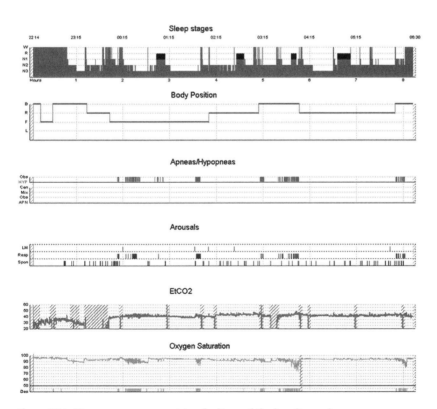

Figure 19.1 Hypnogram summarizing findings of the baseline polysomnogram. Note that the apnea-hypopnea events are mainly present when on the back or supine (B) and the front or prone (F) position.

Outcome

At follow-up 1 week after the sleep study, results were explained in detail to Annie and her family, and an ENT consult was recommended in the hope of a surgical intervention as first line of therapy. She was to follow up in the sleep center 2 months after the surgery. Annie preferred to return to the ENT surgeon who had previously removed her adenoids. The surgeon recommended she improve her compliance with treatment for allergic rhinitis and focus on weight loss. Tonsillectomy, however, was not advised, as she was considered high risk for surgery. Adenoids were deemed not to have regrown.

Annie returned to the sleep center for follow-up only after 3 months had elapsed. She informed us that she had started to attend a medically based outpatient weight loss program in the community but unfortunately had gained 11 more pounds by the end of the 3-month program. Annie's mother was very upset about this, as she had hoped weight loss would be the solution. It was therefore agreed Annie be started on continuous positive airway pressure (CPAP) therapy, and a titration study was ordered. The study was to be done after mask fitting and a 2-week period of acclimation to nightly CPAP at 5 cmH$_2$O.

The titration was well tolerated. At all CPAP settings, the apnea-hypopnea and arousal indices normalized and snoring was eliminated. Additionally, at a CPAP setting of 7 cmH$_2$O, the oxygen saturation was improved along with the airflow contour. CPAP was therefore prescribed at 7 cmH$_2$O (Figure 19.2). She was also encouraged to sleep on her side.

When seen for follow-up 1 month later, it was apparent Annie was not using her CPAP every night. The downloaded PAP machine data showed usage on only about 50% of the nights, with average use of 4 hours per night. She still was napping twice per week after school for an hour or so. It was explained to Annie that daytime sleepiness could potentially be decreased if she were to wear her CPAP consistently. During the discussion, Annie's mother was tearful in the exam room. She expressed concerns regarding Annie's mood and motivation. Based upon this, the family was referred to a clinical psychologist who also regularly worked with children referred to the sleep center. The mother further noted that Annie had not put on any more weight since the last visit. She felt this to be a positive change and did not wish to pursue a consultation with a dietician. Telephone follow-up subsequently suggested improving CPAP compliance. Annie returned to the sleep center over her Christmas break. She looked a little slimmer and wore a grin that told us she was doing well. She carried in a beautiful gift basket for the sleep staff as a token of thanks. Of course, it was full of chocolate, but at least she was giving some away.

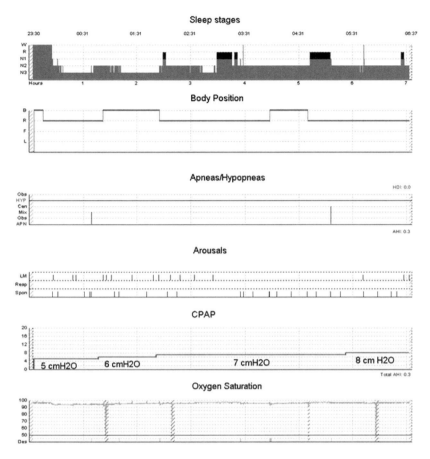

Figure 19.2 Hypnogram summarizing findings of nasal PAP titration. Note, quick response to relatively low pressures in this child.

Discussion

Obese children have a higher risk for OSA than those with normal weight. Studies in northeastern Ohio suggest that obese children were 4 to 5 times more likely to have OSA than normal-weight children. Associations between obesity and AHI have been shown in studies from other countries as well. Adenotonsillar hypertrophy can be a significant contributor, but it may not always be the most important factor in the genesis of OSA and hypoxia in obese children. Other factors, such as restrictive pulmonary dynamics from obesity as well as fatty content of the soft tissues surrounding the upper airway, may play a significant role.

It has nevertheless been suggested that adenotonsillectomy remain the first line treatment for OSA in obese children. Obese children undergoing adenotonsillectomy have a higher incidence of perioperative complications relative to normal-weight children, however. These include intra-operative desaturation, multiple laryngoscopic attempts, difficulty with mask ventilation, and increased length of stay. In Annie's case the surgeon felt the surgical risks outweighed the benefits. Given the favorable positional component of the OSA and relatively low PAP settings, the alternative therapy was successful.

PAP therapy is challenging in children, but it has been successfully implemented and is well-documented in the literature. Patience, encouragement, and education are key. As children grow and develop rapidly, their biophysical profile undergoes rapid changes as well. Accordingly, adequate surveillance with PSG or PAP retitration studies should be planned periodically. Interim office visits to assess compliance with therapy are essential. Referral to a sleep psychologist to help with acclimation, acceptance, and adherence to CPAP therapy can be invaluable.

Bibliography

Dayyat E, Kheirandish-Gozal L, SansCapdevila O, Maarafeya MM, Gozal D. Obstructive sleep apnea in children: Relative contributions of body mass index and adenotonsillar hypertrophy. *Chest.* 2009;136:137–144.

Kirk VG, O'Donnell AR. Continuous positive airway pressure for children: a discussion of how to maximize compliance. *Sleep Med Rev.* 2006;10:119–127.

Nafiu OO, Green GE, Walton S, Morris M, Reddy S, Tremper KK. Obesity and risk of perioperative complications in children presenting for adenotonsillectomy. *Int J Pediatr Otorhinolaryngol.* 2009;73:89–95.

Redline S, Tishler PV, Schlucter M, Aylor J, Clark K, Graham G. Risk factors for sleep-disordered breathing in children: Associations with obesity, race and respiratory problems. *Am J Respir Crit Care Med.* 1999;159:1527–1532.

Tauman, R, Gozal, D. Obesity and obstructive sleep apnea in children. *Paediatr Respir Rev.* 2006;7:247–259.

20
Oral Appliance Lets Teen Sleep Easy

FLAVIA SRESHTA, DDS

Clinical History

Daniel was a 16-year-old young man who was referred for consideration of oral appliance therapy for obstructive sleep apnea (OSA). His sleep problems dated back to 6 years of age, when his mother noticed snoring and difficulty breathing during sleep. He had an adenoidectomy at that time, which controlled his symptoms. However, during puberty his snoring recurred, and by age 14 he developed excessive daytime sleepiness (EDS) and attention and concentration problems. He was diagnosed with attention deficit disorder (ADD) and treated by his pediatrician with Adderall.

When his symptoms failed to improve, Daniel's parents consulted an otolaryngologist who recommended a polysomnogram (PSG). The study revealed an apnea-hypopnea index (AHI) of 20 and oxygen desaturations as low as 83%. He was diagnosed with obstructive sleep apnea syndrome (OSAS) and prescribed continuous positive airway pressure (CPAP) therapy. He used CPAP for nearly 2 years, with remission of snoring and EDS and improvement in school performance. However, at 16 years of age, Daniel was embarrassed by his CPAP machine after his mother insisted he take it with him to a sleepover with friends. He felt different from his friends, who mocked him that night and the next week at school. This prompted his parents to ask Daniel's pediatrician for an alternative solution.

Daniel's sleep history was negative for enuresis, abnormal behaviors in sleep, and symptoms of restless legs syndrome and narcolepsy. His medical history was otherwise unremarkable. His father had OSA. He lived at home with his parents and sibling. He took no medications and did not use tobacco, alcohol, or recreational drugs.

Physical Examination

Daniel's physical exam was remarkable for a narrow face and Angles Class I with overjet of 1.5 mm and overbite of 2 mm (Figures 20.1, 20.2). The tongue size was medium and tongue position was Freidman Grade II (Figure 20.3) with an elevated palatal roof (Figure 20.4). Temporomandibular joint (TMJ) palpation and function was normal. Daniel's body mass index (BMI) was 24.4 kg/m² and his neck circumference was 16 cm. His general and neurological examinations were otherwise unremarkable.

Diagnoses

Obstructive sleep apnea syndrome.
Constricted maxilla, elevated palate, and retrognathic maxillae and mandible.

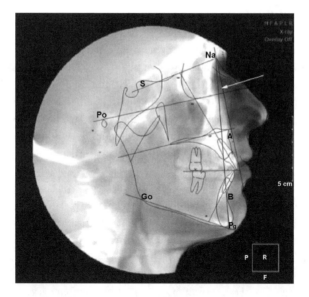

Figure 20.1 Cephalometric Analysis. The SNA and SNB angles represent the anterior-posterior position of the maxilla and mandible respectively to the cranial base. The ANB angle is a comparison of the position of the maxilla and mandible; it is the difference between angles SNA and SNB. (Na) Nasion: The junction of the nasal and frontal bones at the most posterior point on the curvature of the bridge of the nose; (S) Sella: The center of the hypophyseal fossa (sella turcica); (A): Most anterior point of the maxillary apical base; (B): Most anterior measure point of the mandibular apical base. The overjet is indicated by the white arrow. (Go): Junction of the ramus and body of the mandible; (Pg): The Pogonion point, the most anterior point of the chin; (Po): The Porion point located at the external acoustic meatus.

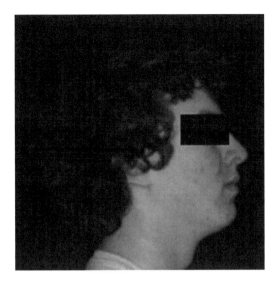

Figure 20.2 Lateral view suggesting retruded mandible.

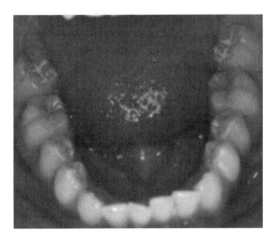

Figure 20.3 Mandibular arch demonstrating retracted tongue.

Outcome

Daniel's normal BMI and neck circumference, along with his age, made him a particularly good candidate for oral appliance therapy. He was fitted with a 2-piece, custom-made mandibular repositioning appliance (MRA) designed to advance the mandible forward. This appliance required dental impressions and bite registration constructed by a dental laboratory. Following an initial 2-week adaptation, the appliance was titrated over 8 weeks. At the 2-week follow-up visit, Daniel was able to wear the MRA almost every night, throughout the

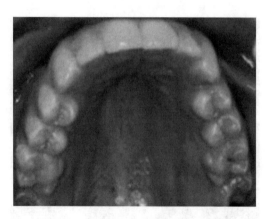

Figure 20.4 Maxillary arch showing elevated palatal roof.

night, without complaints. He reported less fatigue and more energy, and his parents noted improved attention and concentration. At this time, the airway dilator was moved to 6 mm vertical height and 5 mm protrusive movement. At the 4-week follow-up visit, he was advanced to a protrusive position of 7.5 mm with the same vertical height. He was seen at 2-week intervals for further adjustments. At his last follow-up visit, Daniel and his parents reported continued nightly use, better sleep quality, and marked improvement in fatigue, sleepiness, attention, and concentration. He was able to discontinue the use of Adderall. He underwent a PSG 3 weeks later after optimal positioning which revealed a significant reduction in his AHI and abolition of nocturnal oxygen desaturations (Table 20.1).

Table 20.1 Pre- and post-mandibular repositioning device PSG results

	Baseline	MRA
TRT, min	393	435
Sleep efficiency, %	95	94
Sleep latency, min	10.9	9.5
REM latency	102	92
Sleep stage distribution, %		
N1	0.1	5
N2	61.6	65.1
N3	23.4	11
REM	14.8	18.9
Arousal index	19	19
AHI	20	6
SpO_2, mean (nadir), %	96 (83)	96 (93)
Periodic limb movement index	10	0

After optimal positioning of the MRA, Daniel underwent a cone beam computed tomography scan (CBCT) to visualize and quantify his airway in three dimensions with and without the appliance (Figures 20.5, 20.6). Without the MRA, persistent obstruction and marked airway occlusion due to the tongue position was observed (Figures 20.5a, 20.6a). The pharyngeal airway volume

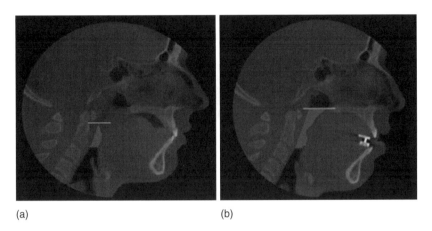

(a)   (b)

Figure 20.5 Cone beam computed tomography (CBCT) sagittal images pre- and post-MRA placement. The upper airway volume is represented by the colored area. The pre-treatment image (a) demonstrates minimal axial space (airway area: 179.2 mm^2, airway volume: 2024.5 mm^3, minimal axial area: 1.5 mm^2). The post-treatment image (b) demonstrates increase in airway area (airway area: 466.5 mm^2, airway volume: 7789.7 mm^3, minimal axial area: 103.0 mm^2).

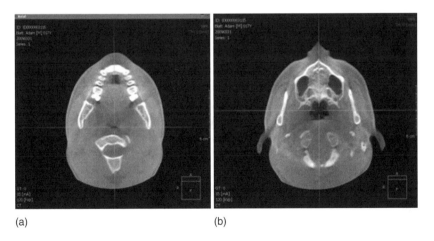

(a)   (b)

Figure 20.6 Cone beam computed tomography (CBCT) axial images pre- and post-MRA placement. Without the MRA, the anteroposterior and lateral dimensions of the upper airway are markedly reduced (a) in comparison to the size of the upper airway when the MRA was in place (b).

was calculated as $2024.5\,\text{mm}^3$ with a minimum axial area, the point of greatest stenosis, calculated as $1.5\,\text{mm}^2$. With the MRA in place, a patent airway was observed with a pharyngeal airway volume of $7789.7\,\text{mm}^3$ and a minimum axial area of $103.0\,\text{mm}^2$ (Figures 20.5b, 20.6b). The appliance improved airway volume and patency in all three axes.

Discussion

Daniel's case illustrates the importance of abnormal craniofacial anatomy in the pathophysiology of OSAS and the role of MRAs as a treatment modality in select cases. As illustrated in the cephalometric analysis (Figure 20.1), the values of Daniel's SNA (77.7°) and SNB (73.2°) angles suggest his maxilla and mandible were retruded as compared with normal values associated with the McKee cephalometric analysis of 82.0° and 80.9° respectively. Daniel's ANB (4.5°) angle was also increased (normal = 1.6°), suggesting a decreased oropharyngeal space. In addition, he had a constricted maxilla, elevated palate, and retracted tongue. His upper airway anatomy resulted in OSAS, causing fatigue, EDS and cognitive difficulties. As a teenager, he preferred the MRA to CPAP therapy, finding it more psychologically and socially acceptable. Not to be underestimated were Daniel's cooperation and collaboration with the clinician in the long-term success of this therapy.

In addition to OSAS, the differential diagnosis for Daniel's presenting complaints included ADD and psychiatric disorders such as depression. His failure to respond to medical therapy for ADD and his marked improvement with treatment of OSAS suggested that his cognitive problems were most likely due to the latter. His pediatrician screened Daniel and his parents for psychiatric disorders and felt that depression was unlikely.

The Angles classification was used to define Daniel's malocclusion based on the relationship of the permanent molars and their locking. Class I is a normal relationship of the jaws with the maxillary first molar occluding in the buccal groove of the mandibular first permanent molar, as observed in Daniel's case. Class II describes a distal relationship of the mandible relative to the maxilla. Class III describes a mesial relationship of the mandible relative to the maxilla.

CBCT was used to quantify Daniel's airway before and after intervention. CBCT allows 3D radiographic images to be obtained in a single rotation. A computer analysis is utilized to provide dimensional analysis of the desired anatomic space. This radiographic method allows for quantification of obstruction and changes in airway volume with a given treatment modality. The patient is analyzed in an upright position, while awake. In Daniel's case, the MRA was shown to improve airway volume and patency in all 3 axes.

MRAs reposition and stabilize the mandible, tongue, and hyoid bone and increase baseline genioglossus muscle activity. These devices increase the size of the airway in the medial-lateral dimension more than in the antero-posterior dimension. They come in 1 piece or 2 and are custom made or prefabricated. The monobloc design rigidly fixes the mandible in an anterior position, while the bibloc design allows some freedom of mandibular movement.

Prior to treatment, the diagnosis of OSAS should be made based on PSG and an evaluation for MRA suitability should be performed (Table 20.2). Patients with mild to moderate OSA who prefer oral appliances to CPAP, those who do not respond to CPAP or are not appropriate candidates for CPAP, and those who fail behavioral intervention—such as weight loss or positional therapy—are acceptable candidates for MRAs. Patients with severe OSA should have a trial of CPAP first. Younger patients with a normal neck circumference and BMI and a mandibular advancement greater than 6 mm are favorable candidates as well.

Acceptable candidates are offered a temporary appliance for a period of 1 to 2 weeks in order to assess patient acceptance and response. A custom-made MRA is then fabricated and gradually titrated over 6 to 8 weeks, aimed at mandibular advancement that yields clinical benefit with minimum side effects, such as daytime tooth discomfort, excessive salivation, and dry mouth. The patient is reassessed monthly until the maximum advancement is achieved, after which a follow-up PSG is performed. Patient adherence, condition of the appliance, and dental health are then re-evaluated at 6-month intervals. If the patient experiences a recurrence or worsening of OSAS symptoms or weight gain, progressive protrusive advancement of the MRA or repeat PSG may be warranted. Routine monitoring by both a sleep specialist and a dentist experienced in MRAs is necessary.

Table 20.2 Indications and prerequisites for mandibular repositioning device

A: Indications
    Patients with mild or moderate OSA
    Patients with severe OSA noncompliant with CPAP
B: Prerequisites
    Absence of significant periodontal disease
    Absence of significant TMJ dysfunction syndrome
    Retrognathia or micrognathia
    Possession of at least 10 viable, well-anchored teeth on both the maxillary and mandibular arches
    No limitation of jaw opening (>25mm)
    Motivated to wear oral appliance

Bibliography

Ferguson KA, et al. Oral appliances for snoring and obstructive sleep apnea: A review. *SLEEP*. 2006;29(2):244–262.

Kushida CA, et al. Practice parameters for the treatment of snoring and obstructive sleep apnea with oral appliances: An update for 2005. *SLEEP*. 2006;29(2): 240–243.

Markland M, et al. Mandibular advancement devices in 630 men and women with obstructive sleep apnea and snoring: Tolerability and prediction of treatment and success. *Chest*. 2004;125(4):1270–1277.

21

Desaturating, but Why?

NATTAPONG JAIMCHARIYATAM, MD, MSc
OMAR MINAI, MD, FCCP

Case History

Christina, a 50-year-old Caucasian office worker, was referred to the pulmonary clinic for evaluation of dyspnea. She reported gradually worsening dyspnea over the previous 6 months that had begun to interfere with daily functioning. Based on a history of coughing, wheezing, and dyspnea on exertion, she was initially diagnosed with asthma, however, treatment did not improve her symptoms. At the time of her evaluation, she complained of shortness of breath with minimal activity (New York Heart Association Functional Class III-IV), daytime easy fatigability, morning headaches, wheezing, and bilateral pedal edema. She experienced dyspnea when ambulating around the house, showering, and even combing her hair. Climbing stairs had become increasingly difficult, and she had recently found herself abstaining from activities she enjoyed, like grocery shopping. She reported frequent snoring but no daytime sleepiness (her Epworth Sleepiness Scale, or ESS, score was 6). She had symptoms of gastroesophageal reflux, including heartburn and a sour taste in the mouth, that sometimes kept her awake at night. She endorsed symptoms of restless legs syndrome (RLS) but denied a family history of RLS, renal disease, anemia, or peripheral neuropathy. Current medications included albuterol and fluticasone/salmeterol inhalers, montelukast 10 mg daily, and esomeprazole 40 mg daily. She was a lifetime nonsmoker.

Physical Examination

Christina appeared in no apparent distress, with a blood pressure of 128/70 mmHg, a heart rate of 80 bpm, a respiratory rate of 22 breaths per minute, and a body mass index (BMI) of 27 kg/m². Her upper airway examination showed crowding of the soft tissue with a Grade III Friedman tongue position and Grade III tonsil size. The lung sounds were clear. Cardiac auscultation revealed a loud pulmonic component of S2 (increased P2) along with a grade 2/6 holo-systolic murmur at the left lower sternal border that increased with inspiration. She had mild bilateral ankle edema. Her examination was otherwise unremark-able. Specifically, there was no evidence of jugular vein distension, oral ulcers, thrush, mucosal telangiectasias, or facial rash.

Evaluation

Pulmonary function test results were normal without evidence of obstructive or restrictive ventilatory defect and a normal diffusion capacity for carbon monox-ide corrected for alveolar volume (Table 21.1) A ventilation-perfusion scan was negative for pulmonary embolism, and computed tomographic scan (CT) of the chest was negative for pulmonary parenchymal disease and pulmonary embo-lism. Her 6-minute walk test revealed a reduction in walk distance at 355 m and lack of exertional oxygen desaturation. Results of laboratory testing revealed a sodium of 142, CO_2 of 24, and a hemoglobin of 17.8 mg/dL.

Christina's echocardiogram revealed normal left ventricular (LV) size and function with a LV ejection fraction (LVEF) of 55%. The right ventricle was dilated with moderate to severely decreased systolic function. There was 2+ to 3+ tricuspid regurgitation and the estimated right ventricular systolic pressure was 100 mmHg. A small patent foramen ovale with right to left shunting was noted by bubble study. Findings on a right heart catheterization demonstrating pulmonary hypertension are summarized in Table 21.2.

Given her history of snoring and fatigue, Christina was referred for a poly-somnogram (PSG). She slept for 300 minutes, including 23 minutes of REM sleep, producing a sleep efficiency of 79%. Sleep latency was 12 minutes. Loud snoring was recorded. She had an apnea-hypopnea index (AHI) of 5 (REM AHI

Table 21.1   Pulmonary function test results

Parameter	Liters	% predicted
FVC (Forced vital capacity)	2.04	64
FEV1 (Forced expiratory volume in 1 second)	1.63	62
FEV1/FVC ratio	0.79	
TLC (Total lung capacity)	4.13	83
RV (Residual volume)	1.92	110
DLCO (diffusion capacity for carbon monoxide)	14.2	65
DLVA (DLCO corrected for alveolar volume)	4.69	94

Table 21.2   Right heart catheterization results

Parameter	Results	Reference Range
mRAP	12	0-5 mmHg
RVP systolic/diastolic	110/20	25/5 mmHg
PAP systolic/diastolic	107/40	16–24/5–12 mmHg
PAP mean	62	9–16 mmHg
PCWP	8	5–12 mmHg
CO	2.98	5–6 L/min
CI	1.66	2.5–3.5 L/min/m²
PVR	18	1–2 Wood units

mRAP: mean right atrial pressure; RVP: right ventricular pressure; PAP: pulmonary artery pressure; PCWP: pulmonary capillary wedge pressure; CO: cardiac output; CI: cardiac index; PVR: pulmonary vascular resistance.

of 9 and NREM AHI of 5) consisting entirely of obstructive apneas. The arousal index was 9. Mean oxygen saturation was 93% awake and 86% during sleep. Oxygen desaturations were more severe in REM sleep, reaching a nadir of 80%. She spent 43% of sleep time with oxygen saturation below 90%. The periodic limb movement (PLM) index was 29 and PLM arousal index was 2. Relevant PSG findings are shown in Figure 21.1. Oxygen supplementation at 2 and then 3 liter/min was introduced toward the end of the study and resulted in a significant improvement in oxygen saturation (Figure 21.1).

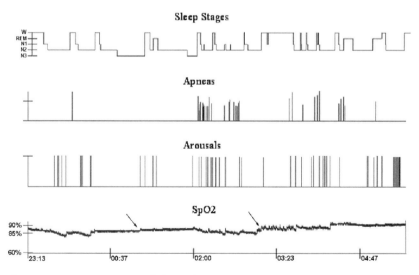

Figure 21.1 Hypnogram revealed significant oxygen desaturation throughout the night, particularly in REM sleep, even in the absence of respiratory events. Oxygen supplementation at 2 and then 3 L/min was introduced toward the end of the study as shown by the first and second arrows, respectively.

Diagnoses

Sleep related hypoxemia due to pulmonary parenchymal or vascular pathology (Table 21.3).
Mild obstructive sleep apnea (OSA).
Restless legs syndrome.
Idiopathic pulmonary arterial hypertension (PAH) with right ventricular dysfunction.
Small patent foramen ovale with predominantly right to left shunt.
Gastroesophageal reflux disease.

Outcome

Christina was initially treated with bosentan (a nonselective endothelin receptor antagonist) along with oxygen supplementation during sleep. This treatment resulted in a modest, though suboptimal, improvement in functional capacity and 6-minute walk test distance. Intravenous treprostinil therapy (a prostacyclin analogue) was added which produced a significant improvement in symptoms and functional capacity (NYHA Class I without chest pain or syncope). At Christina's most recent follow-up visit, her 6-minute walk test distance had increased to 568 m without exertional desaturation. Echocardiogram revealed normal LV function, mild right ventricular hypertrophy, and normal right atrial size, and the estimated right ventricular systolic pressure had improved to 63 mmHg. She felt less fatigued and was finding she had a bit more energy to do the things she most enjoyed.

Table 21.3   ICSD-2 diagnostic criteria for sleep related hypoxemia due to pulmonary parenchymal or vascular pathology

A. Lung parenchymal disease or pulmonary vascular disease is present and believed to be the primary cause of hypoxemia.
B. Polysomnography or sleeping arterial blood gas determination shows at least 1 of the following:
   i. An SpO_2 during sleep of less than 90% for more than 5 minutes with a nadir of at least 85%.
   ii. More than 30% of total sleep time at an SpO_2 of less than 90%.
   iii. Sleeping arterial blood gas with PCO_2 that is abnormally high or disproportionately increased relative to levels during wakefulness.
C. The disorder is not better explained by another current sleep disorder, another medical or neurological disorder, medication use, or substance use disorder.

Discussion

The most notable finding on Christina's PSG was that of sustained oxygen desaturation not explained by discrete apneic or hypopneic events. Obstructive sleep apnea can cause nocturnal hypoxemia, however, desaturations are typically intermittent and temporally related to respiratory events. Christina had sustained oxygen desaturation in sleep, a rare occurrence in patients with OSA, usually limited to severe cases.

The differential diagnosis of sustained nocturnal hypoxemia, as in Christina's case, includes congestive heart failure (CHF), parenchymal lung diseases, such as idiopathic pulmonary fibrosis and chronic obstructive pulmonary disease (COPD), and pulmonary vascular disorders, such as pulmonary embolism and pulmonary hypertension (PH). Pulmonary function evaluation, ventilation-perfusion scanning, lung CT scan, and echocardiography are required to exclude these conditions (Table 21.4). Christina had no evidence of left sided heart failure or pulmonary embolism and her pulmonary function tests were normal. The normal FEV1/FVC ratio excluded COPD, which requires a ratio less than 70%. The normal TLC and RV excluded restrictive lung diseases (such as pulmonary fibrosis where TLC and RV are reduced) and obstructive lung diseases (such as COPD where TLC and RV are increased). The 6-minute walk test has been used extensively to quantify functional capacity and predict survival in patients with cardiac and pulmonary disorders including COPD, interstitial lung diseases, CHF, and PH. In patients with PH, the 6-minute walk test has been shown to be a reliable baseline indicator of PH severity and long-term survival. The echocardiogram and right heart catheterization demonstrated PAH which was felt to be the cause of Christina's nocturnal desaturation.

Sustained nocturnal desaturation previously has been reported in patients with PAH without accompanying OSA. In a study of the prevalence, risk factors, and significance of nocturnal hypoxia in patients with PAH without significant lung disease, we found nocturnal desaturation in approximately 70%

Table 21.4   Differential diagnosis and evaluation for nocturnal hypoxemia

Disorder	Assessment
Obstructive sleep apnea	History, physical examination, PSG
Congestive heart failure	History, physical examination, transthoracic echocardiography
Parenchymal lung disease (e.g., idiopathic pulmonary fibrosis or emphysema)	History, physical examination, pulmonary function testing, lung CT scan
Pulmonary vascular disease (e.g., pulmonary embolism or pulmonary hypertension)	History, physical examination, lung ventilation-perfusion scan, lung CT scan

of cases. Nocturnal hypoxia was more common in older patients with more advanced pulmonary hypertension and right ventricular dysfunction (Figure 21.2). Even though most patients with exertional desaturation were nocturnal desaturators, 60% of PAH patients without exertional hypoxia had nocturnal desaturation. As such, even though exertional desaturation was a good indicator of nocturnal desaturation, lack of exertional desaturation did not exclude the need for nocturnal supplemental oxygen. These findings

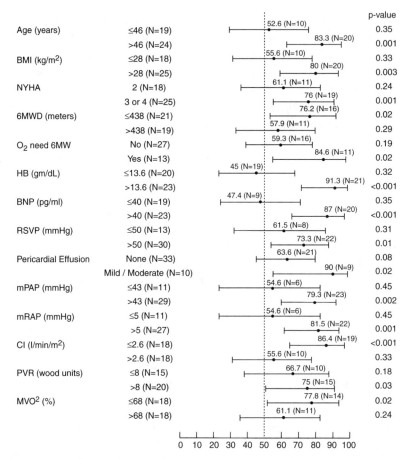

Figure 21.2 Predictors of nocturnal desaturation in patients with pulmonary arterial hypertension. Older patients and those with more functional compromise (higher NYHA FC and lower 6MWD) and severe pulmonary hypertension with right ventricular failure (presence of pericardial effusion on echocardiography; higher BNP, mPAP, mRAP, and PVR; and lower CI and MVO[2]) were more likely to have significant nocturnal desaturation. Reprinted from Minai OA et al. with permission.

6MWD: 6-min walk test distance; HB: hemoglobin; BNP: brain natriuretic protein; RSVP: right ventricular systolic pressure; mPAP: mean pulmonary artery pressure; mRAP: mean right atrial pressure; CI: cardiac index; PVR: pulmonary vascular resistance; MVO[2]: myocardial oxygen consumption.

strengthened the recommendations of the American College of Chest Physicians regarding oxygen supplementation in PAH patients.

The mechanism of nocturnal desaturation in PH is unclear. It is well known that people with normal lungs can desaturate during sleep. In the general population, multiple mechanisms contribute to nocturnal hypoxia, including alterations in ventilation-perfusion, reduced functional residual capacity, reduced respiratory drive, and alveolar hypoventilation. These mechanisms take on added importance in patients with pulmonary disease. It has been suggested that ventilation-perfusion matching is only minimally altered and shunt is uncommon in PAH not associated with congenital heart disease. Therefore, arterial hypoxemia is mild and explained by a low mixed venous oxygen saturation. We previously found that lower FEV1 and FVC and mixed venous oxygen saturation increased the risk of nocturnal desaturation.

Chronic hypoxia can cause increased cardiac output, erythrocytosis, and pulmonary vasoconstriction resulting in sustained elevations in pulmonary arterial pressure and pulmonary vascular resistance, right ventricular failure, and death. Higher hemoglobin among nocturnal desaturators in our study indicated that the hypoxia was chronic. Nocturnal supplemental oxygen is therefore recommended in patients with hypoxia while awake, those well-saturated awake but hypoxic during sleep, and those with complications attributable to sleep hypoxia, such as PH and cardiac arrhythmias. This was clearly the case for Christina.

Nocturnal oximetry should be considered a part of the initial evaluation of patients with PAH without exertional desaturation. Since OSA is a far more common cause of nocturnal desaturation than idiopathic PAH, sleep testing should be routinely performed in nocturnal desaturators. Continuous positive airway pressure therapy is recommended in patients with significant OSA, although patients with apneic episodes restricted to REM sleep may not require treatment. The implications of nocturnal hypoxemia on long-term prognosis in PAH and the utility of long-term oxygen supplementation in improving pulmonary hemodynamics require further study.

Bibliography

Badesch DB, Abman SH, Ahearn GS, et al. Medical therapy for pulmonary arterial hypertension: ACCP evidence-based clinical practice guidelines. *Chest*. 2004;126:35S–362S.

Minai OA, Pandya CM, Golish JA, et al. Predictors of nocturnal oxygen desaturation in pulmonary arterial hypertension. *Chest*. 2007;131:109–117.

Robin ED, Whaley RD, Crump CH, et al. Alveolar gas tensions, pulmonary ventilation and blood pH during physiologic sleep in normal subjects. *J Clin Invest*. 1958;37:981–989.

22

Keeping Up with the 20-Somethings

NATTAPONG JAIMCHARIYATAM, MD, MSc
OMAR MINAI, MD, FCCP

Case History

Carson was a 58-year-old man referred to the sleep disorders center for evaluation of snoring, daytime fatigue, and recurrent awakenings from sleep for the last 3 years. A recent increase in fatigue had begun to interfere with his performance on the assembly line of a metal factory. His co-workers, mostly 30 years his junior, had started to call him "Granddad." His wife reported frequent snoring but had never observed breathing irregularities in sleep. Carson had gained more than 20 lbs in recent years. He was previously a 60-pack year smoker, who had been diagnosed with chronic obstructive pulmonary disease (COPD) 8 years prior. He had episodes of productive cough with fever yearly requiring antibiotics and short courses of corticosteroids, though he had never required mechanical ventilation. He denied shortness of breath with usual exertion.

Carson typically went to bed at 11 p.m. and woke up 7 a.m., often with a dull headache and feeling as if he hadn't slept at all. He was usually able to fall asleep in 5 to 10 minutes other than during COPD exacerbations, when recurrent cough interfered with sleep initiation. He woke up 2 or 3 times most nights between 3 and 7 a.m., choking or gasping for air, but he was able to fall back asleep without difficulty. He usually slept on his back with 1 pillow. He felt sleepy during the day and had started drinking coffee over the course of the day to stay alert. His Epworth Sleepiness Scale (ESS) score was 11. He denied symptoms of restless legs syndrome and abnormal night behaviors.

Carson's medical history was notable for hypertension, Graves' disease (clinically euthyroid), and gastroesophageal reflux disease. His regular medications included theophylline, methimazole, omeprazole, mometasone nasal spray, and formoterol inhaler. He used albuterol inhaler as needed.

Physical Examination

Carson was alert and oriented and in no apparent distress. He had a blood pressure of 125/80 mmHg, a heart rate of 70 beats per minute, a respiratory rate of 18 per minute, and an oxygen saturation of 94% on room air. At 5' 11" tall and 157 lbs, he had a body mass index (BMI) of 23.5 m/kg^2 and a neck circumference of 35 cm. He had a Grade II Friedman tongue position. The tonsils were absent and there was no retrognathia or macroglossia. The cardiac examination revealed a regular rate and rhythm with no murmurs or gallops. He had prolonged expiration with distant breath sounds but no wheezing. His examination was otherwise unremarkable.

Evaluation

Pulmonary function testing revealed a forced expiratory volume in 1 second (FEV1) of 1.91 liters (53% predicted), a forced vital capacity (FVC) of 2.81 liters (61% predicted), and a FEV1/FVC ratio of 0.65. Lung volumes revealed a total lung capacity (TLC) of 6.2 liters (120% predicted) and a residual volume (RV) of 2.4 liters (130% predicted). Diffusion capacity was 13.3 (48% predicted) and 2.76 (69% predicted) when corrected for alveolar volume. These findings were consistent with moderate airflow obstruction, mild hyperinflation due to air trapping, and impaired diffusion due to moderate COPD. An alpha 1 antitrypsin level was normal.

Computer tomography of the chest revealed generalized centrilobular and paraseptal emphysema. Arterial blood gas analysis was abnormal, with pH 7.41, PaO$_2$ 40 mmHg, PaO$_2$ 64 mmHg, and oxygen saturation 93% on room air. This indicated arterial hypoxemia (normal PaO$_2$ should be 80–100 mmHg on room air). An echocardiogram revealed normal left and right ventricular systolic function without chamber enlargement or valvular dysfunction.

Polysomnography (PSG) was performed to assess for sleep related breathing disorders. Key features of the study are shown in Figure 22.1. The total sleep time was 295 minutes, including 12% Stage N1, 52% Stage N2, 13% Stage N3, and 23% REM sleep. The sleep latency was 12 minutes, and sleep efficiency was 71%. There were 17 awakenings, with a total time awake after sleep onset of 109 minutes. The arousal index was 52, and there were 145 stage shifts, suggesting a significant amount of sleep fragmentation. Loud snoring was noted. The apnea-hypopnea index (AHI) was 15, increasing to 56 in REM sleep. During wakefulness, the mean oxygen saturation was 95% with a nadir of 93%. The mean oxygen saturation during sleep was 90% with a minimum of 81%. Carson spent 56% of sleep time with oxygen saturation below 90% and 5% of sleep time with and end-tidal CO$_2$ (EtCO$_2$) above 40 mmHg with a maximum EtCO$_2$

Sleep Stages

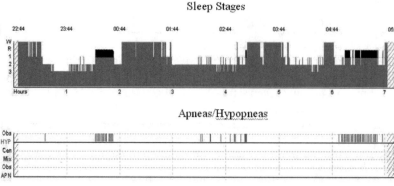

Apneas/Hypopneas

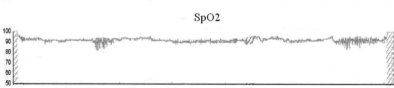

SpO2

Figure 22.1 Hypnogram from the PSG demonstrating persistent hypoxemia throughout the study, even in the absence of respiratory events.

of 44 mmHg. Frequent periodic limb movements were noted during sleep resulting in a periodic limb movement index of 81 and PLM arousal index of 5.

Diagnoses

Sleep related hypoxemia due to lower airway obstruction (moderate chronic obstructive pulmonary disease—(Table 22.1)).
Moderate obstructive sleep apnea syndrome (OSAS).

Outcome

Carson underwent a continuous positive airway pressure (CPAP) titration study during which a pressure of 10 cmH$_2$O normalized the apnea-hypopnea and arousal indices. Oxygen saturation improved from 82%–85% after abolition of respiratory events to 91%–94% with the addition of oxygen 2 liters. His COPD regimen was optimized by adding a long-acting inhaled anticholinergic agent and an inhaled corticosteroid. At follow-up he reported excellent CPAP compliance. This combination regimen produced a significant improvement in his daytime functioning, sleepiness, and fatigue. He reported feeling refreshed upon awakening for the first time in years and reported resolution of morning headaches. Improvements in concentration and stamina at work were observed not

Table 22.1 ICSD-2 diagnostic criteria for sleep related hypoxemia due to lower airway obstruction

A. Lower airway obstructive disease is present (as evidenced by a forced expiratory volume exhaled in one second/forced vital capacity ratio less than 70% of predicted values on pulmonary function testing) and is believed to be the primary cause of hypoxemia.
B. Polysomnography or sleeping arterial blood gas determination shows at least one of the following:
   i. An SpO_2 during sleep of less than 90% for more than 5 minutes with a nadir of at least 85%.
   ii. More than 30% of total sleep time at an SpO_2 of less than 90%.
   iii. Sleeping arterial blood gas with PCO_2 that is abnormally high or disproportionately increased relative to levels during wakefulness.
C. The disorder is not better explained by another current sleep disorder, another medical or neurological disorder, medication use, or substance use disorder.

only by Carson and his younger co-workers, but also by his supervisor, who was pleased with his performance, noting increased speed and accuracy on the job during his most recent evaluation. Both Carson and his wife felt that treating his sleep problems was the key to job security—at least for now.

Discussion

Carson's presenting symptoms included snoring, choking during sleep, daytime fatigue, and recurrent awakenings from sleep. Patients with COPD often complain of difficulty initiating and maintaining sleep, and they are found on PSG to have increased sleep latency, decreased total sleep time, and an increased number of arousals and awakenings. Carson's fragmented sleep could have been due to COPD, OSA, or both. Gastric reflux and medications with stimulant properties, such as theophylline, could also be responsible for or contribute to sleep disruption.

Significant PSG findings in this case include moderate OSAS and persistent nocturnal oxygen desaturation. In addition to sleep related breathing disorders such as OSA and central sleep apnea (CSA), parenchymal pulmonary diseases (COPD and interstitial lung diseases), pulmonary vascular diseases (pulmonary hypertension and pulmonary embolism), and neuromuscular disorders involving the respiratory system should be considered in the differential diagnosis of nocturnal oxygen desaturation. Oxygen desaturation associated with OSA and CSA can be distinguished from respiratory system disorders by clinical history and the presence of periodic alterations in respiratory flow associated with corresponding oxygen desaturations. In contrast, nocturnal oxygen desaturation due to a disorder of the respiratory system is usually more sustained, lasting several minutes or longer, is more pronounced during REM sleep, and can be seen in patients with an awake $PaO_2 > 60$ mmHg. Physiologic hypoventilation may be responsible for the development of nocturnal oxygen desaturation, even in healthy individuals. Factors such as alveolar hypoventilation, maldistribution of ventilation, and increased ventilation-perfusion mismatch may take on a more important role in patients with COPD who have abnormal respiratory mechanics and lower baseline awake oxygenation (Figure 22.2).

An estimated 10%–15% of COPD patients have OSAS, a condition known as the "overlap syndrome." Compared to those with COPD alone, patients with the overlap syndrome tend to have higher ESS scores, lower total sleep time, lower sleep efficiency, and higher arousal indices. In addition, patients with overlap syndrome have more severe nocturnal desaturation, higher prevalence of pulmonary hypertension, and higher mortality when compared to patients with OSAS alone.

Carson's case illustrates the value in treating both OSAS and sustained nocturnal desaturation associated with COPD. In terms of OSA, CPAP therapy

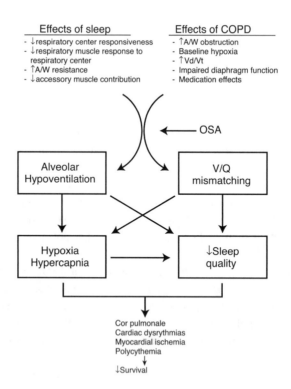

Figure 22.2 Causes of nocturnal oxygen desaturation in patients with COPD and OSA. Reproduced with permission from Krachman S, et al. *Proc Am Thorac Soc.* 2008;5:536–542.

was indicated based on his clinical symptoms and disease severity. The treatment for nocturnal oxygen desaturation is more complex. The use of CPAP itself may improve oxygen saturation during sleep by eliminating respiratory events and increasing the mean airway pressure. However, given the severity of desaturation, this was unlikely to be adequate for Carson, who required optimization of COPD management and supplemental oxygen therapy. Previous studies have shown improved survival with long-term oxygen therapy in hypoxemic COPD patients. However, when it comes to the effects of nocturnal oxygen supplementation on pulmonary hemodynamics and survival, findings are conflicting. This is especially true for patients with isolated nocturnal desaturation. The Global Initiative for Obstructive Lung Disease (GOLD) guidelines recommend the use of nocturnal oxygen therapy in patients with oxygen saturation below 88%, and current practice is to provide supplemental oxygen to hypoxemic patients, especially those with concomitant cor pulmonale or polycythemia. Anticholinergics have been shown to improve nocturnal oxygenation and sleep quality in COPD, and theophylline may improve gas exchange, but they also may reduce sleep quality. Medications such as beta blockers, which may worsen lower airway obstruction, and sedatives such as hypnotics and alcohol, which may decrease respiratory drive with resultant hypercapnic respiratory failure, should be avoided in patients with advanced lung disease.

Bibliography

Ezzie ME, Parsons JP, Mastronarde JG. Sleep and obstructive lung diseases. *Sleep Med Clin.* 2008;3:505–515.

Krachman S, Minai OA, Scharf SM. Sleep abnormalities and treatment in emphysema. *Proc Am Thorac Soc.* 2008;5:536–542.

Sander MH, Newman AB, Haggerty CL, et al. Sleep and sleep-disordered breathing in adults with predominantly mild obstructive airway disease. *Am J Respir Crit Care Med.* 2003;167:7–14.

23

A Teen with Sleep Apnea sans Acid Maltase:
A Tale with a Twist

NATTAPONG JAIMCHARIYATAM, MD, MSc
LOUTFI ABOUSSOUAN, MD
JYOTI KRISHNA, MD

Case History

Ariel was a 17-year-old African-American young woman who was referred for a comprehensive sleep and pulmonary evaluation. She had had muscle weakness due to Pompe disease diagnosed at age 12, as well as restrictive lung disease related to scoliosis. She presented with complaints of snoring and witnessed apneas and had been diagnosed with moderate obstructive sleep apnea syndrome (OSAS) associated with severe oxygen desaturation and hypercapnia 3 years earlier. At that time, a polysomnogram (PSG) showed an apnea-hypopnea index (AHI) of 18.1, minimum oxygen saturation of 79%, and 75% of sleep time was spent with an end-tidal CO_2 (EtCO$_2$) above 45 mmHg. She underwent a bi-level positive airway pressure (bi-level PAP) titration up to 16/12 H_2O, which failed to control apneas, hypopneas, or desaturation. She was nevertheless maintained on a pressure setting of 16/12 cmH$_2$O with a back up rate of 12, and presented to the Cleveland Clinic Sleep Disorders Center for a second opinion.

Her customary bedtime was between 10 and 11 p.m. She awoke around 5 a.m. on weekdays but slept until 11 a.m. on weekends. She occasionally reported morning headache. She was described to be sleepy at times during the day. Daytime naps were taken 2 times a week on weekdays and she always napped 1 time per weekend day for 2 hours, from 3 to 5 p.m.

She had undergone scoliosis surgery due to restrictive lung disease 2 years ago, but there was no history of adenoidectomy or tonsillectomy in the past.

Physical Examination

The patient was in a wheelchair. She was cachectic but alert and pleasant. Her body mass index (BMI) was $10 \, kg/m^2$. Her neck circumference was 25 cm, BP 123/73 mmHg, pulse rate 98/minute and respiratory rate was 16/minute and unlabored. She was afebrile with a resting oxygen saturation of 94%. Her pharynx revealed some crowding of soft tissues defined as Mallampati Grade III, and tonsillar size was Grade II. The chest contour was asymmetric secondary to scoliosis, and the breath sounds were clear but overall diminished on auscultation. The cardiovascular system examination was unremarkable. The abdomen was soft without any palpable organomegaly. She had generalized muscular atrophy and weakness was present symmetrically. She could lift her arms weakly against gravity and there were no cerebellar signs or sensory deficits noted.

Evaluation

Pulmonary Function Studies

The data showed forced vital capacity (FVC) of 0.40 L (12%), forced expiratory volume in first second (FEV1) of 0.37 L (12%), and FEV1/FVC ratio at 0.925. The maximal inspiratory pressure (PImax) was $14.08 \, cmH_2O$ (15%) and maximal expiratory pressure (PEmax) was recorded to be $19.18 \, cmH_2O$ (12%).

Polysomnography

A diagnostic polysomnogram (PSG) was initially planned to obtain baseline data, but Ariel was unable to initiate sleep without her respiratory assist device. Therefore, a bi-level PAP titration study was performed instead. Transcutaneous capnometry ($TcpCO_2$) was requested.

The sleep latency was prolonged at 81.5 minutes, and the REM latency was also prolonged at 398 minutes. Sleep architecture appeared fragmented, with recurrent awakenings and a decreased sleep efficiency of 68.3%. Obstructive sleep apnea (OSA) was seen and only 2 central apneas were noted in REM sleep. Nevertheless, apneas appeared nearly completely controlled at an expiratory positive airway pressure (EPAP) of $16 \, cmH_2O$. At a bi-level PAP setting of 22/16 cmH_2O, the apnea-hypopnea index was 1.1 and the arousal index was 42.9. Snoring was eliminated and the oxygen saturation was maintained above 90% at this setting.

Additionally, significant sleep related hypoventilation was present throughout the study. It was apparent that Ariel had many periods of desaturations that were not associated with OSA events. The hypnogram indicated mirror variation

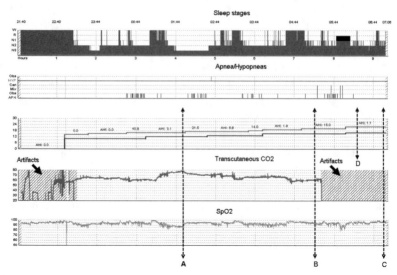

Figure 23.1 Hypnogram reveals mirror variation of oximetry and TcpCO2—i.e., as saturations decrease, there is concomitant elevation of TcpCO2. Additionally, progressive decrease in TcpCO2 is seen as IPAP-EPAP gradient is increased.

A. IPAP/EPAP 16/12, $TcpCO_2$ 78 SpO_2 86.

B. IPAP/EPAP 20/15, $TcpCO_2$ 61, SpO_2 94.

C. IPAP/EPAP 22/16, $TcpCO_2$ signal is lost, but with SpO_2 improving further to 98%, suggesting additional improvement in hypoventilation.

D. Note also control of obstructive apneas at EPAP 16 cmH$_2$O.

of oximetry and transcutaneous CO_2 tracing, suggesting that hypoxemia was more a function of hypoventilation than of typical obstructive sleep apnea alone (Figure 23.1). As the IPAP-EPAP gradient was increased, a progressive decrease in transcutaneous CO_2 was seen (Figure 23.1).

Diagnoses

Obstructive sleep apnea syndrome.
Sleep related hypoventilation/hypoxemia due to neuromuscular and chest wall disorders.

Outcome

Ariel exhibited a combination of OSA and hypoventilation in the setting of severe scoliosis and Pompe disease (acid maltase deficiency). Pulmonary function studies documented the presence of a very severe restrictive pulmonary impairment with associated respiratory muscle weakness. Despite the presence of OSA, recurrent desaturations were predominantly not associated with obstructive respiratory events, but instead reflected mirror variation with TcpCO$_2$ tracing as bi-level PAP pressure settings were manipulated. This would suggest sleep related hypoventilation due to neuromuscular and chest wall disorders as the likely diagnosis (Table 23.1). She was accordingly started on home bi-level PAP. She had trouble tolerating the initially prescribed pressures of 22/16 cmH$_2$O and was decreased to 16/10 cmH$_2$O. Her subsequent course was complicated by an ICU admission for an episode of hypercapnic respiratory failure in the setting of worsening biventricular systolic dysfunction attributed to her underlying muscular disease. Her treatment consisted of intravenous milrinone, diuresis, and nearly continuous use of bi-level PAP. She has since been successfully controlled on an oral vasodilator (enalapril), with only nocturnal use of bi-level PAP at a setting of 16/8 cmH$_2$O. She reports improved energy levels, no orthopnea or paroxysmal nocturnal dyspnea, despite persistent moderate fatigue with activities of daily living.

Discussion

The differential diagnosis of sleep related hypoxemia includes diverse cardiopulmonary disorders including obesity hypoventilation, ventilation-perfusion mismatching, neuromuscular disorders, lower airways obstruction, and pulmonary parenchymal or vascular disease, all of which could worsen in supine position and during sleep (particularly REM sleep). These conditions need to be distinguished from other sleep related breathing disorders, such as obstructive and central sleep apnea syndromes, which can result in hypoxemia during sleep and are usually associated with episodic alterations in flow.

Accordingly, hypoventilation may occur as an isolated nocturnal phenomenon or may present during the day with worsening at night. Daytime arterial blood gas analysis should be obtained to further investigate if the patient needs

Table 23.1 ICSD-2 diagnostic criteria for sleep related hypoventilation/ hypoxemia due to neuromuscular and chest wall disorders.

A. A neuromuscular or chest wall disorder is present and believed to be the primary cause of hypoxemia.
B. Polysomnography or sleeping arterial blood gas determination shows at least 1 of the following:
   i.   An SpO$_2$ during sleep of less than 90% for more than 5 minutes with a nadir of at least 85%.
   ii. More than 30% of total sleep time at a SpO$_2$ of less than 90%.
   iii. Sleeping arterial blood gas with PaCO$_2$ that is abnormally high or disproportionately increased relative to levels during wakefulness.
C. The disorder is not better explained by another current sleep disorder, another medical or neurological disorder, medication use, or substance use disorder.

supportive ventilation during wakefulness. In addition, these patients are at risk for developing pulmonary hypertension and cor pulmonale. Regular cardio-pulmonary evaluation and prompt treatment should be considered.

Treatment includes management of the underlying disease and respiratory support. Night time continuous positive airway pressure (CPAP), especially if there is a significant OSA component, or bi-level PAP are initial options for most patients. Daytime bi-level PAP should also be considered if daytime hypercapnia does not resolve despite adequate use of night time CPAP or bi-level PAP. In the case of per-sistent hypoxemia, oxygen supplementation may be required in addition to PAP.

In Ariel's case, there was additional OSA. This has been noted in 3 out of 13 patients with Pompe disease in one study. Macroglossia and tongue weakness due to fatty metamorphosis had been suggested as possible causes. Whether there is a true association between Pompe disease and OSA is not established, but this combination of OSA and sleep related hypoventilation due to neuromuscular and chest wall disorders nevertheless posed a therapeutic challenge in this particular patient. Note that the titration strategy consisted of increasing the EPAP pressure to a level sufficient to control obstructive apneas (in this case $16\,cmH_2O$), with additional increase in the IPAP-EPAP gradient for control of hypoventilation. A back-up rate on the bi-level PAP device is often prescribed for individuals with neuromuscular disease, and it is set close to the patient's spontaneous breathing rate. The back-up rate is usually prescribed to ensure controlled breathing, par-ticularly if there is concern that neuromuscular weakness will limit triggering of the bi-level PAP device by spontaneous breaths. This was not deemed necessary in Ariel's case. The ICSD-2 encourages the coding of dual diagnoses when criteria for both sleep apnea as well as hypoxemia-hypoventilation conditions are met. This case underscores the importance of capnographic assessment in manage-ment of complex cases with sleep related breathing disorders. Specifically, end-tidal measurements are generally not accurate during PAP titration, and a good trancutaneous signal can be very useful indeed in the appropriate case. Finally, the management plan included advice on adequate sleep time. This was easier for her once appropriate nocturnal respiratory control was achieved.

Bibliography

Bye PT, Ellis ER, Issa FG, Donnelly PM, Sullivan CE. Respiratory failure and sleep in neuromuscular disease. *Thorax.* 1990;45:241–247.

Hill NS, Eveloff SE, Carlisle CC, Goff SG. Efficacy of nocturnal nasal ventilation in patients with restrictive thoracic disease. *Am Rev Respir Dis.* 1992;145:365–371.

Margolis ML, Howlett P, Goldberg R, Eftychiadis A, Levine S. Obstructive sleep apnea syndrome in acid maltase deficiency. *Chest.* 1994;105:947–949.

Mellies U, Ragette R, Schwake C, Baethmann M, Voit T, Teschler H. Sleep-disordered breathing and respiratory failure in acid maltase deficiency. *Neurology.* 2001;57:1290–1295.

24

It's No Joking Matter

CATHERINE GRIFFIN, MD
SILVIA NEME-MERCANTE, MD
NANCY FOLDVARY-SCHAEFER, DO

Case History

Nora was a 36-year-old woman who presented to the sleep clinic complaining of excessive daytime sleepiness (EDS). Her sleepiness began in high school, where she would fall asleep in virtually every class without intent. Her teachers described her as lazy, and her mother was once reprimanded for not making sure she had gotten enough sleep. While she had never had an accident behind the wheel, she admitted to numerous near-misses over the years when she dozed while driving, despite no less than 24 oz of coffee consumption daily. Nora worked for many years as a waitress in a coffee shop. While her co-workers routinely covered for her, often nudging her awake as she leaned against the wall in the kitchen waiting for her orders, in recent months her boss had become irritated by her constant sleepiness, mood swings, and trouble focusing. One month prior to presentation, her work hours were cut due to productivity concerns, placing her health benefits at risk.

On workdays, Nora typically went to bed at 7 p.m. and woke up at 5 a.m. On days off, she could easily sleep until 9 a.m. She rarely made it out with her friends in the evening and was usually absent at family events, choosing to "catch some zzzs" instead. She took daily naps lasting for 1 to 2 hours after work and often spent lunch breaks catnapping in her car. Naps refreshed her for no more than a few hours. She scored 21 on the Epworth Sleepiness Scale (ESS), supporting her complaint of severe EDS.

At 20 years of age, Nora began to experience strange episodes when she laughed or became intensely angry. For a few seconds to minutes, her eyes would close and her speech slurred while her legs felt wobbly, "like jello." These episodes were embarrassing and scary. Once, in a hot tub with friends, she slipped under the water with a chocolate martini in her hand after hearing a funny joke. For several seconds, she sat under water wondering how long it would take for someone to figure out she needed help. Eventually, she was pulled to safety, requiring support for a couple of minutes before she regained her strength.

A few times per month, Nora also experienced episodes of paralysis in the morning after awakening. These were much more disturbing than her laughing spells, as she felt she could not breathe or scream for help, though she tried. A few times per week, before falling asleep she would think she saw a strange person in her room or heard someone calling her, when no one was there. Nora was a vivid dreamer and awoke once or twice a week in a panic, dreaming that someone or something was coming after her. Once she woke up swearing at her sister, with whom she was fighting in her dream. Her sleep history was otherwise unremarkable for witnessed apneas, symptoms of restless legs syndrome, and sleepwalking, though she was told by family that she snored on occasion.

Nora's medical history was notable for hypertension, for which she took diltiazem and hydrochlorothiazide. There was no history of central nervous system infection or significant head injury predating her sleep problems. She lived with her mother and had 6 healthy siblings. She avoided alcohol, tobacco, and recreational drugs. There was no family history of sleep disorders. Her father had died 2 years prior of lung cancer.

Physical Examination

On examination, Nora stood 157.5 cm tall and weighed 67.1 kg with a body mass index (BMI) of 27.2 kg/m². Her neck circumference was 32 cm. She had a blood pressure of 142/86 mmHg, a heart rate of 88 bpm, and a respiratory rate of 14 bpm. She appeared sleepy and yawned frequently. Her upper airway examination was normal with Grade I tonsils and a Friedman tongue position Grade I. The lungs were clear to auscultation. The cardiac examination revealed a normal S1 and S2 without murmur. There was mild edema in the ankles. Her neurological examination was normal.

Evaluation

A polysomnogram (PSG) followed by a multiple sleep latency test (MSLT) was recommended to screen for narcolepsy. Nora was advised to avoid drugs that might influence her sleep or wakefulness for 2 weeks prior to testing and to maintain a consistent sleep-wake schedule. She kept a sleep log for 1 week prior to testing for this purpose. On the overnight study, she slept for 9 hours and 7 minutes and had REM within minutes after sleep onset (Table 24.1). Infrequent hypopneas and periodic limb movements were observed. Eight REM periods were recorded, each fragmented by recurrent arousals and awakenings (Figure 24.1). Muscle tone during REM sleep was atonic. While she did snore, there was no evidence of sleep apnea or frequent periodic limb movements (PLMS). Nora's MSLT showed a mean sleep latency (MSL) of 1.2 minutes with sleep onset REM periods (SOREMPs) in 4 of the 5 nap trials (Figure 24.2).

Table 24.1 Polysomnogram summary

Sleep architecture	
Total recording time (min)	600
Total sleep time (min)	547
Wake time after sleep onset (min)	49
Sleep latency (min)	2.5
REM latency (min)	6
Awakenings	42
Arousals	136
Arousal index	14.9
Stage shifts	175
Sleep stage percentages	
Stage N1	6.8
Stage N2	36.0
Stage N3	31.9
REM	25.3
Respiratory data	
Apneas	0
Hypopneas	16
Total apnea-hypopnea index	1.8
Apnea-hypopnea index, supine	2.3
Apnea-hypopnea index, off supine	0.8
Apnea-hypopnea index, REM	1.3
Apnea-hypopnea index, NREM	1.9
Mean oxygen saturation %	96
Minimum oxygen saturation %	89
Limb movements	
Periodic limb movements	90
PLM index	9.9
PLM associated with arousals	13
PLM-arousal index	1.4

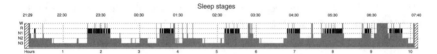

Sleep stages

Figure 24.1 Sleep architecture during the PSG showing multiple REM periods (in black) fragmented by arousals and awakenings.

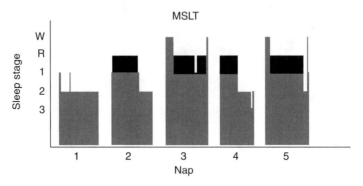

Figure 24.2 MSLT showing SOREMPs in naps 2, 3, 4, and 5. The MSL was 1.2 minutes. This MSLT meets the electrodiagnostic criteria for narcolepsy (MSL < 8 minutes and > 2 SOREMPs).

Diagnoses

Narcolepsy with cataplexy.
Primary snoring.

Outcome

Nora demonstrated the classic signs and symptoms of narcolepsy with cataplexy including EDS, cataplexy, sleep paralysis, and hypnagogic hallucinations. Her PSG and MSLT met the diagnostic criteria for this disorder (Table 24.2). She was educated on the importance of maintaining regular bedtimes and wake times and the value of short, scheduled naps. She was instructed to avoid heavy meals and all drugs that depress the central nervous system (CNS), including alcohol. She was counseled to avoid driving and potentially dangerous activities when feeling drowsy.

Methylphenidate 10 mg, 3 times a day, was initially prescribed for daytime sleepiness. However, she experienced palpitations prompting a change to modafinil 200 mg in the morning. Modafinil was titrated to 600 mg per day with only modest improvement in EDS. Consequently, sodium oxybate 4.5 g per night

Table 24.2 ICSD-2 diagnostic criteria for narcolepsy with cataplexy

A. The patient has a complaint of excessive daytime sleepiness occurring almost daily for at least 3 months.
B. A definite history of cataplexy, defined as sudden and transient episodes of loss of muscle tone triggered by emotions, is present.
C. The diagnosis of narcolepsy with cataplexy should, whenever possible, be confirmed by PSG followed by an MSLT; the mean sleep latency on MSLT is less than or equal to 8 minutes and 2 or more SOREMPs are observed following sufficient nocturnal sleep (minimum 6 hours) during the night prior to the test. Alternatively, hypocretin-1 levels in the CSF are less than or equal to 110 pg/mL or one-third of mean normal control values.
D. The hypersomnia is not better explained by another sleep disorder, medical or neurological disorder, mental disorder, medication use, or substance use disorder.

in 2 divided doses was added and increased by 1.5 g per night every 2 to 4 weeks to a maximum dose of 9 g per night to treat EDS and cataplexy. She responded remarkably to this regimen, with significant improvement in EDS and reduction in the frequency of cataplexy attacks (Figure 24.3). Control of her narcolepsy allowed her to return to working full time in the coffee shop. Her mood improved, and she was able to join her family and friends at social outings again—provided the jokes stayed at home.

Discussion

Narcolepsy is a CNS disorder characterized by severe hypersomnia despite adequate opportunity to sleep. Narcolepsy with cataplexy affects 0.02%–0.18% of the U.S. and Western European populations. Both sexes are affected, with a slight prevalence of males. Narcolepsy can present at any age, but it is infrequently diagnosed in children under 5. Precipitating factors include head trauma, abrupt changes in sleep-wake patterns, sustained sleep deprivation, and viral illnesses. The disorder is associated with the human leukocyte antigen (HLA) subtypes DR2/DRB1*1501 and DQB1*0602, suggesting an autoimmune pathophysiology. Narcolepsy with cataplexy is associated with a deficiency of hypothalamic neurons containing the neuropeptide hypocretin. Hypocretin release is maximal during periods of normal wakefulness and is believed to increase muscle tone through activation of a motor faciliatory system in the locus coeruleus and the raphe nuclei of the brain. More than 90% of patients with narcolepsy with cataplexy have low levels of hypocretin-1 (≤ 110 pg/mL) in cerebral spinal fluid (CSF). Narcolepsy with cataplexy is often

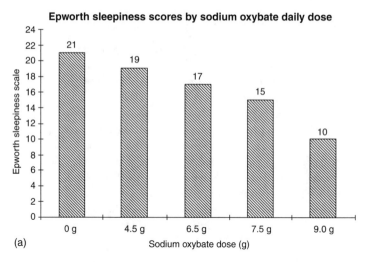

(a)

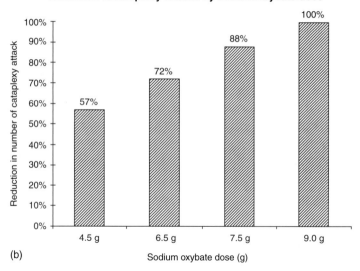

(b)

Figure 24.3 Nora's response to treatment. (a) The nightly administration of sodium oxybate was associated with dose-related reduction in Epworth Sleepiness Scale scores over a 12 week period. (b) The nightly administration of sodium oxybate was associated with dose-related reductions in the number of cataplexy attacks over a 12 week period.

associated with increased BMI, likely due to dysfunction of nearby metabolic control centers.

The hallmark of narcolepsy with cataplexy is severe, unremitting EDS, which is usually the presenting symptom. Excessive daytime sleepiness is followed by the appearance of cataplexy and other dissociated REM sleep events that are due to an unusual tendency to transition rapidly from wakefulness into REM sleep.

Cataplexy is characterized by sudden loss of muscle tone triggered by strong emotions such as laughter, surprise, embarrassment, anger, or fear. The muscle atonia is usually bilateral and can range from mild (knees buckling, jaw dropping) to complete collapse (fall and paralysis) associated with transient loss of deep tendon reflexes. Most attacks are brief in duration, lasting from a few seconds to 1 or 2 minutes, and consciousness remains intact (see video 1). The frequency of cataplexy varies from rare lifetime attacks in some cases to countless daily attacks in others.

Associated features of narcolepsy with cataplexy include sleep paralysis, hypnagogic/hypnopompic hallucinations, and nocturnal sleep disruption. Sleep paralysis refers to episodes of partial or total paralysis during the transition between sleep and wakefulness that occur in 40%–80% of patients with narcolepsy with cataplexy. Episodes are often terrifying and associated with a feeling of suffocation. Hypnagogic/hypnopompic hallucinations are experienced by a similar number of patients. These phenomena may be visual, tactile, auditory, or multisensory and occur as the patient is falling asleep or waking up. Common examples include a visual perception of a strange person in the room or a visual and/or tactile perception of a bug crawling on or near the patient. Nocturnal sleep disruption with frequent, unexplained awakenings occurs in approximately 50% of narcoleptics and may aggravate other symptoms. Narcolepsy can have a profound impact on quality of life. Affected individuals experience academic and occupational underachievement, impaired socialization, and a higher incidence of motor vehicle accidents.

The diagnosis of narcolepsy with cataplexy can be made clinically, but confirmation by overnight PSG followed by an MSLT is recommended when possible. The PSG in patients with narcolepsy typically reveals multiple REM periods fragmented by recurrent arousals or awakenings, a sleep latency of less than 10 minutes, and sometimes an early appearance of REM sleep. Periodic limb movements, sleep apnea, and features of REM sleep behavior disorder are commonly observed.

The MSLT is the gold standard test for the evaluation of narcolepsy as it provides an objective measure of the propensity to fall asleep. A PSG is performed the night before the MSLT to confirm the quantity and quality of sleep and rule out other primary sleep disorders as potential causes of EDS. Stimulants, sedative hypnotics, and other medications that suppress REM sleep and significantly alter sleep architecture should be withdrawn at least 2 weeks prior to testing. Alcohol, caffeine, and tobacco should be avoided for the entire duration of the test, but, most important, for 30 minutes before each trial. Two or more SOREMPs with a MSL of less than 8 minutes are highly suggestive of narcolepsy. However, as many as 25% of patients with narcolepsy have less than 2 SOREMPs on the MSLT and a MSL of less than 8 minutes can be found in up to 30% of normal subjects. Thus, clinical correlation is vital in making the diagnosis.

The differential diagnosis in Nora's case includes the disorders characterized by severe EDS. Narcolepsy with cataplexy is differentiated from narcolepsy without cataplexy by the presence of definite cataplexy. Patients with an MSLT that shows multiple SOREMPs, but no clinical history of cataplexy, should be identified as narcolepsy without cataplexy. Concurrent sleep disorders may exist with narcolepsy with cataplexy, such as obstructive sleep apnea (OSA) and periodic limb movement disorder, and these may contribute to daytime sleepiness. Primary differential diagnoses to consider are idiopathic hypersomnia, recurrent hypersomnia, delayed sleep phase syndrome, behaviorally induced insufficient sleep syndrome, and substance abuse.

In contrast to narcolepsy with cataplexy, idiopathic hypersomnia patients have fewer than two SOREMPs on the MSLT, generally do not feel refreshed after napping, and do not experience cataplexy, sleep paralysis, or sleep related hallucinations. Kleine-Levin Syndrome is a recurrent hypersomnia characterized by episodes of severe sleepiness associated with cognitive and behavioral instability, including excessive food consumption and hypersexual behavior, separated by weeks to months of normal sleep and behavior. In delayed sleep phase disorder (DSPD), there is a consistent pattern of falling asleep and waking up later than preferred. These patients usually have had unsuccessful attempts at regulating sleep-wake times. A key differentiating feature from narcolepsy is that sleep is normal in DSPD and EDS is not present when the affected individual is permitted to maintain his or her own schedule. Patients with behaviorally induced insufficient sleep syndrome generally report short sleep duration and daytime consequences of sleep deprivation, including EDS and fatigue that reverses when adequate sleep is obtained. Substance abuse with alcohol, prescription medications, and recreational drugs can produce disturbed nighttime sleep and EDS. A urine toxicology screen may be performed on the morning of the MSLT in narcolepsy suspects to help exclude this possibility.

Cataplexy is practically pathognomonic for narcolepsy and should be distinguished from cataplexy-like episodes that may be the manifestation of epilepsy, hypotension, cerebral ischemia, psychiatric disorders, or neuromuscular disorders. Typical findings suggestive of cataplexy include an emotional trigger, loss of deep tendon reflexes, abrupt onset, bilateral distribution of weakness, and duration less than 30 seconds. It is essential to consider other causes if there is loss or alteration of consciousness, absence of emotional triggers, unilateral distribution of weakness, pain, or adventitious motor activity.

Optimal management of patients with narcolepsy with cataplexy involves both pharmacologic and nonpharmacologic measures. Patients with narcolepsy should avoid CNS depressants—including alcohol, drugs, and sedating over-the-counter agents—and incorporate healthy lifestyle practices. Scheduled naps and strategic caffeine use can lessen daytime sleepiness. Of paramount importance is the maintenance of a regular sleep-wake schedule and avoidance of sleep deprivation.

Table 24.3 Pharmacotherapy for narcolepsy

Medication	Usual daily dosage	Side effects
Modafinil (Provigil)	100 mg/d to 400 mg/d	Headache, nausea and
Armodafinil (Nuvigil)	150 mg/d to 250 mg/d	nervousness
Methylphenidate (Concerta, Metadate CD, Metadate ER, Methylin, Methylin ER, Ritalin, Ritalin LA, Ritalin SR, Dexmethylphenidate, Focalin, Focalin XR)	10 mg/d to 60 mg/d	Irritability, gastrointestinal distress, anorexia, headache, nervousness, palpitations, high blood pressure, tics, disturbed nighttime sleep
Dextroamphetamine (Obetrol, Biphetamine, Adderall, Adderall XR, Dexedrine, Dexedrine SR, Dextrostat)	5 mg/d to 60 mg/d	Anorexia, increased/ distorted sensations, restlessness, headaches, palpitations, diarrhea, blurred vision, tics,
Methamphetamine (Desoxyn)	5 mg/d to 15 mg/d	insomnia and arrhythmias
Sodium oxybate (Xyrem)	4.5 g/d to 9 g/d	Nausea, fluid retention, dizziness, urinary incontinence, respiratory depression

() Trade names

Wake-promoting medications and anti-cataplexy agents are the primary treatments for patients with narcolepsy with cataplexy (Tables 24.3, 24.4). The ideal wakefulness-promoting agent produces a maximally alert state without side effects or negative impact on one's ability to sleep when desired. Because tolerance can develop over time with stimulant medications, they should be administered in low doses and titrated slowly to obtain the desired effect. Careful monitoring for adverse events, including hypertension and cardiac arrhythmias, is required. Patients should be advised to take drug holidays by avoiding use periodically so as to reduce the development of tolerance.

Treatments for Excessive Daytime Sleepiness

Modafinil Modafinil is approved for the treatment of EDS associated with narcolepsy, OSA, and shift-work sleep disorder. Modafinil acts selectively in the hypothalamus, which regulates sleep and wakefulness. As a result, side effects tend to be mild and short-lived, typically limited to headache, nausea, and nervousness. Women taking oral contraceptives should be advised that modafinil can reduce hormone concentrations, thereby leading to unexpected pregnancy.

Table 24.4 Pharmacotherapy for cataplexy

Medication	Usual daily dosage	Side effects
Sodium oxybate (Xyrem)	4.5 g/d to 9 g/d administered in two nightly doses	Nausea, fluid retention, dizziness, urinary incontinence, respiratory depression
Tricyclic antidepressants		
Imiprame (Tofranil, Janimine)	25 mg/d to 200 mg/d	Dry mouth, blurred vision, urinary retention, constipation,
Clomipramine (Anafranil)	10 mg/d to 200 mg/d	sexual dysfunction, orthostatic
Desipramine (Norpramin, Pertofran)	25 mg/d to 200 mg/d	hypotension
Protriptyline (Vivactil)	5 mg/d to 30 mg/d	
Selective serotonin reuptake inhibitors		
Fluoxetine (Prozac)	20 mg/d to 80 mg/d	Insomnia, sexual dysfunction, anxiety, dizziness, dry mouth
Venlafaxine (Effexor XR)	75 mg/d to 225 mg/d	Nausea, headache, dry mouth, dizziness, insomnia, nervousness

() Trade names

Although modafinil is less potent than traditional stimulants, its low abuse potential and favorable side effect profile have made it a first-line treatment for newly diagnosed narcolepsy patients.

Armodafinil   Approved by the U.S. Food and Drug Administration (FDA) in 2007, armodafinil (R-modafinil) is the longer-lasting isomer of the racemic compound modafinil having a half-life of 10 to 15 hours. The indications are the same as modafinil. Clinical trials demonstrated an enhanced efficacy for wake promotion (wake sustained for a longer time period using doses lower than those of modafinil). The safety profile is similar, and the drug is generally well tolerated. Patients with EDS may prefer the longer duration of action of armodafinil.

Methylphenidate   In use since the 1950s, methylphenidate is approved for the treatment of attention deficit disorder and narcolepsy. Methylphenidate is effective in increasing alertness and is better tolerated than amphetamine agents. Because methylphenidate also increases activity in other parts of the nervous system, untoward side effects are common. These include irritability, gastrointestinal problems, headache, nervousness, palpitations, high blood pressure, and disturbed nighttime sleep.

Amphetamines   Amphetamine and related drugs, such as dextroamphetamine and methamphetamine, increase levels of dopamine, norepinephrine, and serotonin, which are neurotransmitters that sustain alertness and concentration. These drugs also are used illegally as recreational drugs and performance enhancers. Dextroamphetamines have an increased affinity for dopamine receptors in the brain; therefore, they are more effective than amphetamine. The methylated form, known as methamphetamine, has increased CNS penetration, rendering it the most potent in this class. These agents are associated with a variety of side effects, including loss of appetite, increased/distorted sensations, restlessness, headache, palpitations, diarrhea, blurred vision, uncontrollable movements or shaking, insomnia, and arrhythmias. Seizures and psychosis rarely are encountered. With prolonged use and/or high doses, tolerance can develop, therefore increasing the amount of the drug that is needed to maintain wakefulness.

Sodium oxybate   In 2002, the FDA approved sodium oxybate (Xyrem), the first drug specifically approved to treat cataplexy as well as the EDS associated with narcolepsy. This drug is a sodium salt of gamma hydroxy butyrate (GHB). Sodium oxybate also improves the fragmented sleep of narcoleptics. In a double-blind, placebo–controlled study of 228 adults with narcolepsy with cataplexy, treatment with 9 gm of sodium oxybate nightly produced a significant increase in sleep latency on the Maintenance of Wakefulness Test. Dose-related decreases in ESS scores were observed, with median ESS scores decreasing from 19 to 15 with 6 gm and 19 to 12 with 9 gm nightly. Side effects of sodium oxybate are dose dependent. Careful consideration of the sodium load in patients with heart failure, hypertension, or compromised renal function should be considered (a nightly dose of 6 gm contains 1092 mg of sodium, and 9 gm contains 1638 mg of sodium). Deep sedation usually occurs, and therefore household safety needs to be discussed. Other adverse effects include nausea, dizziness, urinary incontinence, and sleepwalking. The consequences of overdose include respiratory depression and coma. The history of GHB is recreational – it was abused as a date-rape drug, which explains why sodium oxybate is tightly controlled and available in the U.S. only through a single central pharmacy. Patients with OSA should not be treated with sodium oxybate unless the sleep apnea is treated and compliance with therapy confirmed.

Treatments for Cataplexy

During the 1970s and 1980s, cataplexy was treated primarily with tricyclic antidepressants (TCAs), such as protriptyline, clomipramine, and imipramine. These drugs remain effective in ameliorating cataplexy, sleep paralysis, and hypnagogic hallucinations, but they produce untoward effects such as dry mouth, blurred vision, and orthostatic hypotension. The selective serotonin reuptake inhibitors (SSRIs), such as fluoxetine, proved to be as effective as TCAs with fewer side effects. Venlafaxine, a medication that increases both serotonin and norepinephrine levels in the brain, appears to be particularly effective in the treatment of cataplexy.

Sodium oxybate is the only drug approved for the treatment of cataplexy. In clinical trials, the frequency of cataplexy significantly decreased over placebo by a median of 44%, 52%, and 62% in patients treated with 4.5 gm, 6 gm, and 9 gm of sodium oxybate, respectively.

In 2000, the discovery of a deficiency in hypocretin/orexin secreting neurons in narcolepsy was a major breakthrough in the field of sleep medicine. More recently, histamine neurons, which are downstream of orexin neurons, were found to be important in controlling arousal, and CSF histamine concentration was reported to be low in subjects with narcolepsy and other hypersomnias of central origin. Consequently, agonists for orexin receptors and histamine H3 antagonists currently are being explored as future therapies for patients with narcolepsy and other forms of hypersomnia.

Bibliography

Black J, Guilleminault C. Medications for the treatment of narcolepsy. *Expert Opin Emerg Drugs*. 2001;6(2):239–247.

Black J, Houghton WC. Sodium oxybate improves excessive daytime sleepiness in narcolepsy. *SLEEP*. 2006;29(7):939–946.

Fujiki N, Ripley B, Yoshida Y, et al. Effects of IV and ICV hypocretin-1 (orexin A) in hypocretin receptor-2 gene mutated narcoleptic dogs and IV hypocretin-1 replacement therapy in a hypocretin ligand deficient narcoleptic dog. *SLEEP*. 2003;6:953–959.

Houghton, WC, Scammell TE, Thorpy M. Pharmacotherapy for cataplexy. *Sleep Med Rev*. 2004;8(5):355–366.

25

When Dormant Issues Awaken, Waking Patients Sleep!

ROXANNE VALENTINO, MD
FARID TALIH, MD

Case History

Jeremy was a 16-year-old boy who presented for evaluation of daytime sleepiness. The sleepiness had been progressive over about 2 years. He was falling asleep in his high school classes and napping 1 or 2 hours per day. His grades had fallen from As and Bs to mostly Cs in 1 academic year.

Jeremy's usual bedtime was 10 p.m. on weekdays and midnight on weekends. His usual wake time was 6:30 a.m. on weekdays and 8 a.m. on weekends. Jeremy denied difficulty falling asleep. In fact, his usual sleep latency was only 1 to 2 minutes. Some nights, he would wake up once to urinate; other nights he would not wake at all until his alarm sounded. He did not feel refreshed in the mornings. His parents described him as a "quiet sleeper" without snoring or abnormal behaviors in sleep. He denied sleep related hallucinations or sleep paralysis. He had experienced buckling of the knees during intense laughter on some occasions, but he had not had any falls. He scored 19/24 on the Epworth Sleepiness Scale (ESS).

Jeremy's medical history was significant for craniopharyngioma diagnosed when he was 11 years old. At that time, the MRI scan showed a well-circumscribed, round mass in the suprasellar region measuring 17x17x14 mm (Figure 25.1). The tumor was excised via standard pterional approach, and his perioperative course was uncomplicated. The postperative MRI scan showed complete resection of the mass with minimal contrast enhancement in the suprasellar cistern, thought to be postsurgical in nature (Figure 25.2). After the

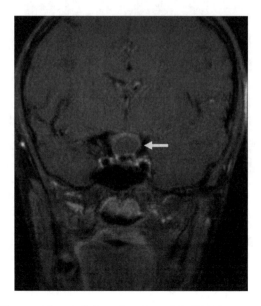

Figure 25.1 MRI scan with gadolinium showing a 17x17x14mm craniopharyngioma. There was a well-circumscribed, round mass in the suprasellar region which demonstrated increased T2 and decreased T1 signal, compatible with fluid content. There was a small, irregular area of decreased signal in the inferior aspect of the mass, compatible with calcification. Following contrast administration, there was rim-like enhancement. The optic chiasm was draped over the mass, which extended into the sella and slightly compressed the pituitary gland.

surgery, Jeremy was treated with hormonal replacement therapy for panhypopituitarism. His medications at the time of initial sleep evaluation included DDAVP, hydrocortisone, dexamethasone, testosterone, growth hormone, and levothyroxine. Subsequent MRI scans had been negative for tumor recurrence. Jeremy denied use of tobacco, alcohol, or illicit drugs.

Physical Examination

Jeremy's examination revealed a healthy-appearing teen with a normal body mass index of 24 kg/m². Head examination was significant for a healed scar in the right frontotemporal area. Neck circumference was 14.0 inches. His oropharyngeal examination showed Grade II tonsils and normal tongue position. There was no retroagnathia. Neurologic examination revealed normal cranial nerve functions, including normal visual fields. Strength, coordination, and deep tendon reflexes were normal in all extremities. His gait was narrow-based and steady.

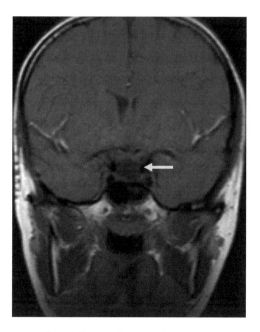

Figure 25.2 MRI scan with gadolinium showing the suprasellar region after resection of craniopharyngioma. The scan showed postoperative changes in the right frontotemporal regions, but the previously seen suprasellar mass was no longer present. There was minimal enhancement seen in the right aspect of the suprasellar cistern, which was thought to be post surgical in nature.

Evaluation

Polysomnography (PSG) followed by a multiple sleep latency test (MSLT) was performed to evaluate severe hypersomnia including a suspicion for narcolepsy. The PSG showed mild obstructive sleep apnea (OSA) with an overall apnea-hypopnea index (AHI) of 5.2. Most of the respiratory events occurred during REM sleep, producing a REM AHI of 10. Sleep efficiency was 93% and total sleep time was approximately 8 hours. The MSLT revealed a mean sleep latency of 2.9 minutes and a sleep-onset REM period (SOREMP) in each nap.

Diagnoses

Narcolepsy due to medical condition (craniopharyngioma, status post resection).
Mild obstructive sleep apnea.
Panhypopituitarism.

Outcome

Jeremy was diagnosed with narcolepsy due to craniopharyngioma resection. His description of muscle weakness triggered by emotion was consistent with cataplexy, and sleep testing met the electrodiagnostic criteria for narcolepsy (Table 25.1). Jeremy was initially treated with methylphenidate 10 mg per day, and he reported some improvement in daytime sleepiness. He was titrated up to 40 mg per day with very good control of his daytime sleepiness. His Epworth Sleepiness Scale improved to 11/24. He did report some appetite suppression, but he did not lose weight, and he denied other side effects. He scheduled one 15- to 20-minute nap into his school day. He was also advised to maintain good sleep hygiene and a regular sleep schedule. He was cautioned to avoid becoming overweight, since this could worsen his degree of sleep apnea. We elected not to treat him with CPAP, but this would certainly remain a consideration for the future. The patient continued to be followed by an endocrinologist with satisfactory monitoring of hormonal replacement therapy.

Discussion

Narcolepsy due to a medical condition is sometimes referred to as "secondary narcolepsy." It can occur with or without cataplexy. Other features of narcolepsy, such as fragmented sleep, sleep related hallucinations, and sleep paralysis may or may not occur. The prevalence of secondary narcolepsy is not known.

Table 25.1 ICSD-2 diagnostic criteria for narcolepsy due to a medical condition

A. The patient has a complaint of excessive daytime sleepiness occurring almost daily for at least 3 months.

B. One of the following is observed:
   i. A definite history of cataplexy, defined as sudden and transient episodes of loss of muscle tone triggered by emotions, is present.
   ii. If cataplexy is not present or is very atypical, polysomnographic monitoring performed over the patient's habitual sleep period followed by an MSLT must demonstrate a mean sleep latency on the MSLT of less than 8 minutes with 2 or more SOREMPs despite sufficient nocturnal sleep prior to the test (minimum 6 hours).
   iii. Hypocretin-1 level in the CSF are less than 110 pg/mL (or 30% of normal control values) provided the patient is not comatose.

C. A significant underlying medical or neurological disorder accounts for the daytime sleepiness.

D. Hypersomnia is not better explained by another sleep disorder, mental disorder, medication use, or substance use disorder.

There are a number of medical conditions that can cause hypersomnia, but not all of them cause a narcolepsy phenotype. It is important from a diagnostic standpoint to separate hypersomnia due to a medical condition from narcolepsy due to a medical condition by the criteria above. The second diagnostic "division" is to distinguish the subtype based upon presence or absence of cataplexy.

As a rule, secondary narcolepsy with cataplexy can be caused by structural lesions in the posterolateral hypothalamus. Some examples of conditions that can cause secondary narcolepsy with cataplexy are: (1) tumors, (2) sarcoid, (3) multiple sclerosis plaques, (4) stroke, (5) anti-Ma2 brainstem encephalitis, (6) Nieman-Pick type C, and (7) Coffin-Lowry disease.

Other conditions that can cause secondary narcolepsy, but are usually not associated with cataplexy, include: (1) myotonic dystrophy, (2) Prader-Willi syndrome, (3) head trauma, (4) Parkinson's disease, and (5) multiple system atrophy (MSA).

In this case, the differential diagnosis included sleepiness due to OSA. Ideally, sleep apnea should be adequately treated prior to diagnosing narcolepsy. We thought it was unlikely that the mild degree of sleep-disordered breathing could account for the profound symptoms and MSLT findings in this case. Another possibility was that the patient had narcolepsy with cataplexy that was unrelated to the history of craniophayngioma. This is a reasonable consideration, since narcolepsy often presents during the teen years and the tumor excision was about 5 years prior to the reported onset of sleepiness. HLA typing for narcolepsy (DQB1-0602 subtype) would have been interesting in the sense that a negative test would support our suspicion that the narcolepsy was due to his medical condition rather than representing a separate and unrelated condition. For Caucasians with "primary" narcolepsy with cataplexy, the HLA marker sensitivity is 85%–100%, so a negative test still does not rule out the condition. In this case, the patient's parents did not consent to the test, so it was not performed.

Craniopharyngiomas are epithelial tumors derived from Rathke's cleft, which is the embryonic precursor to the adenohypophysis. Tumors can occur anywhere along the course of the craniopharyngeal duct which extends from the pharynx to the sella turcica and third ventricle. Males and females have a similar incidence of craniopharyngioma. There is a bimodal age distribution, with the first peak at age 5 to 10 years and the second peak at 40 to 60 years. In pediatrics, craniopharyngiomas are the most common intracranial tumor of nonglial origin and account for 54% of all sellar and prechiasmatic tumors. Craniopharyngiomas are generally benign, slow-growing tumors and present with headaches, visual field disturbances, and/or endocrine derangements. Occasionally they can metastasize.

After resection of craniopharyngioma, hypothalamic damage leading to loss of hypocretin secreting cells can cause a narcolepsy phenotype. It is important to recognize, however, that there are other possible causes of hypersomnia in these cases. The other considerations include inadequate supplementation of hormones (i.e., thyroid or adrenal) and sleep related breathing disorder. In fact, any lesion affecting the hypothalamus can cause obesity related to hormonal imbalance; therefore, sleep apnea should be considered as an important cause for hypersomnolence. In pediatric populations following craniopharyngioma resection, the incidence of obesity is about 50%. One study showed that in 10 obese children with previous craniopharyngioma resection, only 2 had OSA, whereas 4 had a narcolepsy phenotype.

Bibliography

Kryger MH, Roth T, Dement WC. *Principles and Practice of Sleep Medicine.* 4th ed. Philadelphia, PA: Elsevier Saunders; 2005.

Marcus CL, Trescher WH, Halbower AC, Lutz J. Secondary narcolepsy in children with brain tumors. *SLEEP.* 2002;25(4):435–439.

Muller HL, Muller-Stover S, Gebhardt U, et al. Secondary narcolepsy may be a causative factor of increased daytime sleepiness in obese childhood craniopharyngioma patients. *Journal of Pediatric Endocrinology and Metabolism.* 2006;19 Suppl1:423–429.

Snow A, Gozal E, Malhotra A, et al. Severe hypersomnolence after pituitary/hypothalamic surgery in adolescents: clinical characteristics and potential mechanisms. *Pediatrics.* 2002;100(6):e74.

26

Basic Instincts: Hungry, Sleepy, and Misbehaving

CRAIG BROOKER, MD
PRAKASH KOTAGAL, MD

Case History

Chad was a 16-year-old boy who presented to the sleep center for bouts of excessive sleepiness. His first episode occurred when he was 15 years old. It was early December, and he had been feeling ill with a cough, headache, fever, and body aches during his final exams. For his viral illness he took some Benadryl and codeine, which were shortly followed by unusual behavior. The normally shy and timid Chad became hyperactive and started acting like a clown. Afterwards, he asked if he actually acted like that and when it was confirmed, he burst into tears. Over subsequent hours he became very sleepy and fearful. He began to sleep nearly all day, was difficult to arouse, and became aggressive and irritable. On Christmas Day his parents forced him out of bed to join them for a steak dinner, but he could not figure out how to use the fork and knife to eat it. A total of 10 days after the onset of the episode, Chad was back to his baseline for behavior and sleep requirements.

Three weeks later a similar episode occurred. This time, Chad awoke in the middle of the night and turned on all of the lights in the house because he was afraid, for unclear reasons, He insisted on sleeping in his parents' bed, something he had not done since he was 5. Thereafter, he was difficult to rouse, and when awakened, he became aggressive. This odd behavior persisted for 7 days and subsequently normalized just as mysteriously. Four weeks after this episode, he sensed yet another episode coming on when he was headed to church. He quickly fell asleep during the service and towards the end woke up and started blowing kisses at girls in church, something he had never done before. In the hours that followed, he grew sleepy, difficult to arouse, and aggressive. This time Chad was admitted to the hospital for observation. His behavior continued to be aggressive, inappropriate, and out of character, once calling one of the nurses "bitch" for no apparent reason. After 2 more days of sleeping excessively, he snapped out of the episode and returned back to his baseline behavior and sleeping pattern.

At his visit to the sleep center, Chad described that when he was at baseline he usually went to bed around 11:30 p.m. and got up at 6:30 a.m. on weekdays and 9 a.m. on weekends, generally feeling refreshed. He generally fell asleep within 15 minutes and rarely ever woke up at night. He occasionally snored lightly, but this was the exception, not the rule. Rarely did he nap, except after a late Friday night out with his friends. Between episodes, he denied excessive daytime sleepiness (EDS) and had an Epworth Sleepiness Scale score of 2. During episodes, however, he described a dream-like mentation with insatiable desire to sleep and almost persistent irritability. He also vaguely remembered that every time he woke up during the episode that he had a voracious appetite and increased libido.

Chad had no significant past medical history or family history of hypersomnia. He had no recent head trauma, headache, diplopia, or speech problems, nor had he ever had a seizure.

Physical Examination

Chad weighed 144 lbs (65.4 Kg) and was 6'0" (183 cm) tall, resulting in a body mass index of 19.5 kg/m². His vital signs were within normal limits and without evidence for orthostatic hypotension. He had a Grade I Friedman tongue position. The neck circumference was 13.5 inches (34.3 cm). There was no nasal congestion or retrognathia. The cranial nerves were intact and there was no papilledema. His motor exam revealed muscle power of 5/5 throughout. Sensory exam was intact to light touch, pinprick, vibration, and proprioception. The deep tendon reflexes were 2/4 throughout with down-going toes and no Hoffman's sign. His gait was normal with a negative Romberg sign.

Evaluation

MRI scan of the brain was normal. Two EEGs during the episode were significant only for diffuse slowing. No interictal epileptiform abnormalities or seizures were recorded. Blood count, metabolic panel, glucose, thyroid, and urine toxicology studies were unremarkable. Epstein-Barr virus and cytomegalovirus titers were negative and pituitary hormone panel was unremarkable.

In order to better characterize his sleep disorder a polysomnogram (PSG) was performed. The PSG was significant for early onset of REM sleep 21.5 minutes after sleep onset but was otherwise unremarkable (Table 26.1). A multiple sleep latency test (MSLT) was performed at the beginning, toward the end, and after the hypersomnia episode. During the hypersomnia episode, MSLT showed sleep-onset REM period (SOREMP) in 2 naps with a mean sleep latency of 3.2 minutes, indicating severe hypersomnolence (Figure 26.1). The second MSLT toward the end of the episode showed only one SOREMP and a mean sleep latency of 7.7 minutes (patient did not fall asleep during the fifth nap) which paralleled the clinical improvement. Finally, a third MSLT was done later during an asymptomatic period which was normal with a mean sleep latency of 15.4 minutes.

Table 26.1 Chad's polysomnogram during symptomatic episodes and asymptomatic intervals

Parameter	Episode	Interval
Total sleep time (TST), min	423	352
Sleep efficiency (%)	91.7	89
Stage N1 (%TST)	5.2	5.4
Stage N2 (%TST)	61.4	46.5
Stage N3 (%TST)	14.0	27.0
Stage REM (% TST)	19.4	21.0
Sleep latency, min	5.5	34.0
REM latency, min	21.5	47

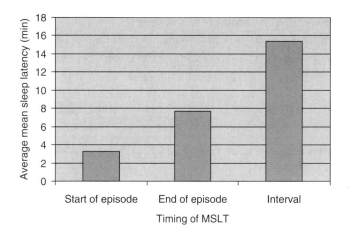

Figure 26.1 Mean sleep latency during and at the end of the symptomatic periods and during the asymptomatic interval.

Diagnosis

Recurrent hypersomnia—Kleine-Levin syndrome.

Outcome

Chad went on to have a total of 4 episodes, the last of which was very mild, before complete resolution of his symptoms. He was not treated with medications.

Discussion

Based on recurrent episodic hypersomnia with behavioral changes and cognitive abnormalities with normal behavior and sleep requirements between episodes, Chad met ICSD-2 criteria for Kleine-Levin Syndrome (Table 26.2).

The differential diagnosis of Kleine-Levin syndrome in women includes the other recurrent hypersomnia recognized by ICSD-2, namely menstrual-related hypersomnia, in which recurrent episodes of sleepiness begin around menarche and continue monthly the week before menses and resolve quickly with menses. Other diagnostic considerations include narcolepsy, idiopathic hypersomnia with (or without) long sleep time, behaviorally induced insufficient sleep syndrome, and hypersomnia due to medical condition, drug or substance.

Kleine-Levin syndrome is a rare, recurrent hypersomnia first reported by Kleine in 1925. With fewer than 200 case reports, the symptoms were poorly described until 2005, when Arnulf et al did a meta-analysis of 186 case reports from 1962 to 2004. In 2008, the same investigators reported findings of clinical data and blood samples in 108 patients diagnosed with Kleine-Levin syndrome based on worldwide networking of sleep centers. Data relied primarily on extensive survey, first to confirm the diagnosis and then to further describe it. Additionally, these patients were compared to a matched control group. Based on their data, Kleine-Levin syndrome is represented 3 times more often in

---

Table 26.2 ICSD-2 diagnostic criteria for recurrent hypersomnia

A. The patient experiences recurrent episodes of excessive sleepiness of 2 days to 4 weeks duration.
B. Episodes recur at least once a year.
C. The patient has normal alertness, cognitive functioning, and behavior between attacks.
D. The hypersomnia is not better explained by another sleep disorder, medical or neurological disorder, mental disorder, medication use, or substance use disorder.

Caucasians and 6 times more often in Ashkenazi Jews than expected. Additionally, 89% of patients recall an event closely associated to the onset of the first episode including infection (72%, 25% with cold-like syndrome with fever), alcohol use (23%), sleep deprivation (22%), unusual stress (20%), physical exertion (19%), traveling (10%), head trauma (9%), and marijuana use (6%).

Episodes generally involved sleeping for prolonged periods of time with intense dreaming and difficulty waking. While awake, most patients reported cognitive impairment in multiple modalities including impaired speech (94%), concentration (91%), reading (75%), memory (66%), coordination (66%, causing 3 broken limbs in the 108 patients), and ability to make a decision (66%). Similarly, "altered perception" was ubiquitously reported including a "dreamy state" in 81%, derealization (63%), mind-body disconnect (52%), altered taste (50%), voices sounding distant (36%), altered smell (35%), and blurred vision (23%). Meningeal and autonomic symptoms occurred in 89% including fever (68%), photophobia (59%), headache (48%), sweating (46%), and nausea (18%). Psychological changes were diverse including irritability (65%), frustration (55%), depressed mood (53%), anxiety (45%), compulsions (36%), delusions (35%), and hallucinations (27%). Hyperphagia (66%) resulted in significant weight gain of 4.6 ± 3.1 kg/episode. Half of the patients reported increased sexual drive and sexual disinhibition, though this was more common in males. All of these symptoms resolved after the episodes. Notably, mean depression scores between controls and Kleine-Levin patients outside of an episode showed no significant difference. Clinical course duration was on average 13.6 years amounting to an average of 237 incapacitating days per patient. This duration of disability is longer than previously believed, making this syndrome less benign than previously thought.

The pathophysiology of Kleine-Levin syndrome is unclear. Basic motor, cerebellar, and sensory systems are generally intact, but sleep and higher-level functions are altered. This, combined with the diverse symptoms, suggests widespread brain abnormalities involving the thalamus, hypothalamus, and fronto-temporal areas.

Klein-Levin patients at initial presentation should undergo a careful neurological examination as well as EEG to exclude seizure activity, MRI to assess for structural abnormalities, complete metabolic panel, and toxicology screen. Although sleep studies are not always performed, we find them useful to exclude other causes of hypersomnolence and to demonstrate the return to normalcy in between episodes.

There are no controlled trials of pharmacologic treatment in Klein-Levin syndrome. It is difficult to draw firm conclusions from anecdotal case reports. A Cochrane review concluded that stimulants may improve sleepiness but do not help other symptoms. The use of several antiepileptic drugs has been attempted by various investigators including carbamazepine, valproate, gabapentin, and phenytoin, with some success in attenuating or preventing future attacks.

Lithium was found to be effective in up to 40% of subjects, but antidepressants are felt to be generally ineffective. Co-morbid sleep disorders should be treated and known precipitants, such as stress, sleep deprivation, and alcohol and drugs, should be avoided or minimized.

Bibliography

Arnulf, I, Lin L, Gadoth N, et al. Kleine-Levin syndrome: A systematic study of 108 patients. *Ann Neurol.* 2008;63:482–493.

Arnulf, I, Zeitzer JM, File J, et al. Kleine-Levin syndrome: a systemic review of 186 cases in the literature. *Brain.* 2005;128:2763–2776.

Oliveira MM, Conti C, Saconato H, Fernades do Prado G. Pharmacologic treatment for Klein-Levin syndrome. *Cochrane Database Syst Rev.* 2009;15:CD006685.

Rosenow F, Kotagal P, Cohen B, and Wyllie E. Multiple sleep latency test and polysomnography in diagnosing Kleine-Levin syndrome and periodic hypersomnia. *JClin Neurophys.* 2000;17:519–522.

27

An Over-the-Counter Recipe for Getting through Medical School

NATTAPONG JAIMCHARIYATAM, MD, MSc
KUMAR BUDUR, MD, MS

Case History

Adrian was a 47-year-old female physician who presented to the sleep disorders center with the chief complaint of long-standing excessive daytime sleepiness (EDS). She was sleepy since her college days and vividly remembered dozing off during lectures. She slept through classes in medical school and seriously contemplated giving up her dream of becoming a doctor. She denied sleep problems in childhood. In the morning, she felt refreshed, and she generally did not take naps. In college, she started taking naps lasting for 1 to 2 hours almost daily despite 8 to 9 hours of sleep at night. Naps were not refreshing. There was no history of preceding viral infection or head trauma. She had used pseudoephedrine, caffeine, and vigorous exercise for years to help her stay awake. She decided to seek treatment after federal regulations on over-the-counter cold preparations changed, and medications she found effective were no longer readily available.

At the time of presentation, Adrian reported a typical bedtime of 11 to 11:30 p.m. and wake time of 7:30 a.m. After waking up, she felt better, but not refreshed. On weekends, she went to bed at 10 to 10:30 p.m. and slept until 8 to 8:30 a.m. She usually took less than 10 minutes to fall asleep. She woke up 1 or 2 times every night to go to the restroom but was able to go back to sleep in less than 5 minutes. She never had difficulty falling or staying asleep. She estimated a total sleep time at night of 8 to 9 hours on weekdays and 9 to 10 hours on weekends.

She was a partner at a busy family practice group and worked as a family practitioner. She did all day outpatient clinics 5 days a week. She went to work at 8:30 a.m. and the workday usually ended by 6 pm. Despite feeling very sleepy, she did not think daytime sleepiness interfered with daytime functioning as long as she kept busy. However, on rare occasions when she had few minutes to relax, she readily dozed off to sleep. She napped for as long as 2 hours, 2 or 3 days per week after work. On weekends, however, she took 2 to 3 naps each day, each lasting for 1 to 2 hours, but she still felt tired and sleepy. She regularly dozed off to sleep at traffic lights for many years but denied any near-accidents or accidents.

Adrian denied cataplexy, hypnagogic or hypnopompic hallucinations, and sleep paralysis. She did not snore or have witnessed apnea. She denied symptoms of restless legs syndrome and parasomnias.

Medical history was notable for hypothyroidism that was under control with levothyroxine. There was no family history of sleep disorders. She denied any psychiatric problems, including major depressive disorder.

She denied use of alcohol or illicit drugs or abuse of prescription medications. As mentioned, she did abuse over-the-counter pseudoephedrine for many years to help her stay awake during the daytime. She drank 3 to 4 eight-oz cups of coffee per day, but this did not have any effect on her sleepiness. Adrian was married for 17 years and had 2 teenaged children. She denied any marital or financial problems. However, she did report some friction with her husband and children, mainly during the weekends because of her sleeping most of the time.

The Epworth Sleepiness Scale (ESS) score was 18/24, Fatigue Severity Scale (FSS) score was 54, and the Beck Depression Inventory (BDI) score was 0.

Physical Examination

Adrian's BMI was 24.3 kg/m^2 and she had a pulse of 76 per minute; blood pressure was 122/84 mmHg and the respiratory rate was 14. Her short- and long-term memory was intact. The physical examination was unremarkable, except for Grade III Friedman tongue position.

Evaluation

Adrian completed a sleep log that showed a sleep-wake pattern consistent with the history (Figure 27.1).

A polysomnogram (PSG) followed by multiple sleep latency test (MSLT) were done to exclude any nocturnal causes of daytime sleepiness and further evaluate the severity of daytime sleepiness. The PSG showed a total sleep time of 368 minutes with a sleep efficiency of 89%. Sleep latency was 12 minutes, and REM latency was 138 minutes. The apnea-hypopnea index was 3 and the arousal index was 13. The mean oxygen saturation was 96% with a minimum

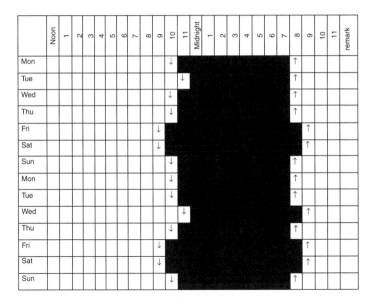

Figure 27.1 Sleep log shows sleep-wake times that are consistent with the reported sleep pattern. The patient averaged 8 to 9 hours of sleep on weekdays and 9 to 10 hours on weekends.

oxygen saturation of 91%. The MSLT showed a mean sleep latency of 5.9 minutes and no sleep onset REM periods (SOREMPs).

Diagnosis

Idiopathic hypersomnia without long sleep time (Table 27.1).

Outcome

Adrian was started on a wake-promoting agent, modafinil, to treat EDS. The starting dose was 200 mg every morning. She was informed about the role of scheduled naps that could potentially help her during the day but because of the nature of her job, this was not an option. She was informed about driving-related safety and other precautions related to EDS. Specifically, she was advised not to drive if she felt sleepy. She was also instructed on the potential for errors (like prescription errors) were she to get drowsy while at work. Adrian acknowledged the potential for sleep/fatigue-related errors. She tolerated the medication well and did not report any side effects. Four weeks later she noted some improvement for most of the day but continued to feel sleepy and tired mainly in the late afternoon. The dose of modafinil was increased to 400 mg per

Table 27.1 ICSD-2 criteria for idiopathic hypersomnia without long sleep time

A. The patient has a complaint of excessive daytime sleepiness occurring almost daily for at least 3 months.
B. The patient has normal nocturnal sleep (greater than 6 hours but less than 10 hours), documented by interview, actigraphy, or sleep logs.
C. Nocturnal polysomnography has excluded other causes of daytime sleepiness.
D. Polysomnography demonstrates a major sleep period that is normal in duration (greater than 6 hours but less than 10 hours).
E. An MSLT following overnight polysomnography demonstrates a mean sleep latency of less than 8 minutes and fewer than 2 SOREMPs. Mean sleep latency in idiopathic hypersomnia has been shown to be 6.2 ± 3.0 minutes.*
F. The hypersomnia is not better explained by another sleep disorder, medical or neurological disorder, mental disorder, medication use, or substance use disorder.

* **Note:** A mean sleep latency of less than eight minutes can be found in up to 30% of the general population. Both the mean sleep latency on the MSLT and the clinician's interpretation of the patient's symptoms, most notably a clinically significant complaint of sleepiness, should be taken into account in reaching the diagnosis of idiopathic hypersomnia without long sleep time.

day and she felt much better at this dose. She did not report any side effects at the higher dose, and it did not impair her ability to initiate and maintain asleep at night. She felt awake and alert all day and discontinued her naps. She felt that her quality of life, including her relationship with her husband and children, had also improved now that she was not feeling tired and sleepy all the time.

During her most recent visit for follow-up, she did not report any problems (ESS was 7/24; FSS was 5/63) on 400 mg of modafinil every morning.

Discussion

Adrian was diagnosed with idiopathic hypersomnia without long sleep time given the presence of EDS, habitual sleep duration of 8 to 9 hours per night, and long, unrefreshing naps. Her PSG and MSLT confirmed this diagnosis. In patients with severe daytime sleepiness like Adrian, one of the first diagnoses to consider is narcolepsy without cataplexy. However, some aspects of her history were not typical of narcolepsy including unrefreshing nocturnal sleep, long and unrefreshing naps, and the absence of hypnagogic or hypnapompic hallucinations, sleep paralysis and SOREMPs on the MSLT. The other diagnoses to consider are:

(1) Behaviorally induced insufficient sleep syndrome: This was unlikely because the patient is getting adequate sleep every night, and daytime sleepiness persisted despite getting at least 9 to 10 hours of sleep on weekends.

(2) Hypersomnia due to medical condition or drug/substance use: This was unlikely, since the only other medical condition the patient had was hypothyroidism, which was treated, and there was no history of other somnogenic drugs or substance use.

(3) Hypersomnia not due to substance or known physiological condition should be considered in patients with personality disorder or psychiatric conditions, and these were not noted in Adrian.

(4) Idiopathic hypersomnia without long sleep time is differentiated from idiopathic hypersomnia with long sleep time mainly by the duration of the major sleep period. In idiopathic hypersomnia with long sleep time, the major sleep period is greater than 10 hours. The symptoms of idiopathic hypersomnia can sometimes mimic narcolepsy without cataplexy. However, in idiopathic hypersomnia, although the mean sleep latency is less than 8 minutes (similar to narcolepsy), the number of SOREMPs is less than 2 (whereas in narcolepsy, there are usually 2 or more SOREMPs).

Idiopathic hypersomnia without long sleep time is characterized by constant and severe EDS with unrefreshing naps, a normal or slightly prolonged (but total sleep time less than 10 hours) major sleep period, and great difficulty waking up from sleep. The etiology is not known, but it may be familial with an autosomal dominant mode of inheritance. The age of onset is usually before 25 years and, once established, the disorder is more often stable, although spontaneous remissions are sometimes reported. Little is known about the prevalence and epidemiological features of this disorder. The diagnosis of Idiopathic hypersomnia without long sleep time is confirmed by sleep laboratory testing. The PSG shows either a normal or slightly prolonged nocturnal sleep period (greater than 6 and less than 10 hours) and a sleep efficiency of 85% or higher. In addition, sleep related breathing disorders and periodic limb movement disorder should either be absent or adequately treated before making this diagnosis. The MSLT shows a mean sleep latency of less than 8 minutes and fewer than two SOREMPs.

The management of idiopathic hypersomnia is similar to that of narcolepsy and consists of behavioral modifications to optimize sleep. Pharmacotherapy with the wake-promoting medication, modafinil, is found to be effective, although some reports indicate that the response is not as robust as seen in patients with narcolepsy. Stimulant medications such as methylphenidates and amphetamine salts are also effective. Advice on how to deal with day-to-day functioning is also very important. First and foremost, from a safety standpoint, advising patients about driving and other related precautions is important. Obtaining adequate nocturnal sleep and preventing sleep deprivation is critical.

Bibliography

Aldrich MS. The clinical spectrum of narcolepsy and idiopathic hypersomnia. *Neurology.* 1996;46:393–401.

Billiard M. Diagnosis of narcolepsy and idiopathic hypersomnia. An update based on the international Classification of Sleep Disorders, 2nd ed. *Sleep Med Rev.* 2007;11:377–388.

28

Another Cup of Joe for Jacquie

NATTAPONG JAIMCHARIYATAM, MD, MSc
KUMAR BUDUR, MD, MS

Case History

Jacquie was a 48-year-old nurse who presented with excessive daytime sleepiness (EDS), fatigue, and concentration problems that were interfering with her ability to function on the job. Her symptoms started 2 years prior but became worse over the past 6 months. She attributed this to recent major life events, including divorce and the death of her mother. She had a set of 9-year-old twins and a full-time job as a nurse practitioner, and she worked from 8 a.m. until 5 to 6 p.m. She went to bed by 11:30 p.m. to midnight and woke up at 5 to 5:30 a.m. Before going to bed at night, she did house work, tackled paperwork left over from her work day, or paid bills. Once in bed, she was able to fall asleep within 10 minutes, barely able to finish a paragraph or 2 in the novel that had become a fixture at her bedside. She woke up for no apparent reason 2 or 3 times per night, but she was always able to go back to sleep within minutes. After waking in the morning, she rarely felt refreshed, but forced herself to exercise everyday for 1 hour, after which she got her children ready for school and drove to work. Over the past 6 months, she began dozing off in meetings at work and caught herself almost falling asleep charting during patient visits. She was having trouble keeping her eyes open at stoplights behind the wheel and on a few occasions could not remember the drive home. She drank a pot of strong coffee every morning at work to keep herself awake and another 3 or 4 caffeinated beverages in the afternoon. She estimated a total sleep time of 5 to 5.5 hours on weekdays. On weekends, she slept until 10 a.m. and felt markedly refreshed after 10 to 11 hours of sleep. She scored 15 on the Epworth Sleepiness Scale (ESS) and 58 on the Fatigue Severity Scale (FSS).

Jacquie denied cataplexy, hypnagogic hallucination, or sleep paralysis. She reported snoring but denied waking up from sleep gasping for air or choking. Her ex-husband had never complained of snoring or apneic events, although friends who observed her sleep described her breathing being shallow in sleep. She denied symptoms of restless legs syndrome and parasomnias.

Jacquie was diagnosed with major depressive disorder, moderate in severity, and prescribed bupropion after her divorce, but she was in remission for the past 18 months. At the time of her presentation to the sleep center, she denied depressive symptoms. Her family history was negative for significant medical, psychiatric, and sleep disorders. She denied smoking and recreational drugs and drank a glass of wine every 2 to 3 weeks.

Physical Examination

Jacquie appeared tired but had a normal mental status. Her body mass index (BMI) was 28 kg/m². The upper airway exam was notable for a Grade III Friedman tongue position. The neurological exam was remarkable for a mild postural tremor. The rest of the examination was normal.

Evaluation

Jacquie completed a sleep diary prior to her initial visit that corroborated her reported sleep history (Figure 28.1). A polysomnogram (PSG) was done to screen for sleep apnea given her history of snoring, shallow breathing, spontaneous awakenings at night, upper airway crowding, and elevated BMI. It showed a total sleep time of 410 minutes, resulting in a sleep efficiency of 96%. The sleep latency was 2 minutes and the REM latency was 103 minutes. She spent 11.7% of sleep time in Stage N1, 60.2% in N2, 10.2% in N3 and 17.9% in REM sleep. Light snoring was noted. The apnea-hypopnea index was 0.6, and arousal index was 19.5. The minimum oxygen saturation was 94%. The periodic limb movements index was 1.9 and periodic limb movement arousal index was 0.

Diagnosis

Behaviorally induced insufficient sleep syndrome (Table 28.1).

Outcome

Jacquie's EDS was attributed to sleep deprivation due to behaviorally induced insufficient sleep. She was advised she would have to make major changes in her

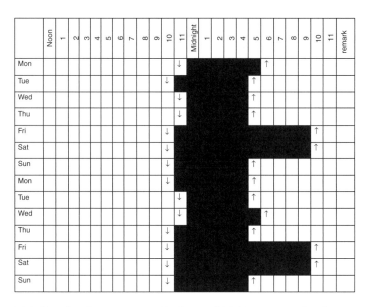

Figure 28.1 Sleep log showing a usual bedtime of 11:30 p.m. to midnight on weekdays and a wake up time of 5 to 5:30 a.m. The average sleep time was 5 to 6 hours on weekdays and 10 to 11 hours on weekends.

Table 28.1 ICSD-2 criteria for behaviorally induced insufficient sleep syndrome

A. The patient has a complaint of excessive daytime sleepiness or, in prepubertal children, a complaint of behavioral abnormalities suggesting sleepiness. The abnormal sleep pattern is present almost daily for at least 3 months.

B. The patient's habitual sleep episode, established using history, a sleep log, or actigraphy, is usually shorter than expected from age-adjusted normative data.

C. When the habitual sleep schedule is not maintained (weekends or vacation time), the patient will sleep considerably longer than usual.

D. If diagnostic polysomnography is performed (not required for diagnosis), sleep latency is less than 10 minutes and sleep efficiency is greater than 90%. During the MSLT, a short mean sleep latency of less than 8 minutes (with or without multiple SOREMPs) may be observed.

E. The hypersomnia is not better explained by another sleep disorder, medical or neurological disorder, mental disorder, medication use, or substance use disorder.

daily schedule to ensure a minimum of 7 to 8 hours of sleep each night. While it was hard for her to accomplish this, due to the nature of her job and social commitments, she acknowledged that the amount of sleep she was getting was not sufficient. She was informed of the risks of sleep deprivation, including motor vehicle accidents and errors on the job and about the warning signs of sleepiness and counter-strategies (Table 28.2). She decided to cut back on

Table 28.2 Signs and symptoms of excessive sleepiness

Warning signs of drowsiness
- Falling asleep or yawning in sedentary situations
- Feeling restless and irritable
- Having to check work repeatedly
- Difficulty concentrating or staying on task
- Increased reaction time
- Inconsistent performance
- Poor decision making
- Reduced short-term memory
- Decreased ability to learn
- Anxiety

Signs of drowsy driving
- Trouble focusing on the road
- Difficulty keeping the eyes open or closing the eyes at stoplights
- Nodding
- Yawning repeatedly
- Drifting from the lane
- Missing signs or exits
- Not remembering driving the last few miles

Signs of severe sleepiness
- Reduced head control
- Nystagmus
- Hand tremors
- Blurred vision
- Intermittent dysarthria
- Ptosis
- Visual hallucinations

---

exercise by 30 minutes per day and reduced the amount of time she spent on work at home in the evening. With these modest changes, she was able to sleep 60 minutes earlier and wake up 30 minutes later than her usual sleep schedule and got approximately 7 hours of sleep every night. She felt more alert and efficient at work and noticed the she slept 1 hour less on weekends. Her caffeine consumption declined considerably, as did her ESS (now 8) and FSS (now 4) scores. At her last visit, 6 months later, Jacquie had maintained a sleep duration of at least 7 hours per night and continued to feel more alert and productive.

Discussion

Jacquie's sleep history is not unlike that of many adults who voluntarily restrict sleep in order to fulfill the commitments of everyday life, a condition known as behaviorally induced insufficient sleep syndrome. She reported an average sleep duration of only 5 to 6 hours during the work week, and she caught up on sleep on the weekends. Her total sleep time on weekdays was significantly less than what is required by the majority of the population, and her symptoms (EDS fatigue, difficulty with concentration) were the result of sleep deprivation. The findings on the PSG supported this diagnosis.

The differential diagnosis of EDS is extensive. In Jacquie's case, diagnostic considerations included:

(1) Narcolepsy without cataplexy. The EDS was significant enough to consider a diagnosis of narcolepsy. However, the history was not typical. Jacquie felt much more alert after increasing sleep times on the weekends, and she did not have hypnagogic or hypnapompic hallucinations or sleep paralysis.

(2) Hypersomnia not due to substance or known physiological condition (also known as hypersomnia associated with mental disorders or nonorganic hypersomnia, NOS) should be considered in patients with psychiatric conditions. While Jacquie did have a history of depression, her depression was in remission, and even if she had had residual symptoms, it would have been unlikely to cause the degree of daytime sleepiness and fatigue reported.

(3) Idiopathic hypersomnia without long sleep time. This diagnosis was thought to be unlikely, since Jacquie was sleeping less than 6 hours most nights and did not have long, unrefreshing naps often associated with this condition.

Sleep deprivation is very common in modern society and results from behaviors that curtail total sleep time as well as medical and psychiatric disorders and substance abuse. The consequences of sleep deprivation are vast and include alterations in physical, mental, and cognitive functioning. In terms of physical health, inadequate sleep (most commonly defined as less than 6 hours per day) is associated with an increased risk of obesity, insulin resistance and Type II diabetes. Mental health problems can worsen with sleep deprivation—for example, relapse of mania in bipolar disorders. Numerous studies have shown that sleep deprivation affects concentration, memory, and judgment; several of these studies were done in medical professionals, pilots and military personnel. The National Highway Traffic Safety Administration expert panel on Driver Fatigue and Sleepiness reports that in 1996 about 56,000 crashes and 1550 deaths were cited by the police to be due to driver drowsiness and fatigue. Humans underestimate sleepiness and overestimate alertness even when extremely sleepy. A study involving anesthesia residents showed that more than half of the time, subjects did not perceive themselves to be sleepy even when they fell asleep during the multiple sleep latency test. More than two-thirds of those who fell asleep believed that they had not.

Awareness of the signs and symptoms of sleep deprivation (Table 28.2) and lifestyle changes make it possible to effectively manage this all too common problem. The most effective countermeasure for sleep deprivation is to get adequate sleep (7 to 9 hours) before anticipated sleep loss and avoid starting out the day with a sleep debt. Other effective strategies include taking scheduled brief naps lasting no more than 20 to 30 minutes, caffeine, exercise, sleep hygiene, and addressing any primary sleep disorders, if present, such as sleep apnea, restless legs syndrome and narcolepsy.

Bibliography

Dinges DF, Pack F, Williams K, et al. Cumulative sleepiness, mood disturbance, and psychomotor vigilance performance decrements during a week of sleep restricted to 4-5 hours per night. *SLEEP.* 1997;20:67–77.

Howard SK, Gaba DM, Rosekind MR, et al. The risks and implications of excessive daytime sleepiness in resident physicians. *Acad Med.* 2002;77(10):1019–1025.

Komada Y, Inoue Y, Hayashida K, Nakajima T, Takahashi K. Clinical significance and correlates of behaviorally induced insufficient sleep syndrome. *Sleep Med.* 2007;9:851–856.

National Highway Traffic Safety Administration. http://www.nhtsa.dot.gov/people/injury/drowsy_driving1/Drowsy.html; accessed 4-12-10

Roehrs T, Zorick F, Sicklesteel J, Witting R, Roth T. Excessive daytime sleepiness associated with insufficient sleep. *SLEEP.* 1983;6:319–325.

Spiegel K, Knutson K, Leproult R et al. Sleep loss: a novel risk factor for insulin resistance and Type 2 diabetes. *J Appl Physiol.* 2005;99:2008–2019.

29

Tackling Teenage Hypersomnia: "Joint" Partners Required

JENNIFER SCIUVA, MSN, PNP

KUMAR BUDUR, MD, MS

JYOTI KRISHNA, MD

Case History

Life had recently really changed for 17-year-old Mike. Until the age of 15, he was an outgoing, athletic teenager who had no problem keeping up with his busy schedule. His GPA during his freshman year of high school was 4.0 despite active involvement in sports and other extracurricular activities. However, over the past two 2 years he felt increasingly sleepy and tired during the day. He was dozing off unintentionally at school, and he was not able to keep up with his busy schedule. From being a clean-cut, trimly dressed young man, his appearance was now slightly disheveled. He was unable to wake up for school in the morning and maintain alertness during classes, so his mother decided it would be best for him to be homeschooled. Mike typically went to bed at 10:30 p.m. and was able to sleep within 15 to 20 minutes. He denied problems falling or staying asleep and woke up at 6:30 a.m. not feeling refreshed. He felt sleepy within 2 to 3 hours after waking up and took 3 to 5 brief naps, each lasting 10 to 20 minutes, throughout the day. In the evenings, he took a 2-hour nap from 5 to 7 p.m. Naps were modestly helpful at best. His Epworth Sleepiness Scale (ESS) score was 17 and Fatigue Severity Scale (FSS) score was 52. There was no history of infection or head injury prior to the onset of his sleep symptoms, nor was there any history of snoring, witnessed apneas, restless legs symptoms, cataplexy, hypnagogic hallucinations, or sleep paralysis. Mike's mother reported that he was "different," in that he stopped talking about his friends or school activities even when he was still attending regular school.

His father had brushed off this change as "normal teenage stuff." His mother was perplexed at the gradual deterioration in Mike's health and brought him to the sleep center for an assessment.

Mike's past medical history was significant for seasonal allergies. Although he denied use of illicit drugs, Mike confidentially shared that he had experimented with alcohol. The family history was negative for sleep disorders. Mike lived at home with his parents and younger brother. His parents worked full time and there was limited supervision at home.

Physical Examination

Mike was a well-built, muscular adolescent with a body mass index of $27.6\,kg/m^2$. His appearance was somewhat disheveled, with ungroomed hair and unironed clothes. He appeared sleepy and his eyes were slightly red, but pupils were of normal size and reactive to light. His upper airway exam showed Grade I Friedman tongue position and Grade II tonsillar size. The rest of the physical examination was normal except for mild dysmetria and gait instability, which Mike attributed to feeling sleepy.

Evaluation

A polysomnogram (PSG) followed by Multiple Sleep Latency Test (MSLT) were ordered to determine the etiology and severity of excessive daytime sleepiness (EDS), especially with the view to screen for narcolepsy. The PSG showed no evidence of sleep related breathing disorder. Total sleep time was 478 minutes, with a sleep efficiency of 92%. The apnea-hypopnea index was 1.2, and the arousal index was 2. There were no periodic limb movements in sleep. The MSLT showed a mean sleep latency of 6.5 minutes and no sleep onset REM periods (SOREMPs). The urine toxicology screen done on the morning of the MSLT was positive for cannabinoids.

Diagnosis

Hypersomnia due to drug or substance (abuse) (Table 29.1).

Outcome

Mike and his parents returned 1 week after sleep testing to discuss the results and begin treatment. Although not required in the case of a minor, in order to

Table 29.1 ICSD-2 criteria for hypersomnia due to drug or substance

Hypersomnia due to drug or substance (abuse)

A. The patient has a complaint of sleepiness or excessive sleep.
B. The complaint is believed to be secondary to current use, recent discontinuation, or prior prolonged use of drugs.
C. The hypersomnia is not better explained by another sleep disorder, medical or neurological disorder, mental disorder, or medication use.

Hypersomnia due to drug or substance (medications)

A. The patient has a complaint of sleepiness or excessive sleep.
B. The complaint is believed to be secondary to current use, recent discontinuation, or prior prolonged use of medication.
C. The hypersomnia is not better explained by another sleep disorder, medical or neurological disorder, mental disorder, or substance use disorder.

keep his trust, Mike's permission was obtained prior to discussing the results of urine drug screen with his parents. The discussion with the family centered mainly on the positive drug screen for cannabinoids. The relationship between drug use and sleep problems was discussed at length, after which Mike readily admitted to using marijuana over the past 2 years. What started as intermittent use for fun had evolved into a regular habit. He had developed tolerance to marijuana, which required him to escalate use to get the same relaxing effect. He admitted to using up to "7 or 8 joints" throughout the day to prevent feelings of irritability and agitation. His parents were shocked at this revelation but remained positive and supportive. Mike and his parents were keen to try wake-promoting medications to help him stay alert and function better during the day. Caution was emphasized regarding prescription of a stimulant medication while Mike was actively using marijuana. However, the family was informed that medication options would be considered if Mike continued to have problems with EDS despite being abstinent from marijuana. This would mean that he would need to have future abnormal MSLT testing that confirmed ongoing EDS in the context of negative urine toxicology screens and adequate sleep hygiene. Mike was referred to the Alcohol and Drug Rehabilitation Center at the Cleveland Clinic.

Mike attended several sessions of counseling with a therapist specializing in drug abuse treatment. He abstained from further use of marijuana and returned for follow-up 2 months later, at which time his mother jubilantly stated, "I have got my child back." A confident, sociable young man was sitting in the exam room. Mike was doing well; his daytime sleepiness had decreased significantly, and he did not complain of fatigue. His ESS and FSS scores reduced to 3 and 14, respectively. He was motivated and helpful at home and in his neighborhood. The family was looking forward to his future and planning to re-enroll him in a public high school for the next school year. He was confident he would be able to stay away from drugs and expressed willingness to continue therapy as long as necessary. A repeat urine drug screen was negative.

Discussion

Mike's case illustrates an unfortunately common sleep disorder in adolescents and young adults—hypersomnia due to substance abuse. Although some clues to this diagnosis (unkempt appearance, altered behavior, reddened sclerae, and incoordination) were present, other diagnoses to be considered include:

(1) Narcolepsy: The history was not typical, in that naps were not necessarily refreshing and he did not have a history of cataplexy, sleep paralysis, or hypnagogic hallucinations. Although the mean sleep latency was less than 8 minutes, no SOREMPs were noted.

(2) Idiopathic hypersomnia: Hypersomnia despite what appeared to be adequate sleep at night was a consideration. The mean sleep latency and lack of SOREMPs also supported this diagnosis. However, based upon a high index of suspicion, drug abuse needed to be excluded first.

(3) Behaviorally induced insufficient sleep syndrome: This diagnosis was unlikely given that Mike was getting about 8 hours of sleep on most nights.

(4) Hypersomnia due to mental disorders: This was another diagnostic possibility, but unlikely, since Mike denied any psychiatric symptoms.

There is a bi-directional relationship between substance abuse and sleep disturbances. Sleep problems such as insomnia increase the risk of alcohol and sedative abuse while sleep disorders that cause EDS, such as narcolepsy or idiopathic hypersomnia, themselves increase the risk of stimulant abuse. Similarly, substance abuse can lead to both insomnia and EDS, depending on the substance abused. Drug abuse is not uncommon. According to the National Survey on Drug and Health in 2007, 7.6% of Americans older than 12 years met the criteria for alcohol abuse or dependence, and the prevalence of illicit drug use in the same year was as high as 14.5%. In another study involving patients admitted to an alcohol/drug rehabilitation center, more than 90% reported poor quality sleep, more than half had symptoms of sleep apnea, and one-third experienced symptoms suggestive of restless legs syndrome.

Sleep laboratory testing is not necessary to diagnose hypersomnia due to drug or substance unless a concomitant sleep disorder is suspected. It is best to delay sleep testing until the patient is abstinent from substance abuse. In Mike's case, a PSG and MSLT were performed as he initially denied drug use. One should interpret sleep testing cautiously in patients using recreational drugs and alcohol. The results will vary depending on the substance abused and the time of last intake. In general, it is best to stop all the drugs that can influence the MSLT for a minimum of 2 weeks, or at least 5 half lives of the substance. This includes medications such as selective serotonin reuptake inhibitors (SSRIs) that can result in false positive identification of REM sleep by their ability to cause rapid eye movements in NREM sleep. In addition, SSRIs can suppress REM sleep. Similarly, most sedatives, muscle relaxants, and antiepileptic drugs can cause sedation and decrease the mean sleep latency. Conversely, stimulant medications can increase the sleep latency. A urine drug screen, although not mandatory, should be considered in all patients suspected of abusing prescription or illicit drugs.

A high index of suspicion is needed to diagnose patients such as Mike. When suspected, a detailed history (often in private after parental permission, if the patient is a minor), a good rapport with the patient, assurance of confidentiality to the extent possible, and urine toxicology screen are required. Although discussion of signs and symptoms of abuse of various drugs is outside the scope of this chapter, some of the signs and symptoms of marijuana abuse are listed in Table 29.2. The patient's motivation to get better and stay abstinent from drug abuse is critical to ensure a good outcome. In this case, Mike's determination to stay away from drugs and his parents' support were keys to success. Mike saw a therapist specializing in substance abuse treatment on a regular basis and was able to stop marijuana abuse. Depending on the nature and the severity of substance abuse, sometimes a formal psychiatric assessment and/or inpatient assessment is indicated. It is also important to note that some patients have co-existing sleep and substance abuse disorders, in which case both require treatment.

Table 29.2 Marijuana: signs and symptoms of abuse

- Red eyes
- Drowsiness
- Lack of interest or motivation
- Impaired thinking
- Apathy
- Poor coordination
- Inappropriate laughter
- Anxiety, panic
- Distorted perceptions, including hallucinations
- Hunger, thirst

Bibliography

Bootzin, R.R. & Stevens, S.J. Adolescents, substance abuse and the treatment of insomnia and daytime sleepiness. *Clin Psych Review.* 2005;25:629–644.

Mahfoud Y, Talih F, Streem, D, Budur K. Sleep disorders in substance abusers: How common are they? *Psychiatry.* 2009;6(9):38–42.

U.S. Department of Health and Human Services. Substance Abuse and Mental Health Services Administration. 2007 National Survey on Drug Use and Health; http://dx.doi.org/10.3886/ICPSR23782

30

More Stimulants, Please

CARLOS RODRIGUEZ, MD

Case History

Brian was a 20-year-old college student who presented to the sleep center with a history of excessive daytime sleepiness (EDS) for the past 2 years. He believed he needed more stimulant medication than his physician was willing to prescribe. He reported difficulty paying attention in class and would doze during lectures, while studying and on several occasions while driving, although he denied ever being involved in a motor vehicle accident. He reported sleeping between 5.5 and 8.5 hours per night and had difficulty awakening in the morning. He typically went to bed between midnight and 1 a.m. and would fall asleep within minutes. Whenever he went to bed earlier, he would lie in bed awake, unable to fall asleep before midnight. On weekends, he preferred to go to bed at 3 a.m. and sleep in until 11 a.m. or noon. He used 2 alarm clocks, often relied on his roommate to wake him up in the morning for school, and felt groggy and confused for 1 hour after awakening. He did whatever he could to avoid having to be awake in the morning and preferred late afternoon and evening classes so that he could sleep in. He felt most alert and productive from 9 p.m. to midnight. He was missing morning classes regularly and worried that he would not make it through the semester without help.

Brian reported sleeping well at night without any awakenings but felt unrefreshed in the morning. He took 2- to 3-hour naps at least 3 days per week, but if anything felt worse instead of better after napping. He scored 15/24 on the Epworth Sleepiness Scale (ESS) and 23/63 on the Fatigue Severity Scale (FSS). His roommate complained of his loud snoring. There was no history of witnessed apneas, and Brian denied gasping for air during sleep, nocturia, leg jerks and restless legs symptoms, tooth grinding, and heartburn at night. About 1 year prior to presentation, he had an episode as he was falling asleep in which he could not move or speak for about 1 minute. He described this as "terrifying" and said that it resolved as quickly as it seemed to set in. He denied cataplexy and sleep related hallucinations, depression, appetite changes, and a history of head injury or flu-like illnesses prior to the onset of his sleep symptoms. He was not related to anyone with similar complaints. Brian's medical history was notable for allergic rhinitis, for which he used fluticasone. He took no regular medications and did not smoke or use recreational drugs. He drank no more than 1 beer on the weekends.

Brian had a polysomnogram (PSG) a few months prior to presentation and was diagnosed with primary snoring. The total sleep time was 379 minutes, and sleep architecture was relatively normal (N1 7%, N2 52%, N3 19%, REM 22%). There were no periodic limb movements (PLMS), and the apnea-hypopnea index (AHI) was 1.6. This was followed by a multiple sleep latency test (MSLT) that showed a mean sleep latency (MSL) of 6.8 minutes (sleep latency of 1, 2, 7, 10, and 14 minutes respectively, in each of the 5 naps) and sleep onset REM periods (SOREMPs) in naps 1 and 2 of the 5-nap study. His complete blood count, metabolic panel, liver function tests, and thyroid stimulating hormone were normal. He was diagnosed with narcolepsy without cataplexy and started on modafinil 100 mg every morning, which improved his EDS by an estimated 40%. He believed he could function normally with a higher dose of medications and requested "more stimulants, please."

Physical Examination

Brian appeared a bit sluggish but was awake with normal mental status, affect, and language. His body mass index (BMI) was 24 kg/m^2 and his neck circumference was 15.25 inches. His upper airway exam revealed a mild deviated nasal septum to the right, absent tonsils, and a Grade II Friedman tongue position. His general and neurological exams were otherwise normal.

Evaluation

Due to concerns that Brian may have been misdiagnosed, he was advised to hold the modafinil for 2 weeks and repeat the sleep testing. He completed a sleep log for 2 weeks immediately beforehand (Figure 30.1). This sleep log was used to time the PSG and MSLT appropriately in accordance with his usual sleep and wake times. Based upon this sleep schedule, the PSG began at 1 a.m. and he awoke at 9 a.m. the following morning. The MSLT naps were conducted at 11 a.m. and 1, 3, 5, and 7 p.m. The PSG revealed a total sleep time of 433 minutes, sleep efficiency of 88%, sleep latency of 9 minutes, REM latency of 138 minutes, and supine sleep time of 25%. Sleep architecture was normal

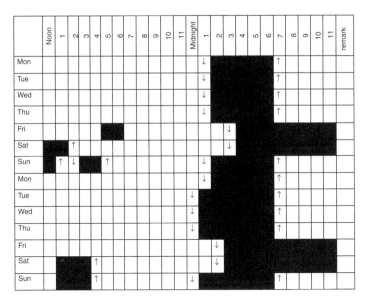

Figure 30.1 Sleep log. The sleep log was very similar to his reported sleep durations. He usually went to bed at 12:30 to 12:45 a.m. on weekdays and was awake at 6 a.m. The total sleep time on weekdays was 5 to 5.5 hours. On weekends, he went to bed at 2:30 a.m. and would sleep until 11:45 a.m. The total sleep time on weekends was 10 to 10.5 hours.

(N1 9%, N2 55%, N3 15%, and REM 21%). The AHI was 3 and the PLM index was 1. The MSLT showed an MSL of 11.9 minutes with no SOREMPs. Urine toxicology screen on the day of the MSLT was negative.

Diagnosis

Circadian rhythm sleep disorder, delayed sleep phase type (delayed sleep phase disorder [DSPD]).

Outcome

The results of the sleep study and the diagnosis and treatment options were explained to Brian. He was glad that he did not have narcolepsy, and he was committed to getting better. He was educated about sleep hygiene and encouraged to keep a structured sleep-wake schedule with awakening in the morning at 7 a.m. on weekdays and no later than 8 a.m. on weekends. He was instructed to avoid bright light exposure in the evenings and at night and, optimize light exposure in the morning. He started phototherapy using a light box emitting

10,000 lux for 60 minutes every morning from 7:30 to 8:30 a.m. The light box was placed on the table where he worked on his homework in the mornings after showering and dressing. This was a change in his routine that was difficult to comply with because he was very sleepy in the mornings. In addition, he started melatonin 0.3 mg every night at 7 p.m.

Brian was seen for follow-up 1 month later and reported a significant improvement in daytime sleepiness. He was able to comply with the sleep hygiene, phototherapy, and melatonin therapy. He was falling asleep by 11 p.m. and waking at 7 a.m. on weekdays. He discontinued the modafinil, as his EDS was virtually resolved. After adjusting to his new schedule, he felt refreshed in the mornings, was able to concentrate at school, and no longer napped in lectures.

Discussion

Brian's case illustrates the diagnostic considerations in patients with EDS and pitfalls in the interpretation of the MSLT in sleepy patients. Brian's EDS and findings on MSLT led to an erroneous diagnosis of narcolepsy without cataplexy. However, he lacked some of the cardinal features of narcolepsy and had historical features concerning for other disorders. In particular, his sleep duration, especially on weekdays, was inadequate and he felt less sleepy on weekends after getting more sleep, suggesting that insufficient sleep was partly to blame for his sleepiness. In addition, he was able to sleep well through the night but had difficulty falling asleep and waking up in the morning and was most alert late in the evenings. This is suggestive of a circadian rhythm sleep disorder rather than narcolepsy.

One way of conceptualizing the differential diagnosis of EDS is to consider 3 categories: (1) sleep fragmenting disorders, (2) disorders of insufficient or inappropriately timed sleep, and (3) central hypersomnias (Table 30.1).

Among the sleep fragmenting disorders, the primary consideration in Brian's case was obstructive sleep apnea syndrome, given the history of loud snoring and EDS. This possibility was ruled out, given that his PSG revealed only snoring. The use of a nasal transducer during the recording makes upper airway resistance syndrome unlikely, but the optimal method of ruling out this condition is with the use of an esophageal manometry.

Behaviorally induced insufficient sleep syndrome was a consideration, but in this condition the total sleep duration is usually less than 6 hours, and patients do not have any difficulty falling asleep at night. While Brian did not sleep enough during the school week, he was not able to fall asleep until at least midnight or 1 a.m.

Among the central hypersomnias, idiopathic hypersomnia without long sleep time needed to be considered. This diagnosis was supported by the history of sleep drunkenness (having great difficulty waking up in the morning with

Table 30.1 Differential diagnosis of excessive daytime sleepiness

A. Disorders of sleep fragmentation
   Sleep related breathing disorders
   Periodic limb movement disorder
   Restless legs syndrome with PLMS
   Environmental sleep disorder
   Other sleep fragmenting disorders (bruxism, sleep related GERD)
B. Disorders of insufficient or inappropriately timed sleep
   Behaviorally induced insufficient sleep syndrome
   Insomnias
   Circadian rhythm disorders
C. Central hypersomnias
   Narcolepsy (with and without cataplexy and secondary to medical conditions)
   Recurrent hypersomnias (i.e. Kleine-Levin and menstrual-related)
   Idiopathic hypersomnias (i.e., with and without long sleep time)
   Hypersomnia due to a medical condition
   Hypersomnia due to a drug or substance
   Hypersomnia not due to a substance or known physiologic condition

sleepiness, confusion, and slowed mentation); the presence of normal and uninterrupted nocturnal sleep; long unrefreshing daytime naps; and onset prior to age 25. However, this is a diagnosis of exclusion and it requires an MSLT demonstrating a MSL of less than 8 minutes and fewer than 2 SOREMPs. When the MSLT was done per protocol to test for EDS in an individual with a shifted sleep schedule, it was normal.

The other consideration was narcolepsy without cataplexy, which was Brian's initial diagnosis. The historical features that supported this diagnosis at least superficially included onset of EDS at a young age with daytime napping, sleep paralysis, and an initial MSLT showing a MSL of 6.8 minutes with 2 SOREMPs. However, Brian had only a single episode of sleep paralysis, which is a nonspecific symptom that can be experienced by normal individuals. Patients with narcolepsy tend to experience this on a more regular basis. Furthermore, Brian did not exhibit recurrent awakenings from sleep, which are commonly seen in patients with narcolepsy. The MSLT result was falsely positive for narcolepsy when performed without consideration of his regular sleep time. In fact, the first nap trial was performed at 7 a.m. and the second trial at 9 a.m., times when Brian had a propensity for REM sleep because it corresponded to the last third of his nocturnal sleep period, when REM sleep predominates. The presence of SOREMPs during the first 2 naps is a red flag and suggests the possibility of DSPD. According to the Practice Parameter for the Clinical Use of the MSLT and MWT, the first nap trial of the MSLT should be delayed for 1.5 to 3 hours after the final awakening on the PSG. When conducted properly, Brian's second MSLT clearly ruled out narcolepsy.

Table 30.2 ICSD-2 criteria for delayed sleep phase disorder

A. There is a delay in the phase of the major sleep period in relation to the desired sleep time and wake-up time, as evidenced by a chronic or recurrent complaint of inability to fall asleep at a desired conventional clock time together with the inability to awaken at a desired and socially acceptable time.
B. When allowed to choose their preferred schedule, patients will exhibit normal sleep quality and duration for age and maintain a delayed, but stable phase of entrainment to the 24-hour sleep-wake pattern.
C. Sleep log or actigraphy monitoring (including sleep diary) for at least 7 days demonstrates a stable delay in the timing of the habitual sleep period.*
D. The sleep disturbance is not better explained by another current sleep disorder, medical or neurological disorder, mental disorder, medication use, or substance use disorder.

*Note: In addition, a delay in the timing of other circadian rhythms, such as the nadir of the core body temperature rhythm or dim-light melatonin onset (DLMO) is useful for the confirmation of the delayed phase.

Another important diagnostic possibility is substance- or medication-induced hypersomnia. This is an important consideration, given the patient's age. Testing with a urinary toxicology screen during the MSLT can help reduce the likelihood that a substance or medication is the source of the hypersomnia.

Brian exhibited the typical sleep and wake times characteristic of delayed sleep phase disorder (Table 30.2). When permitted to sleep on his preferred schedule, as he did on weekends, he had normal nocturnal sleep without awakenings, and daytime sleepiness was not a problem. On weekdays, he was forced to go to sleep and wake up earlier because of school commitments. Since he could not fall asleep earlier, he found himself struggling to wake up without adequate sleep (sleep drunkenness) and experienced symptoms of sleep deprivation, including poor concentration and an episode of sleep paralysis. If afforded an opportunity to take later classes, he would have gladly done so. The Horne-Ostberg morningness-eveningness questionnaire may assist in the identification of patients with DSPD (see Appendix).

Bibliography

Litner MR, et al. Practice parameter for the clinical use of the Multiple Sleep Latency Test and the Maintenance of Wakefulness Test. *SLEEP.* 2005;28(1): 113–121.
Reid KJ, Zee PC. Circadian disorders of the sleep-wake cycle. In: Kryger MH, et al, eds. *Principles and Practice of Sleep Medicine.* Philadelphia, PA: WB Saunders; 2005:691–696.

31

How Shall I Wake? Let Me Count the Alarms

WILLIAM NOVAK, MD

Case History

Cathy, a 32-year-old medical professional, presented to the sleep disorders center with a complaint of excessive daytime sleepiness (EDS). This was particularly problematic on weekdays, during which she was scheduled to start work at 8 a.m. Despite the use of 4 clock radio alarms, 2 television alarms, and at least 1 phone call from her mother, who was living halfway across the country, she rarely ever made it to work on time, often sleeping until 9 a.m., if not later.

She reported that when arriving to work in the morning, typically 2 hours after her scheduled start time, she was sleepy and "barely productive." Feeling, "useless," she often took an early lunch break around 11 a.m., during which she would take a 1-hour nap in her car while parked in the lot of a local fast food restaurant. After returning to work around noon, she felt some improvement in energy level and productivity, but would have to stay at work until 10 p.m. on most nights to catch up on the day's activities. She felt she got more work done after her co-workers went home for the day.

Cathy's day ended with her arriving home around 11 p.m. She stated that her preference would be to go directly to bed. Yet, despite her desire to fall asleep between 11 p.m. and midnight, she typically found herself surfing the Internet or watching TV before finally going to sleep between 2 and 3 a.m. She denied feeling worried, nervous, or anxious and stated that she just didn't feel tired at that time of the night.

On weekends, when free of work responsibilities, she would fall asleep at the same time, but she tended to sleep until the late morning, if not the early afternoon. On these days she felt a bit more awake.

Cathy's daytime sleepiness had been present for at least 4 years but she denied sleep paralysis or hallucinations, cataplexy, snoring, witnessed apneas, bruxism, restless legs, limb movements, and parasomnias. Her primary care physician performed an extensive evaluation including labs and imaging to rule out infectious etiologies, multiple sclerosis, epilepsy, anemia, and endocrine disorders—the workup was normal. Trials of modafinil (Provigil), dextroamphetamine (Adderall), and methylphenidates (Ritalin XL, Concerta) did not improve her sleepiness.

The past medical history was significant for migraines (resolved at the time of her sleep presentation) and seasonal allergies. She had had a tonsillectomy and adenoidectomy due to recurrent streptococcal infections in childhood. She denied use of tobacco, alcohol, or illicit drugs and had no family history of sleep disorders.

Review of systems was negative, including for symptoms of depression and thyroid problems. At the time of her evaluation, her Epworth Sleepiness Scale (ESS) score was 21/24 indicating severe EDS.

Physical Examination

The vital signs were unremarkable including a BMI of $24.1 \, kg/m^2$ and neck size of 14 inches. Her general physical exam was also unrevealing including a Friedman Grade 1 tongue position, Her neurologic examination was normal.

Evaluation

Cathy brought a completed sleep log to her first sleep center appointment (Figure 31.1). Given her history and sleep log findings suggesting both delayed sleep and wake times, Cathy was advised to wear an actigraph for 2 weeks (a noninvasive method of monitoring rest/activity cycles). She understood this was an objective attempt to better understand her sleep-wake cycle and confirm her own observations. The actigraph tracing confirmed her history (Figure 31.2).

Diagnosis

Circadian rhythm sleep disorder, delayed sleep phase type.

Outcome

The goal of Cathy's treatment was to advance her sleep times such that she would go to sleep by 11 p.m. and in turn be able to wake by 7 a.m. This would

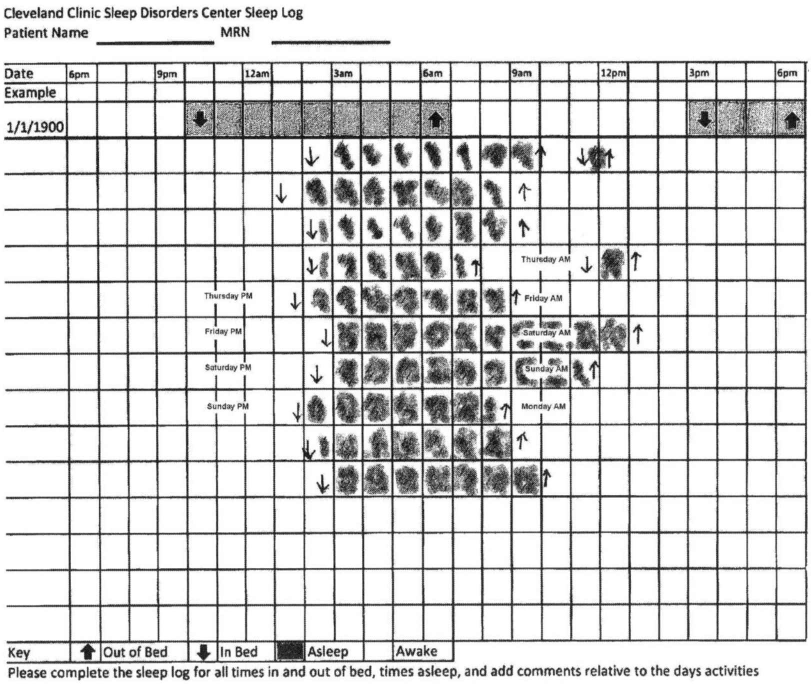

Cleveland Clinic Sleep Disorders Center Sleep Log
Patient Name _____ MRN _____

Figure 31.1 Sleep log shows a typical sleep time of approximately 2 a.m. and a wake time of 9 a.m., longer on the weekends. The patient brought this to the initial visit. The sleep log record began on a Sunday and continued for 10 days.

continue to provide for approximately 8 hours of sleep per night, and also allow her to be more awake in the morning hours, increasing her work productivity and improving her overall daytime functioning.

Treatment options included chronotherapy, a behavioral technique in which the patient's bedtime is systematically delayed, which follows the natural tendencies of human biology. However chronotherapy is difficult to implement as it takes several days and sometimes weeks to complete, and the possibility of quickly reverting back to a delayed sleep phase pattern is high. It also results in patients having varying sleep and wake times during the therapy itself that can interfere with their daytime/social activities.

Instead, the following treatments were initiated:

(1) Exogenous melatonin (1 mg) which was to be taken at 7 p.m. nightly or 4 to 5 hours prior to Cathy's goal sleep onset time of 11 p.m.
(2) Bright light (10,000 lux) or blue light therapy used in the morning hours for approximately 30 minutes each day.

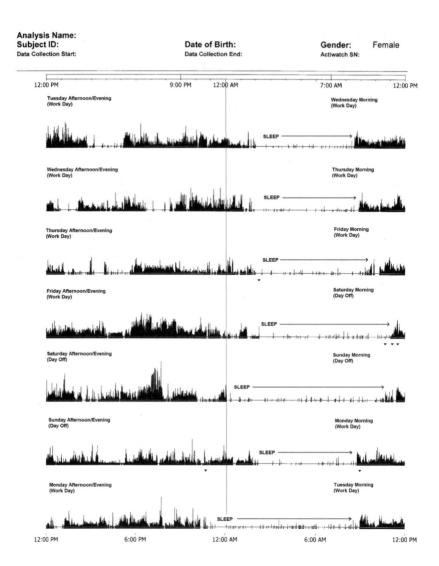

Analysis Name:
Subject ID: Date of Birth: Gender: Female
Data Collection Start: Data Collection End: Actiwatch SN:

Figure 31.2 The actigraph tracing confirms the patient history. The typical sleep time is 2 a.m. and wake time is 9 a.m. Although the sleep log and actigraph were recorded at different times, the sleep-wake pattern is consistently delayed.

(3) Behavioral changes including:

Waking up at the same time daily

Increasing daylight exposure in the morning (opening blinds/curtains/windows and bright light treatment upon waking). It should be noted that individuals with delayed sleep phase type circadian disorder will typically describe their bedrooms as dark, as they make attempts to eliminate any signs of morning sunlight (to the extreme of hanging dark garbage bags over the windows)

Decreasing light exposure at night (not working in brightly lit environments, trying to reduce room lighting to 60 watts);

Modifications to improve sleep hygiene such as avoiding caffeinated products, alcohol, sleeping pills, and nicotine, that can adversely affect sleep quality; maintaining a cool, quiet, and comfortable bedroom; and avoiding activities before bedtime that are stimulating, such as exercise, computer games, and TV.

Cathy was seen in again in the sleep clinic approximately 45 days following initiation of therapy. She reported having an easier time waking in the morning, using only one alarm clock and waking at 7 a.m. daily. She found herself to be more productive at work, and was now leaving work by 6 p.m. nightly. While her social schedule did not always allow her to be home by her desired sleep onset time of 11 p.m., she was now typically falling asleep by midnight. Perhaps most impressive was the improvement in her ESS, which was decreased to 7/24.

Discussion

Daytime sleepiness can be due to various etiologies: central hypersomnia, obstructive sleep apnea, sleep deprivation, etc. (discussed in detail in Chapter 30). In Cathy's case, sleepiness, by history, was more prominent during the morning hours and was not persistent throughout the day. She became more productive at work during the late afternoon and evening hours and even had difficulties falling asleep at night (sleep onset insomnia). Her history, sleep logs, and actigraphy supported the diagnosis of a circadian abnormality—delayed sleep phase type (Table 31.1).

Actigraphy is a useful means by which delayed sleep phase type and other circadian abnormalities can be objectively identified. Actigraphy is a noninvasive method of monitoring rest/activity cycles using a wrist watch-type device worn on the wrist of their nondominant arm, or another extremity, including a leg. Within the device is a sensor (accelerometer) which measures gross motor activity. Actigraphs are useful for determining sleep-wake patterns over extended periods of time, often for 1 to 2 weeks. Actigraphy can also be used in the evaluation of insomnia and sleep related movement disorders such as restless legs syndrome, and to objectively assess the effectiveness of pharmacologic, behavioral, phototherapy, and chronotherapy when treating a circadian disorder. Additional features include: (1) user input: the patient presses a button on the device to indicate a specific event (lights out at bedtime, waking in the morning), and (2) sensors that allow for monitoring of environmental factors (temperature, ambient light).

Table 31.1 ICSD-2 diagnostic criteria for delayed sleep phase disorder

A. There is a delay in the phase of the major sleep period in relation to the desired sleep time and wake-up time, as evidenced by a chronic or recurrent complaint of inability to fall asleep at a desired conventional clock time together with the inability to awaken at a desired and socially acceptable time.

B. When allowed to choose their preferred schedule, patients will exhibit normal sleep quality and duration for age and maintain a delayed, but stable phase of entrainment to the 24-hour sleep-wake pattern.

C. Sleep log or actigraphy monitoring (including sleep diary) for at least 7 days demonstrates a stable delay in the timing of the habitual sleep period.*

D. The sleep disturbance is not better explained by another current sleep disorder, medical or neurological disorder, mental disorder, medication use, or substance use disorder.

*Note: In addition, a delay in the timing of other circadian rhythms, such as the nadir of the core body temperature rhythm or dim-light melatonin onset (DLMO) is useful for the confirmation of the delayed phase.

Chosen Treatment Options

Light Therapy Early-morning exposure to bright light tends to lead to alertness in the mornings and advanced sleep onset at night; it does so by manipulating the timing and levels of endogenous melatonin. When ganglion cells lining the retina that contain the pigment melanopsin are exposed to light, a neural signal is sent via the retinohypothalamic pathway to the suprachiasmatic nucleus, which in turn inhibits the release of endogenous melatonin. Environmental light may be inadequate, especially during the winter months. Thus, artificial light is used to consistently expose patients with delayed sleep phase type to light early in the morning. This morning light in turn manipulates the timing and levels of melatonin. In those with delayed sleep phase, the onset and offset of melatonin levels are delayed, and exposure to bright light in the morning helps to restore the appropriate onset and offset of melatonin. Studies have supported the use of bright light boxes that emit approximately 10,000 lux of white light. There is also data to support blue-light therapy (light in the spectrum range of approximately 480 nm). Modern light therapy should not emit ultraviolet radiation; confirmation with the light manufacturer is recommended. In most cases, the patient sits in front of the light at a specified distance for approximately 30 to 60 minutes in the morning. The exact timing of light therapy should be based on the patient's minimum body temperature, which can be determined by sleep history, sleep logs, or actigraphy. The minimum body temperature occurs approximately 3 hours before the patient's preferred wake time (usually weekend wake times are best as the patient has no morning responsibilities).

Bright-light therapy administered after the time of minimum body temperature will advance both sleep and wake times, while that administered before will result in their delay. While bright-light therapy can advance the patient's sleep-wake times when used in the morning, it needs to be avoided during the evening and at night, when it acts to delay sleep-wake times.

Exogenous Melatonin   Melatonin is secreted by the pineal gland, and it drives an individual to sleep. Secretion occurs when it is dark and is suppressed by exposure to light. The use of exogenous melatonin can regulate sleep and help promote sleep onset. A series of studies supports the use of melatonin in treating delayed sleep phase disorder. Studies indicate that the time of melatonin administration is critical to its efficacy (the earlier given, the more effective). Endogenous melatonin is released 3 to 4 hours prior to actual sleep onset. Thus, it is usually recommended that exogenous melatonin be given at least 3 to 4 hours before the goal time of sleep onset. There is no consensus regarding the dose of melatonin for delayed sleep phase syndrome, and while many prefer a lower dose (0.1 mg) some prefer a relatively higher dose (1 to 3 mg). The dose used in clinical research ranges from 0.1 to 3 mg. The doses most commonly found in retail stores include 1 and 3 mg. Synthetic melatonin is recommended to ensure consistency of ingredients. Melatonin is contraindicated in some medical conditions, including, but not limited to, autoimmune disorders, orthostatic intolerance, certain malignancies, and pregnancy. Some studies have also indicated worsening of mood disorders. Thus, a patient's past medical history needs be reviewed before initiating treatment. There is no consensus on the duration of melatonin therapy, although some recommend no longer than 6 months.

Bibliography

Morgenthaler T, Alessi C, Friedman L, et al. Practice parameters for the use of actigraphy in the assessment of sleep and sleep disorders: an update for 2007. *SLEEP*. 2007 Apr 1;30(4):519–529.

Mundey K, Benloucif S, Harsanyi, et al. Phase-dependent treatment of delayed sleep phase syndrome with melatonin. *SLEEP* 2005;28(10):1271–1278.

Weitzman ED, Czeisler CA, Coleman RM, et al. Delayed sleep phase syndrome: A chronobiological disorder with sleep-onset insomnia. *Arch Gen Psych*. 1981; 38(7):737–746.

32

A Machinist Who Could Not Take Shift Work Anymore

KUMAR BUDUR, MD, MS

Case History

Joe was a 36-year-old man who worked night shifts as a machinist for the past 3 months. He had held the same job but worked first shift for 4 years before going to nights. He did relatively well when he first went on nights, but over the past 2 months, he had noticed that it was getting increasingly difficult for him to stay awake at night and fall asleep during the day. He made an appointment at the sleep clinic because he did not want others to see him sleeping on the job and feared he might lose his job. Joe was a good employee and everyone at work liked him. However, in recent months, his supervisor brought to his attention some errors he had made assembling machine parts. Initially, Joe could not believe he was to blame, since he had done that step on the assembly line thousands of times over the years. Now, however, he was beginning to wonder if his supervisor was right. He had been feeling tired at work and sometimes felt so sleepy that he almost dozed off. He realized that it could be dangerous to fall asleep on the job. During his shift, he had an hour break from 2 to 3 a.m. During this time, he usually took a nap but did not feel refreshed afterwards. One month prior to presentation, he took a week off from work to rest and was able to sleep through the night for 7 hours, feeling well rested in the morning. When he returned to work, he asked his supervisor if he could get back on first or second shift, but his request was denied.

Joe worked 5 nights a week. His shift started at 11 p.m. and ended at 8 a.m. It typically took an hour to get home after work. He would eat breakfast and get to bed by 10 a.m. It took nearly an hour to fall asleep. He would typically wake up at 2 p.m., either spontaneously or from the phone ringing, and would have trouble falling back to sleep. He watched TV in bed and sometimes ate a snack.

He felt anxious and worried about not being able to go back to sleep, felt tense and nervous. He would also get angry and frustrated when he couldn't sleep and sometime even took a jog around the block hoping to get tired. On most days, he was able to go back to sleep in 60 to 90 minutes and get another 2 to 3 hours of sleep. He spent some time watching TV in the evening after he woke up and then would take a shower and eat dinner before heading off to work again at 10 p.m. He was single and had no children. On weekends, he would watch movies all night with his friends and sleep from 6 a.m. until midafternoon.

Joe denied medical or psychosocial stressors that could have contributed to his sleep problem. He did not snore and denied symptoms of restless legs, narcolepsy, and parasomnias. His medical history was significant for a right leg fracture 2 years prior, resulting from a fall on the job, and gastroesophageal reflux, which was controlled with lansaprozole. He took no other medications other than a multivitamin. There was no family history of significant medical, psychiatric, or sleep disorders. He did not smoke or use recreational drugs, though he drank 6 to 8 beers on Saturday and Sunday nights. He drank one cup of coffee every evening after dinner.

His Epworth Sleepiness Scale (ESS) score was 14 and his Fatigue Severity Scale (FSS) score was 55.

Physical Examination

Joe appeared tired during the assessment. His body mass index was 26.2 kg/m^2. The upper airway exam showed a Freidman tongue position Grade I. The remainder of his examination was unremarkable.

Evaluation

Joe maintained a sleep diary for 2 weeks that showed a sleep-wake pattern consistent with the history obtained in the sleep clinic (Figure 32.1).

Diagnoses

Circadian rhythm sleep disorder, shift work type.
Psychophysiological insomnia.

Outcome

Joe was diagnosed with shift work sleep disorder and psychophysiological insomnia. He was educated about the general principles of good sleep hygiene and

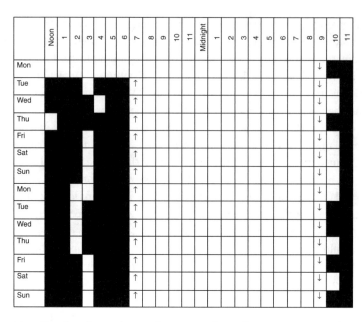

	Noon	1	2	3	4	5	6	7	8	9	10	11	Midnight	1	2	3	4	5	6	7	8	9	10	11

Figure 32.1 Sleep log shows sleep-wake pattern that is fairly consistent with the history of difficulty falling and maintaining sleep. Majority of the days it took him about 60 to 90 min to fall asleep after he went to bed. He is up for about 60 minutes after he woke up at 2 p.m. (but sometimes at 1 p.m.). His total sleep time averaged around 7 hours a day.

given the following recommendations in order to optimize the quality and quantity of sleep after working the night shift:(1) limit exposure to bright light/sunlight in the morning by wearing sunglasses on the drive home from work and limiting light exposure in the house, (2) take a warm bath prior to going to bed, (3) keep the bedroom dark by using heavy, lined curtains, (4) use an eye mask and ear plugs to reduce light and environmental noises, (5) keep the bedroom temperature cool (65–68°F), and (6) establish sleep rules with family and friends so as to minimize disturbances.

He was also told to avoid operating machinery and driving when drowsy and to use his break time at work to nap when sleepy. He agreed to try these recommendations and return for a follow-up visit in 6 weeks. At his next visit, he reported that he had complied with most of the recommendations. He was able to make the room darker and minimize interruptions during the day by friends. He was sleeping for 7 to 8 hours with fewer awakenings during the day. However, he continued to feel tired and sleepy at work and routinely took a 30-minute nap most nights. He worried he might lose his job due to persistent suggestions by his supervisor that the quality of his work was slipping. As a result, he was prescribed modafinil 200 mg to be taken an hour before the start of his shift. When he returned 4 weeks later, he reported a marked improvement in alertness on the job and had taken a nap during his break no more than 3 times the entire month since his last visit. He tolerated the medication and had no trouble falling asleep in the morning. Even his supervisor noticed that things had improved. His ESS and FSS scores were 5 and 11 respectively, both within normal limits.

Discussion

Joe met all the ICSD-2 criteria for shift work sleep disorder (Table 32.1). In addition, he also had symptoms of psychophysiological insomnia such as inability to go back to sleep with associated anxiety and frustration suggestive of hypearousability and some conditioned difficulty with going back to sleep. Although psychophysiological insomnia contributed to some of the symptoms, it is unlikely to account for all of the problems Joe was experiencing. Other diagnostic considerations included behaviorally induced insufficient sleep syndrome, psychophysiological insomnia, and idiopathic insomnia. Behaviorally induced insufficient sleep syndrome was unlikely, because it appeared that he was able to get about 7 hours of sleep on most days and he functioned well with similar number of hours of sleep in the past. The fact that Joe felt refreshed and functioned well until 3 months prior, and experienced an improvement in sleepiness over a recent vacation, made idiopathic hypersomnia unlikely.

Circadian rhythm sleep disorder, shift work type, or shift work sleep disorder, is thought to affect about 10%–20% of shift workers. Shift work is becoming increasingly common due to the growth of the service industry, advancements in the information technology, and globalization of the economy. It is estimated that about 1 in 5 employed Americans work mostly during the evenings, nights, or on rotating or highly variable schedules.

Shift work is associated with a variety of challenges resulting from the complex interaction of circadian desynchronization (fatigue, poor concentration, impaired digestion); sleep factors (sleep deprivation, difficulty falling/staying

---

Table 32.1 ICSD-2 criteria for circadian rhythm sleep disorder, shift work type

A. There is a complaint of insomnia or excessive sleepiness that is temporally associated with a recurrent work schedule that overlaps the usual time for sleep.
B. The symptoms are associated with the shift-work schedule over the course of at least 1 month.
C. Sleep log or actigraphy monitoring (with sleep diaries) for at least 7 days demonstrates disturbed circadian and sleep-time misalignment.
D. The sleep disturbance is not better explained by another sleep disorder, medical or neurological disorder, mental disorder, medication use, or substance use disorder.

---

asleep, excessive sleepiness); and social factors (marital issues, child care, relationship and intimacy problems). Many shift workers experience a constant struggle to maintain sleep and wake when they are out of sync with the innate circadian rhythm. This is in contrast to jet lag, in which the body usually synchronizes with the new time zone within a few days. In normal individuals, core body temperature starts to decline at around 9 p.m. and reaches a nadir at 5 to 6 a.m., then gradually increasing. The level of alertness follows the core body temperature rhythm, resulting in a gradual decline in alertness at night and increasing alertness during the day (Figure 32.2). Night shift workers have to work against these internal rhythms. As core body temperature and alertness decline, they must be maximally alert and as the level of alertness and core body temperature begin to rise, they need to go to sleep.

Although about 20% of the working population is employed in shift work, only a fraction (10%–20%) of them are affected by shift work sleep disorder. Risk factors for shift work sleep disorder include age greater than 50 years, a history of sleep or gastrointestinal disorders, alcohol or substance abuse, heavy domestic workload, holding multiple jobs, and chronic medical problems such as epilepsy, diabetes, or cardiac problems. Similarly, there are certain factors associated with the work environment that can increase the likelihood of shift work sleep disorder. These include working more than 5 third shifts in a row or more than four 12-hour shifts in a row; weekly rotations; backward rotations; and 12-hour shifts involving critical monitoring tasks or heavy physical tasks.

Shift workers should be educated about the strategies shown to be helpful in mitigating the effects of shift work. Of paramount importance is to get adequate

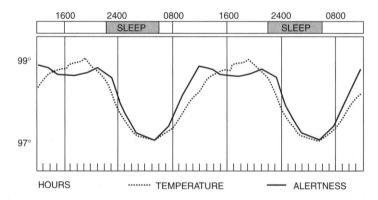

Figure 32.2 Circadian rhythm of core body temperature and alertness. Time (00:00 to 24:00 h) on X-axis and temperature (in Fahrenheit) on Y-axis. Note that the core body temperature decreases gradually as the night progresses and the level alertness also falls, closely following the core body temperature levels. During the daytime, the core body temperature increases and so does the level of alertness. The lowest point of alertness is around 4 to 6 a.m.

sleep before a night shift so that the individual does not start a shift in a sleep deprived state. Adequate sleep can be ensured by avoiding bright light exposure before going to sleep; keeping the bed room dark, quite and cool; eating adequately; and taking a warm bath before going to sleep. Most patients find it useful to inform friends and family not to disturb them during the major sleep period. Similarly, alertness at night can be optimized by a bright and well-lit workplace, napping during break time, and use of moderate amounts of caffeine. Preserving occupational and driving safety is of utmost importance. Shift work also has implications for relationships and personal commitments. It helps for shift workers to develop a plan to ensure adequate time for family and social activities.

Modafinil is the only medication approved by the U.S. Food and Drug Administration for shift work sleep disorder. It is a wake-promoting agent that is usually administered at a dose of 200 mg before the night shift. In clinical trials, modafinil 200 mg resulted in improvement from baseline in mean ($\pm$SEM) night-time sleep latency (SL: time from lights-off to sleep onset) compared to placebo (1.7 ± 0.4 vs. 0.3 ± 0.3 minutes; $P = 0.002$), and a fewer number of patients on modafinil reported accidents or near-accidents while commuting home compared to those who were on placebo (29% vs. 54%; $p < 0.001$). In addition, patients on modafinil felt better symptomatically, and it did not affect their ability to sleep during the day. It is important to note that although a statistically significant improvement in wakefulness was noted with modafinil compared to placebo, subjects on modafinil were still sleepy (mean sleep latency of 3.8 minutes on modafinil 200 mg compared to 2.1 minutes at baseline). Sometimes hypnotics are prescribed for a short duration, if difficulty falling and/or staying asleep during the day is a major problem. However, hypnotic medications for shift work sleep disorder are not well studied and their utility is not well established.

Bibliography

Costa G. Shift work and occupational medicine: an overview. *Occupl Med.* 2003; 53:83–88.

Czeisler CA, Walsh JK, Roth T, Hughes RJ, et al. Modafinil for excessive sleepiness associated with shift-work sleep disorder. *NEJM.* 2005;353:476–486.

33

Why Humans Don't Have Wings

WILLIAM NOVAK, MD

Case History

Jim, a 38-year-old business executive, complained of difficulties falling asleep at night and excessive daytime sleepiness (EDS). Jim was not new to the sleep disorders center. He was first seen 2 years prior for the same concerns. He underwent an overnight polysomnogram (PSG) and was diagnosed with moderate obstructive sleep apnea syndrome (OSAS), for which he was prescribed continuous positive airway pressure (CPAP) therapy based upon an overnight titration study. He was compliant with therapy and doing well until 3 to 4 months prior to presentation, when his symptoms recurred. Since his sleep testing, Jim had no changes with regard to his medical history or medications. He had hypertension and had taken a diuretic for several years. He had no significant weight change and denied snoring, gasping, or choking in sleep using CPAP. He denied sleep related anxiety and rumination about sleep loss, an urge to move his legs, or discomforts suggestive of restless legs syndrome, leg jerks at night, cataplexy, sleep paralysis, sleep related hallucinations, and abnormal behaviors in sleep. He did not use caffeine, alcohol, or illicit drugs.

What had changed since Jim's last evaluation were his responsibilities at work. While his hours, from 9 a.m. to 5 p.m., were the same, his job now entailed travel from Cleveland, Ohio to the West Coast of the United States once per week, where he would spend 2 days and 1 or 2 nights. He had been making these trips for the past 4 months, about the same duration as his relapsing sleep symptoms. On further reflection, he thought the insomnia and daytime sleepiness were worse when he was home. When he traveled to the West Coast, he was able to fall asleep by 11 p.m. Pacific Time (3 hours behind Eastern Time), and he did not feel tired in the morning when he woke up at 8 a.m. At home, however, he rarely found himself falling asleep by midnight and longed to sleep until the late morning hours. After about the fourth consecutive night at home, his sleep seemed to improve—he was able to get to sleep a bit earlier and was more awake the next day. However, before long, he was back on the runway, heading out west again. He scored 17/24 on the Epworth Sleepiness Scale (ESS) at the time of his initial visit, 2 days after returning from the West Coast. He wondered whether he should take a sleeping pill at night or a stimulant during the day like so many of his fellow travelers were doing.

Physical Examination

Jim had a body mass index of 29.3 kg/m^2, pulse of 74, and blood pressure of 132/68 mmHg. His upper airway examination revealed a Friedman tongue position Grade III. His neck circumference was 17.5 inches. The physical and neurological examinations were otherwise unremarkable.

Diagnoses

Circadian rhythm sleep disorder: jet lag type.
Obstructive sleep apnea.

Outcome

Jim was diagnosed with jet lag disorder. The goal of treatment was to maintain synchronization of the internal sleep-wake cycle with his ever-changing external cues. Making this somewhat difficult was the frequency of time zone changes per week (east to west to east, with a time difference of 3 hours). It was recommended that Jim make the following behavioral changes:

(1) During his time on the West Coast, if outside, he should wear sunglasses with side shields to limit daylight exposure after 4 p.m. Pacific Time (corresponding to 7 p.m. back home). The goal of this recommendation was to avoid daylight exposure, which could result in a delay of his sleep-wake cycle when back home. It was also recommended that he keep the blinds down and curtains closed in his office and hotel room during these hours.
(2) When on the West Coast, he was to set his alarm for 5 a.m. Pacific Time in an attempt to maintain his 8 a.m. Eastern Time usual wake-up time.
(3) When on the West Coast, and when possible at home, he was to try and maintain his home sleep time by going to bed no later than 8 p.m. Pacific Time.

(4) He was to use light therapy (10,000 Lux for 30 minutes) at home and during travel. However, when on the West Coast, he was advised to use it no later than 6 a.m. Pacific Time, the equivalent of his 9 a.m. home use.

(5) He was instructed to avoid naps on the airplane and after arriving at his destination.

(6) He was to use melatonin 1 mg at 4 p.m. Pacific time on the West Coast and 7 p.m. Eastern Time when returning home. He would take this daily as long as he continued to travel cross-country (multiple time zones) on a regular basis.

Approximately 30 days later, at his return office visit, Jim reported a significant improvement in symptoms. On the West Coast, he was in bed by 8 to 8:30 p.m. and asleep by 9 p.m. Pacific Time. At home on the East Coast, even on the night after returning home, he was able to fall asleep by 10 to 11 p.m. and wake up at 7 to 8 am without difficulty. While he felt taking melatonin daily was an inconvenience, he recognized this was much preferred to being awake all night and sleepy all day. His ESS score was 7/24.

Discussion

Jet lag is a temporary condition that some people experience following travel across several time zones in a short period. The result is that the traveler's internal clock becomes "out of synch" with the external environment. Thus, he has a difficult time maintaining his typical sleep-wake cycle in the new location. Actual changes in environmental entraining factors, such as the time of day and amount of daylight exposure, along with local time schedules, result in a desynchronization of the sleep-wake cycle. Symptoms of jet lag disorder include insomnia, daytime sleepiness and fatigue, headaches, changes in mood, decreased mental performance, and autonomic symptoms such as gastrointestinal irritability. Key to the diagnosis is the complaint of insomnia or EDS associated with transmeridian travel across at least 2 time zones (Table 33.1).

Table 33.1 ICSD-2 diagnostic criteria for circadian rhythm sleep disorder, jet lag type

A. There is a complaint of insomnia or excessive daytime sleepiness associated with transmeridian jet travel across at least 2 time zones.
B. There is associated impairment of daytime function, general malaise, and symptoms such as gastrointestinal disturbance within 1 to 2 days after travel.
C. The sleep disturbance is not better explained by another current sleep disorder, medical or neurological disorder, mental disorder, medication use, or substance abuse disorder.

The degree of circadian disruption typically is dependent on the number and rapidity of time zone changes. It is also dependent on the individual's own ability to adapt, with some reporting relatively little if any sleep disruption and others, like Jim, having significant symptoms. Patients with circadian rhythm disorders are at risk for jet lag syndrome, likely due to abnormal endogenous circadian cycles or responses to light cues.

Symptoms of jet lag are usually worse when traveling west to east rather than east to west, as it is easier for most individuals to delay the sleep-wake cycle than to advance it. For most individuals, advancement in the sleep-wake cycle occurs at about 1 to 1.5 hours per day, while delay is about 2 hours per day. For this reason, Jim had little difficulty on the West Coast. However, upon returning home to the East Coast, it would take several days before his sleep-wake cycle normalized.

When treating jet lag, an attempt is made to adapt to the new time zone as soon as possible. If, as in Jim's case, one is in the new time zone for a short period of time (1 to 2 days), an attempt should be made to maintain the predominant sleep-wake cycle (making adaptations to the new time zone's environment to make it similar to that of the patient's normal sleep-wake cycle at home). While the time of flight and naps may help the individual better adjust to time zone changes, these are rarely options for business travelers. Likewise, flight options are often limited, and transportation delays make it hard to plan ahead for jet lag. Some individuals have successfully minimized the effects of jet lag by preparing themselves for the new sleep-wake schedule, especially when traveling across multiple time zones. These individuals advance or delay the sleep-wake cycles gradually over a period of several days prior to travel. For the reasons mentioned above, these measures are not always successful or practical.

The use of melatonin in jet lag is not well established, with some finding it helpful while others have shown no benefit. The benefits of melatonin are likely derived by its sleep-promoting properties. The timing of melatonin administration is thought to be more important than the dose – as in this case, 1 mg of melatonin 3 to 4 hours prior to the goal bedtime may hasten the adjustment of the sleep-wake cycle.

In cases in which individuals are frequently flying back and forth between the West and East Coasts, or if only on one coast for 1 to 2 days maximum, treatment should focus on circadian and environmental adaptation to maintain the individuals home sleep-wake cycle. This includes behavioral changes that prevent entraining factors such as light from adjusting the circadian rhythm: avoiding light when it would otherwise be dark at home by means of blinds, curtains, and sunglasses; and use of light therapy in an attempt to simulate the daylight hours of home when it is otherwise dark in the new time zone.

While treatment for jet lag disorder can be frustrating, as it takes effort on the traveler's part, those who comply—like Jim—are pleased with the results. Each case of jet lag disorder will be unique with respect to frequency and number of time zone changes, and symptom severity. The treatment must be customized to the individual.

Bibliography

Arendt J, Stone B, Skene D. Jet lag and sleep disruption. In: Kryger MH, Roth T, Dement WC., eds. *Principles and Practice of Sleep Medicine*. 3rd ed. Philadelphia, PA: WB Saunders;2000:591–599.

Haimov I, Arendt J. The prevention and treatment of jet lag. *Sleep Med Rev.* 1999;3:229–240.

34

The Case of Hobbling José

ASIM ROY, MD
SILVIA NEME-MERCANTE, MD
NANCY FOLDVARY-SCHAEFER, DO

Case History

José was a 35-year-old, right-handed Hispanic man who presented to the sleep clinic with his wife reporting violent behaviors in sleep for 15 years following his immigration to the United States. At 11:30 p.m. one night 2 months prior to presentation, José jumped from his third-storey bedroom window, fracturing both his legs. He vaguely recalled thinking he was escaping a house fire. Fortunately, he didn't "rescue" his 3-year-old son, who was sleeping soundly in an adjacent room, although apparently he had tried to do so. Instead of grabbing the boy, he had tossed a bedside lamp out the window before taking the plunge. He thought he must have mistaken the lamp for his son, who normally shared the bed with him and his wife. After the fall, he required surgery to stabilize a right femoral fracture and was transferred to a rehabilitation facility. One night when he was admitted, he had an altercation with an attendant as he wandered outside his room asleep. He was wrestled to the ground after it appeared that he was trying to choke the attendant. This prompted transfer to a psychiatric ward, where he was evaluated and discharged a few days later without further treatment. He was noticeably shaken when recounting these events.

José's broken legs were a wake-up call to his wife, who insisted he finally seek medical attention. During his initial visit, the couple recalled numerous examples of abnormal, threatening, and dangerous night behaviors, including several occasions on which he "attacked" his wife as she tried to coax him back to bed. Once, while dreaming that 3 men carrying knives were chasing him, he grabbed a razor blade and awoke to hear his wife screaming as he held it against her neck. He had less dramatic episodes 2 to 3 times per week in which he would wander outside his bedroom asleep or wake up confused, typically within a couple hours of sleep onset but, rarely, as late as 4 a.m. José's mother first observed this behavior in his early childhood, but episodes were infrequent, occurring once or twice per year and never resulting in injury. By his late teens, they had increased in frequency and were sometimes associated with a bad dream. He generally would not respond during episodes and had little to no recollection of what had transpired.

José's sleep history was otherwise relatively unremarkable. He would go to bed at 9:30 p.m. and wake up at 7:30 a.m., usually feeling refreshed. He had mild daytime sleepiness that he attributed to medications. He snored a bit, but his wife had never witnessed apneic episodes. He denied sleep paralysis, hypnagogic hallucinations, cataplexy, or leg restlessness at night.

Review of his medical history revealed normal birth and development. José had had a single febrile seizure, at 3 years of age, and several concussions in his teenage years, none with loss of consciousness. He had been diagnosed with depression several years prior to presentation and was taking quetiapine and nefazodone with relatively good control. As a young adult, he abused alcohol and drugs, but he had been free of all substance use for several years. His older son had nightmares in childhood and had wandered around the house in sleep on 1 or 2 occasions.

Physical Examination

On examination, José had a blood pressure of 128/76 mmHg, heart rate of 72 bpm, respiratory rate of 14 breaths/minute, and a body mass index of 25 kg/m^2. The upper airway examination revealed mild turbinate hypertrophy, Grade I tonsils and Grade II Friedman tongue position. The general and neurological examinations were normal, with the exception of mild pitting edema of the distal left lower extremity and a cast on the right leg. He hobbled with a single crutch under his right arm.

Evaluation

A polysomnogram (PSG) with video and expanded EEG was performed. There was no evidence of sleep apnea or periodic limb movements, although snoring was recorded. He slept for 284 minutes, resulting in a sleep efficiency of 68%. The majority of sleep consisted of Stages N1 and N2, with only a few minutes of REM and N3 sleep, punctuated by frequent arousals and awakenings. No abnormal behaviors were observed, and no epileptiform discharges or seizure patterns were recorded.

Due to persistent disruptive night behaviors despite treatment, long-term video EEG (VEEG) monitoring was performed for 5 days in the epilepsy monitoring unit. The waking EEG showed a background rhythm of 9 Hz and intermittent generalized slow activity was observed. Sleep structures were symmetric. While muscle tone was normal in REM sleep, arousals from slow-wave sleep were observed, one associated with clinical arousal and mumbling without ambulation. The evaluation failed to reveal any evidence of epilepsy.

Diagnoses

Disorder of arousal during NREM sleep–sleepwalking and confusional arousals. Primary snoring.
Depression.

Outcome

José and his wife were informed of the importance of securing a safe sleep environment for patients with sleepwalking and other types of arousal disorders. This included alerting devices, like alarms or bells on doors, so that the family would awaken should José wander in his sleep, and locks on windows on the upper levels of their home. In addition, they were advised to secure knives, razors, and other potentially dangerous items. He was reminded to avoid alcohol and recreational drugs and to maintain healthy sleep patterns so as to minimize sleep deprivation. He was advised to sleep on the ground floor if possible, and he began to sleep in the family's spare bedroom. Given concerns regarding his substance abuse history and co-morbid depression, decision making for pharmacotherapy was undertaken in collaboration with José's psychiatrist and psychologist. Trials of several tricyclic antidepressants and benzodiazepines, including clonazepam, initially reduced the frequency and intensity of his night behaviors. However, the benefits waned with time. Antiepileptic drug trials with gabapentin and carbamazepine did not improve José's condition.

Due to the persistence of episodes and the history of a febrile seizure and closed head injuries, both risk factors for epilepsy, magnetic resonance imaging (MRI) of the brain was performed. This revealed a cystic lesion in the right inferior temporal region without enhancement, suggestive of a low-grade glioma (Figure 34.1). Despite the lack of epileptiform activity on EEG and a low suspicion of epilepsy, concerns regarding progression of the temporal tumor prompted a craniotomy and a right inferior temporal lesionectomy. The pathology revealed a dysembryoplastic neuroepithelial tumor, a lesion commonly associated with pharmacoresistant seizures. Not surprisingly, José's spells continued. But over the ensuing few years, optimization of depression management, stress reduction,

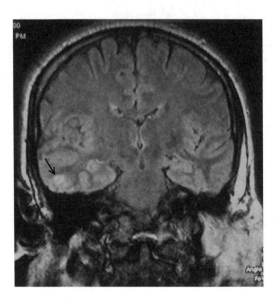

Figure 34.1 Coronal MRI of the brain at the level of the hippocampal body showing a circumscribed area of heterogeneous hyperintensity in the right inferior temporal gyrus (arrow) suggestive of a low-grade glioma. The lesion did not enhance on the gadolinium study. The pathology revealed a dysembryoplastic neuroepithelial tumor.

and strict adherence to good sleep hygiene and safety measures resulted in a marked decline in sleepwalking episodes. At his most recent follow-up visit, José and his wife were pleased to report that no dangerous or disturbing incidents had recurred.

Discussion

José's case illustrates the spectrum of complex behaviors seen in partial-arousal parasomnias characterized by abnormal behaviors associated with sudden partial arousal from slow-wave sleep. While classified as sleepwalking, sleep terrors, or confusional arousals for nosological purposes, these behaviors often co-exist in the same patient. José had frequent episodes of sleepwalking and confusional arousals that were usually uneventful. However, on occasion these were associated with dream enactment and vocalization, similar to that observed in REM sleep behavior disorder (RBD), raising concern about injury to himself and to those in his immediate surround. As in this case, most episodes of sleepwalking occur in the first third of the sleep period, when slow-wave sleep predominates (Tables 34.1 and 34.2). The frequency of sleepwalking episodes varies considerably from case to case, ranging from isolated, rare occurrences to multiple

Table 34.1 ICSD-2 diagnostic criteria for sleepwalking

A. Ambulation occurs during sleep.
B. Persistence of sleep, an altered state of consciousness, or impaired judgment during ambulation as demonstrated by at least 1 of the following:
    i. Difficulty in arousing the person.
    ii. Mental confusion when awakened from an episode.
    iii. Amnesia (complete or partial) for the episode.
    iv. Routine behaviors that occur at inappropriate times.
    v. Inappropriate or nonsensical behaviors.
    vi. Dangerous or potentially dangerous behaviors.
C. The disturbance is not better explained by another sleep disorder, medical or neurological disorder, mental disorder, medication use, or substance use disorder.

Table 34.2 ICSD-2 diagnostic criteria for confusional arousals

A. Recurrent mental confusion or confusional behavior occurs during an arousal or awakening from nocturnal sleep or a daytime nap.
B. The disturbance is not better explained by another sleep disorder, medical or neurological disorder, mental disorder, medication use, or substance use disorder.

episodes per night. Events may cluster for several nights, followed by remission for weeks to months. Sleepwalking and confusional arousals are commonly precipitated by sleep deprivation, emotional or physical stress, fever, co-morbid psychiatric and neurological disorders, and medications (Table 34.3).

Sleepwalking is a common disorder, affecting roughly 15% of children and 4% of adults, with peak prevalence between ages 8 and 12. In the majority of cases, sleepwalking and confusional arousals begin in the first decade of life and remit spontaneously in late childhood or adolescence, although onset in adulthood does occur. Childhood-onset sleepwalking continues into adulthood in about 20% of cases. Sleepwalking has a strong genetic predisposition, increasing in relation to the number of affected parents.

The differential diagnosis of abnormal sleep related behaviors without awareness or with partial awareness includes the NREM arousal disorders, RBD, epileptic seizures, sleep related dissociative disorder, sleep apnea syndromes with recurrent arousals, confusion and automatic behavior, and malingering. Among 100 consecutive adults with repeated sleep related injury investigated with PSG, sleepwalking/sleep terrors and RBD were the most common diagnoses, reported in 54 and 36 cases, respectively. The diagnosis of dissociative disorder was made in 7 cases, with the remainder representing nocturnal seizures (N = 2) and sleep apnea (N = 1).

Table 34.3 Precipitants of sleepwalking and disordered arousals

Sleep deprivation
Sleeping in unfamiliar environments
Physical/emotional stress
Febrile illnesses
Bladder distention
Environmental stimuli (light, noise)
Primary sleep disorders (sleep apnea, restless legs syndrome)
Hyperthyroidism
Psychiatric disorders (depression, anxiety, bipolar disorder)
Co-morbid neurologic disorders (migraine, stroke, encephalitis, head injury)
Alcohol or substance use
Drugs (phenothiazines, lithium carbonate, anticholinergic agents, sedative hypnotics, antihistamines, anticonvulsants)

The differentiation of seizures and parasomnias is challenging, due to the overlapping features of nocturnal frontal lobe epilepsy (FLE) and disorders of arousal, shared precipitating factors, and limitations of scalp EEG. Seizures arising from deep or midline structures, such as the mesial frontal and orbitofrontal regions, are often brief in duration and characterized by large, repetitive proximal movements (hypermotor activity) obscuring the EEG recording. Even in the absence of excessive muscle artifact, the ictal EEG (EEG recording during the seizure) in FLE often fails to demonstrate a localized or lateralized ictal pattern, and the interictal EEG (EEG recording in the seizure free period) is often normal or shows epileptiform discharges that appear widespread due to rapid propagation to the contralateral hemisphere. As a result, the clinical manifestations, frequency of episodes, pattern of occurrence and state from which episodes emerge, particularly in combination with video analysis of a typical event, are often more useful than the EEG. In contrast to parasomnias, seizures are stereotyped, each episode exhibiting similar, if not identical, behavioral features, often consisting of dyskinetic, dystonic, or tonic movements. Seizures are usually abrupt in onset and offset, usually less than 1 minute in duration, and can emerge from any sleep stage, most commonly during sleep-wake transitions or light NREM sleep. Frontal lobe seizures tend to have a higher frequency than sleepwalking and confusional arousals, often occurring in clusters multiple times per night.

The Frontal Lobe Epilepsy and Parasomnias (FLEP) Scale has been proposed as an adjunct to the clinical history and laboratory testing in the differentiation of frontal lobe seizures and parasomnias (Table 34.4). The FLEP scale has been shown to have high positive and negative predictive values, however, misdiagnosis can occur in as many as one-third of patients, especially in cases of RBD. A score of 0 or less is very unlikely to be seen in epilepsy, whereas, patients scoring 3 or greater generally have epilepsy. Additional testing including VEEG

Table 34.4 Frontal Lobe Epilepsy and Parasomnia (FLEP) Scale

Age at onset	< 55 y	0
	≥ 55 y	−1
Duration of a typical event	< 2 min	+1
	2–10 min	0
	10 min	−2
Typical no. events/night	1 or 2	0
	3–5	+1
	>5	+2
Time of night events occur	30 min of sleep onset	+1
	Other times	0
Definite aura	Yes	+2
	No	0
Wander outside bedroom	Yes	−2
	No (or uncertain)	0
Complex, directed behaviors	Yes	−2
	No (or uncertain)	0
Dystonic posturing, cramping, tonic limb extension	Yes	+1
	No (or uncertain)	0
Stereotypy of events	Highly stereotyped	+1
	Some variability/uncertain	0
	Highly variable	−1
Event recollection	Lucid recall	+1
	No or vague	0
Speech during event	No sounds/single words only	0
	Coherent with incomplete/no recall	−2
	Coherent with recall	+2

monitoring or PSG is generally necessary in borderline cases (scores of +1 to +3). José's FLEP score was −5 (−2 for wandering outside bedroom; −2 for complex, directed behaviors; and −1 for highly variable behaviors lacking stereotypy), supporting the diagnosis of an arousal disorder.

In José's case, the history of sleep related injury and risk of harm to his family posed by persistent episodes necessitated a swift and definitive diagnosis. Sleep apnea and nocturnal seizures were excluded by PSG and VEEG evaluations, and while he had experienced episodes of dream enactment, he did not have excessive sustained or phasic EMG activity in REM sleep, which would have supported the diagnosis of RBD. Consequently, parasomia overlap disorder, in which RBD and an arousal disorder co-exist in a given patient, was also excluded.

Given José's co-morbid depression, it was also important to exclude dissociative disorder and malingering. Sleep related dissociative disorders are characterized by disruption in the usually integrated functions of consciousness, memory, identity, or perception of the environment that occur during wakefulness in the transition to sleep or after awakening. Most affected individuals have dissociative episodes during the day and a history of severe psychiatric disturbances, including physical or sexual abuse, suicide attempts, major depression, and post traumatic stress disorder. Since José's depression had been well-controlled with medical therapy and a confusional arousal had been recorded during the VEEG evaluation, both dissociative disorder and malingering were felt to be unlikely. The clinical history and evaluation were most suggestive of a NREM arousal disorder.

In most cases, the diagnosis of disorders of arousal from NREM sleep is based on clinical history alone, and laboratory evaluation is not routinely indicated. However, PSG should be considered in patients with potentially injurious night behaviors or behaviors otherwise disruptive to the bed partner or household members. PSG should also be considered for cases with atypical features or features suggestive of nocturnal seizures, daytime consequences such as sleepiness, and failure to respond to appropriate therapy. In addition, PSG should be performed when co-morbid primary sleep disorders such as sleep apnea are suspected, the treatment of which may potentially reduce the frequency of episodes. The EEG during sleepwalking often shows a build-up of hypersynchronous, rhythmic delta or theta activity that may precede the behavioral arousal. Patients with arousal disorders may have slow-wave sleep arousals on PSG in the absence of abnormal behaviors. Sleep deprivation for 24 hours prior to testing has been shown to increase the yield of recording a typical episode. Conversely, a normal PSG does not rule out the diagnosis of an arousal disorder.

Seizure recognition during routine PSG is hindered by the limited number of channels dedicated to EEG, particularly in patients with frontal lobe seizures, which are most often confused with the arousal disorders. The detection of epileptiform activity in the sleep laboratory is greater with expanded EEG montages and video analysis. Therefore, to optimize the differentiation of seizures and parasomnias, the PSG montage should be expanded to include more extensive EEG and EMG monitoring in conjunction with high-quality video. Studies should be performed by technologists with skills in performing focused patient interviews at the time of the suspected event. They should also have experience in clinical and EEG seizure recognition. In José's case, routine PSG was combined with VEEG including the 21 electrodes of the International 10–20 Electrode System.

In the vast majority of cases, treatment of arousal disorders centers around maintaining a safe sleeping environment, free of dangerous or sharp objects. Doors and windows should be secured and glass windows covered with heavy draperies. Patients should avoid precipitating factors and maintain a regular sleep schedule so as to avoid sleep deprivation. It is important that family members are provided instruction on minimizing interactions with the patient during sleepwalking episodes, as attempts to wake the patient, especially when done forcefully, can trigger a violent, aggressive response. Treatment of co-morbid sleep and psychiatric disorders should be optimized. Stress reduction, psychotherapy, and hypnosis may be useful in select cases. For injurious or disruptive behavior, pharmacotherapy should be considered. There are no controlled trials investigating medications in the treatment of parasomnias. Benzodiazepines, most notably clonazepam, and antidepressants reduce the frequency and severity of episodes in some cases.

Bibliography

Derry CP, Davey M, Johns M, et al. Distinguishing sleep disorders from seizures: Diagnosing bumps in the night. *Arch Neurol.* 2006;63:705–709.

Foldvary-Schaefer N, De Ocampo J, Mascha E, Burgess R, Dinner D, Morris H. Accuracy of seizure detection using abbreviated EEG during polysomnography. *J Clin Neurophysiol.* 2006;23:68–71.

Schenck CH, Milner DM, Hurwitz TD, Bundlie SR, Mahowald MW. A polysomnographic and clinical report on sleep-related injury in 100 adult patients. *Am J Psych.* 1989; 146:1166–1173.

Schenck CH, Pareja JA, Patterson AL, Mahowald MW. Analysis of polysomnographic events surrounding 252 slow-wave sleep arousals in thirty-eight adults with injurious sleepwalking and sleep terrors. *JCNP.* 1998; 15(2):159–166.

Zucconi M, Ferini-Strambi L. NREM parasomnias: arousal disorders and differentiation from nocturnal frontal lobe epilepsy. *Clin Neurophysiol.*111, Suppl 2. 2000;S129.

35

Young, Terrified, and Does Not Even Know It!

ANNA IRWIN, MD

JYOTI KRISHNA, MD

Case History

Six-year old Jamie hated early mornings. When her mother dressed her for school, she cried and tried to sneak back to bed. In school, she was grouchy and sleepy. Starting at the age of 3, Jamie would wake up and scream at night. At first, these episodes occurred a few times per week, but then her bouts became more frequent. The timing of these episodes was fairly consistent. Almost every night around 1 a.m., Jamie screamed out and sat up in bed crying. She looked frightened, as if she had just seen a ghost. Her eyes were partially open, her breathing was labored, and she was covered with sweat. Sometimes she moved aimlessly around the bed and tugged on her blankets. She appeared to be confused and did not recognize her mother when she tried to comfort her. On occasion, she moved her mouth as if she were sucking on a popsicle. She was rarely awake enough to talk, and when being hugged, she did not hug back. Her crying subsided gradually and within 30 minutes Jamie returned to sleep. Once asleep, Jamie did not wake up again except for the occasional need to urinate, at which time she came to her mother's bedroom and asked for help. In the mornings, Jamie would not recall these episodes.

Jamie's mother had taken a job as a nurse aide at a local hospital one and a half years prior, causing Jamie to have an irregular sleep schedule. Second-shift duties rarely allowed mother to get home before 11 p.m., and it was Jamie's grandmother who usually put her to bed. Jamie's bedtime routine consisted of a nightly bath and a story time. Sometimes she was allowed to watch TV for 30 minutes before going to bed. Quite often, Jamie stayed up waiting for her mother, and because of this her bedtime varied between 9 and 11 p.m. When Jamie's grandmother was successful in putting her to bed early, it took her an average of 1.5 hours to fall asleep. Once in bed, Jamie got up a number of times to drink water, use the bathroom, or ask her grandmother whether she truly needed to go to school the next day. Once asleep, she did not exhibit any snoring, leg jerking, tongue biting, or bed-wetting behavior.

Jamie's wake-up time was 7 a.m., except for the weekends, when she was allowed to sleep as late as she wanted and usually did not wake up until 9 a.m. During the day, she complained of being sleepy and fell asleep in the car on the way to and from school. She was not allowed to drink any caffeinated beverages, but she did drink 8 oz of chocolate milk every evening. Jamie's parents had been separated for the past 3 years, and she enjoyed visiting her father every other weekend. Three nights per week, Jamie shared her bed with her younger stepsister, whom she adored and in whose presence Jamie seemed to sleep much better.

Jamie's medical history was remarkable for occasional constipation, ear infections, and mild asthma. She was delivered without complications at 40 weeks via C-section, weighing 9 lb, 7 oz. Her physical development had been normal, but her mother described her as being "slower" than her other children. Her teachers described her as a shy, quiet, and somewhat uninterested child, but denied any significant behavioral or academic problems. Jamie's mother had been struggling with bipolar disorder and obesity. Her father had obstructive sleep apnea (OSA). As a child, he had frequent episodes of sleepwalking that persisted into his adulthood, albeit infrequently.

Physical Examination

In the sleep clinic, Jamie was a pale, skinny, and painfully shy child who clung to her mother and did not speak with the examiner. Her vital signs and physical and neurological exams were normal. Specifically, her cranio-facial morphology was unremarkable, without evidence of retrognathia or nasal abnormality. Her tonsils were small without erythema or exudates. Her tongue was proportional to her mouth with a Friedman Grade I position.

Diagnoses

Sleep terrors.
Behavioral insomnia of childhood.

Outcome

Jamie was diagnosed with parasomnia disorder, most consistent with sleep terrors. The diagnosis was complicated by bedtime anxiety, as well as behavioral insomnia of childhood of the limit setting type. As a result of this visit, Jamie's mom was educated on sleep terrors and was reassured that this problem was unlikely to persist into adulthood. She was provided with a handout on healthy sleep habits. She was instructed on scheduling consistency with a goal of providing the child with enough sleep, which would be helpful in decreasing sleep terror episodes, and the importance that Jamie adhere to a bedtime routine. At first, her bedtime was set at 10:30 p.m. to ensure that she was adequately tired and likely to fall asleep quickly. When this was achieved, Jamie's bedtime was to be advanced by 15 minutes every few days until she was used to falling asleep at 9 p.m. or earlier. Jamie's wake-up time was to be maintained at around 7 a.m. regardless of the day of the week.

Since the frequency of sleep terrors was of concern and the timing of their occurrence fairly predictable, a trial of scheduled awakenings was recommended. Mother was to briefly wake Jamie up 15 to 30 minutes before the anticipated episode, and then allow her to resume sleep.

When Jamie was seen for a follow-up visit 8 weeks later, her mother reported a more alert child during the day. The terrors seemed to occur about 3 times per week rather then nightly. Her mother felt that sleep-scheduling consistency was particularly helpful, but she did not like scheduled awakenings, as she felt that they disrupted sleep for the entire family. Given her medical background, her mother expressed a desire to schedule Jamie for sleep testing. She worried the popsicle-sucking movements Jamie exhibited might be a sign of seizures. She also expressed an interest in her child attending psychotherapy sessions to address sleep related anxiety.

Two weeks later Jamie underwent a polysomnogram (PSG) with expanded electroencephalography (EEG) montage to rule out primary sleep disorders, such as OSA and nocturnal seizure activity. The study revealed multiple chewing episodes during stage N3 sleep followed by microarousals. In addition, she had an episode of crying emerging from stage N3 sleep during which Jamie sat up in bed for about 1 minute and was tachypneic and tachycardic. On respiratory monitoring, there was no significant breathing disorder noted. Her study was consistent with the diagnosis of sleep terrors. The EEG revealed no epileptiform activity (Figure 35.1).

Discussion

The clinical picture provided by Jamie's mother was consistent with the diagnosis of sleep terrors, also known as pavor nocturnus or night terrors (Table 35.1). The most prominent characteristic of sleep terrors is a sudden arousal from sleep that is associated with an intense yell or cry occurring in the first part of the night. Activation of sympathetic nervous system manifesting as tachycardia, tachypnea, diaphoresis, and mydriasis are common. Other characteristics

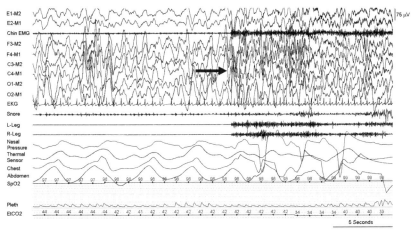

Figure 35.1 A 30-second polysomnogram tracing from the patient captured during a sleep terror. Note the abrupt arousal from Stage N3 (arrow) with no precipitating limb movement or respiratory event. Tachycardia (130 bpm) is evident during the arousal. The full EEG montage is not shown here for brevity (see text for discussion).

Table 35.1 ICSD-2 diagnostic criteria for sleep terrors

A. A sudden episode of terror occurs during sleep, usually initiated by a cry or loud scream that is accompanied with autonomic nervous system and behavioral manifestations of intense fear.

B. At least 1 of the following associated features is present:
   i.   Difficulty in arousing the person.
   ii. Mental confusion when awakened from an episode.
   iii. Amnesia (complete or partial) for the episode.
   iv. Dangerous or potentially dangerous behaviors.

C. The disturbance is not better explained by another sleep disorder, medical or neurological disorder, mental disorder, medication use, or substance use disorder.

include confusion through the entire episode, inconsolability, and poor recollection of the event the morning after. It is important to recognize that while these features are pathognomonic of childhood sleep terrors, they are not always true for adults. In fact, older patients can experience sleep terrors in any NREM stage of sleep, and patients can have fuzzy recollection of the event. Sleep terrors typically peak in the early elementary school ages and resolve by middle school age.

The differential diagnosis of sleep terrors is broad, including other NREM parasomnias, such as sleepwalking and confusional arousals (common in children), as well as REM sleep disorders, such as nightmares and REM sleep behavior disorder (very rare in children). Unlike in Jamie's case, nightmares tend to occur in the latter part of the night, are associated with the REM cycle, and are marked by vivid recollection of terrifying dreams. There is a lot of anxiety upon complete awakening that often follows the episode. Nightmares are not associated with much motor movement. On the other hand, the lines between sleep terrors, confusional arousals, and sleepwalking are blurry, as one disorder can often occur in conjunction with another, since all of these entities arise from deep NREM sleep (see videos 1–3).

Confusional arousals, unlike sleep terrors, have less autonomic involvement and lack the abrupt onset with a scream or yell. They may begin with moaning or stirring and then progress to more dramatic verbal-motor agitation. There is a strong genetic component with a better than 50% chance of occurrence if both parents had arousal parasomnias, according to some studies. In Jamie's case, her father was a sleepwalker as a child and into his adult years.

It is important to recognize that underlying OSA can trigger episodes of sleep terrors. Other triggers for NREM parasomnias include sleep deprivation, neuroactive medications like sedatives and antihistamines, fever, stress, and periodic limb movements in sleep. External stimuli such as noise or touch may also trigger episodes (see video 2). In addition, nocturnal frontal lobe epilepsy, which occurs almost exclusively in sleep and is characterized by stereotyped motor behavior, should be considered in the differential diagnosis. Certainly, clinical suspicion for nocturnal seizures masquerading as parasomnia is higher if there are stereotypical behaviors, prior history of seizures, or multiple arousal episodes per night. Given Jamie's family history of OSA as well as high maternal anxiety for possible epilepsy, a PSG including an 18-channel EEG with video was performed. In patients who present with a clinical picture typical for sleep terrors, PSG is not necessary, since it is unusual to capture such episodes in a sleep laboratory. This makes home videos that capture sleep terrors particularly helpful in making correct diagnosis.

Concomitant psychiatric disorders such as anxiety, nocturnal panic attacks, or post traumatic stress disorder need to be identified and treated. In Jamie's case, a referral to a sleep psychologist was made to address her bedtime anxiety. There is no known direct association between psychiatric disorders and childhood sleep terrors.

The diagnosis of sleep terrors is often distressing to the entire family, but it is mostly benign and does not warrant aggressive pharmaceutical intervention. It does not help to try to intervene by awakening the child during the episode or to discuss it the next morning. The authors have elicited detailed descriptions of the episodes that the child "recalled" as a result of breakfast-table discussions, making distinction from REM parasomnias that much more difficult! Besides, discussions of this nature may unnecessarily reinforce that "something is wrong" with the child.

The mainstays of therapy for sleep terrors involve reassurance, adequate sleep time, regular sleep schedule, treatment of secondary triggers like OSA, safety precautions, and, if episodes are predictable, a trial of scheduled awakenings.

The latter involves disturbing the patient's sleep just enough to cause stirring and arousal without total awakening. The parent is asked to do this several minutes prior to the predicted event. In Jamie's case, this proved to be unacceptable to the family.

If safety concerns arise, such as combative behavior or concomitant sleepwalking, safeguarding the bedroom may be necessary. Patients' families should be counseled on such measures as putting locks or alarms on doors and windows, reducing the height of patient's bed, separating the patient from their bed partner/sibling, and installing gates at stairwells. Particularly resistant cases can be tried on benzodiazepines or tricyclic antidepressants.

Jamie and her mother were seen in clinic 6 months following her PSG. Happily, mother reported decreased bed-related anxiety, and though Jamie's sleep terror episodes had not completely resolved, they were now occurring less than once per week. When these episodes did occur, they were less distressing on her family due to better understanding of the diagnosis, its prognosis, and the reassurance that these were not seizure related.

Bibliography

Bornemann MA, Mahowald MW, and Schenck CH. Parasomnias: Clinical features and forensic implications. *Chest*. 2006;130: 605–610.

Mason TBA, Pack A. Pediatric parasomnias. *SLEEP*. 2007;30(2):141–151.

Mindell JA, Owens JA. A clinical guide to pediatric sleep: Diagnosis and management of sleep problems in children and adolescents. Lippincott Williams & Wilkins, Philadelphia; 2003.

36

Catch Me if You Can

SILVIA NEME-MERCANTE, MD

ALON AVIDAN MD, MPH

Case History

Philip was a 62-year-old, right handed man who was referred to the sleep disorder center for evaluation of recurrent episodes of confusion and violent behaviors during sleep. His sleep history was uneventful until 7 years prior, when his wife first noticed episodes of talking and groaning in his sleep, sometimes accompanied by unusual body movements. For the first 2 years, the frequency of these events, which were inconsequential, was about once a month. However, five years prior to presentation, his night behaviors became more dramatic. His wife recalled the first violent episode, when she woke up to find him sitting at the edge of the bed facing the bedside table with the lamp on the floor and blood dripping from his left eyelid. He was shouting and sweating profusely. Once she was able to calm him down, he told her he was dreaming a man was chasing him while he was jogging at a park. He decided to hide behind a tree and planned to jump his aggressor as he passed in an effort to catch him. Over time, his episodes became more violent and frequent, occurring 2 to 3 times per week, typically 2 to 3 hours after sleep onset. Afterwards, he was usually able to provide a detailed account of his dreams. While he reported that his actions had never injured his wife, she nevertheless moved to the guest room, fearing harm.

Philip maintained a regular sleep schedule during weekdays and weekends. He went to bed by 10 p.m., fell asleep in 5 minutes, and usually woke up by 7 a.m. He often woke up feeling unrefreshed, though he did not take naps during the day. His Epworth Sleepiness Scale score was 5 and Patient Health Questionnaire-9, an index of depression, was normal at 3. He and his wife denied oral trauma, urine or stool incontinence, and convulsive movements during episodes. There was no history of cataplexy, hypnagogic hallucinations, sleep paralysis, snoring, choking at night, or symptoms of restless legs syndrome.

One year before presentation, Philip began to experience episodes of confusion during the day, and his wife noticed trouble with his memory. Once, while driving home alone from the grocery store, he forgot how to get back home and could not recall his address when he waved down a police officer for assistance. His wife recounted other times when Philip had trouble getting the right words out, writing, or driving to a familiar location. She felt he was becoming increasingly dependent on her, withdrawn, and emotionally and socially detached.

His past medical and psychiatric history was unremarkable. He denied caffeine alcohol, tobacco, and illicit drug use. He was not taking any regular medications. He worked as an investment banker, but his hours had been cut substantially due to what his boss called "recent performance deficiencies." His mother had a history of Alzheimer's disease, diagnosed at 70 years of age.

Physical Examination

The general examination was normal. Philip's body mass index was $25 \, \text{kg/m}^2$ and his neck circumference was 17 inches. The upper airway examination revealed patent nares and a Grade II Friedman tongue position with no retrognathia.

His neurological examination revealed intact long- and short-term memory. He scored 29/30 on the Mini Mental Status Exam. His speech was fluent. Comprehension, naming, and repetition were intact. Examination of the cranial nerves was normal. His motor exam revealed normal tone, bulk, and strength bilaterally, with no tremor or involuntary movements. Coordination and sensation of pinprick, vibration, and proprioception were intact. The deep tendon reflexes were 2/4 and symmetric. Plantar stimulation was flexor. The gait was normal.

Evaluation

Prior to his presentation in the sleep center, Philip underwent an evaluation for his usual night behaviors and daytime confusion. Brain MRI was normal, without evidence of hydrocephalus, infarction or atrophy. Electroencephalogram (EEG) revealed a normal background rhythm of 8 Hz and no epileptiform activity. Thyroid stimulating hormone, complete metabolic panel, rapid plasma reagin, vitamin B12, vitamin E, zinc, and folate were normal.

To further investigate his complaints, a diagnostic polysomnogram (PSG) utilizing expanded EEG and a neuropsychological evaluation were performed.

The PSG showed a total sleep time of 413 minutes and a sleep efficiency of 84%. The sleep latency was 13 minutes, and rapid eye movement (REM) sleep latency was 379 minutes. Sleep stage percentages included 35% N1, 63% N2, and 2% REM with no N3 sleep recorded. The arousal index [AHI] was elevated at 32, but there was no evidence of sleep apnea (apnea-hypopnea index [AHI] was 0.1) or periodic limb movements (PLMS; the PLM arousal index was 0.6). The EKG revealed normal sinus rhythm and the EEG was normal. During the brief period of REM sleep, preservation of submental electromyogram (EMG) tone and limb twitching were observed (Figure 36.1). The next morning, he did not recall whether he dreamt during the night.

Neuropsychological testing revealed an average Full Scale IQ with average verbal intellectual abilities and low-average nonverbal intellectual skills. There was evidence of mild disruption to frontal-striatal circuits, with fairly prominent visual constructional deficits, basic auditory attention span, processing speed, and mental flexibility. Phonemic word fluency test was impaired, and copy of a complex geometric figure was notable for a highly disorganized and

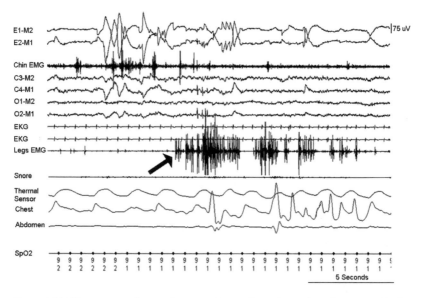

Figure 36.1 The arrow indicates the point during REM sleep when the patient had abnormal dream-enactment behavior. Note the persistence of elevated EMG activity in the tibialis anterior (TA) muscles during REM suggesting REM sleep without atonia. Channels are: electro-oculogram (left: E1-M2, right: E2-M1), chin electromyogram (EMG), electroencephalogram (left central, right central, left occipital, right occipital), 2 ECG channels, limb EMG (left-right TA), snore channel, nasal-oral airflow, respiratory effort (thoracic, abdominal), and oxygen saturation (SpO$_2$). Modified from Avidan, AY, Sleep Disorders in the Elderly, Primary Care: Clinics in Office Practice on Sleep Disorders. *Sleep Medicine* 2005;32(2):563–586. With permission from Elsevier.

piecemeal approach to the task. Memory difficulties primarily reflecting problems with the organizational aspects of memory characteristic of a frontally based memory disturbance were reported.

Diagnoses

REM-sleep behavior disorder (RBD).
Mild cognitive impairment with neuropsychological pattern highly suggestive of diffuse Lewy body disease.

Outcome

Philip was diagnosed with RBD and started on 0.5 mg clonazepam at bedtime. Home safety precautions were implemented, including the removal of potentially dangerous objects from the bedroom and placement of a cushion around the bed. Almost immediately after starting treatment, the frequency of nocturnal spells decreased to 1 per month. At a follow-up visit 6 months later, his wife reported worsening of his daytime symptoms, particularly problems with memory, concentration, restlessness, increased anxiety, and visual hallucinations and illusions. He was exhibiting delusional thinking, holding the belief that people were in the house when nobody was there. The clonazepam was discontinued, and the hallucinations and illusions resolved. He was switched to lorazepam 1 mg at bedtime, which controlled his dream enactment. Despite improvements in sleep quality, his cognitive decline progressed, which prompted him to take an early retirement.

Discussion

Illustrated here is a classic case of RBD, a REM sleep parasomnia that usually emerges later in life, typically after age 50. The presenting complaint in RBD is typically recurrent dream-enacting behaviors that have the potential, in about one-third of cases, to result in injury to the affected individual or the bed partner (see video 1). Spells occur about 2 hours after sleep onset, which coincides with the onset of REM sleep. The diagnosis of RBD is made in patients with REM sleep without atonia in the chin or limb EMG on PSG and either sleep related injurious, potentially injurious or disruptive behaviors documented by history or abnormal REM sleep behaviors documented on PSG. There must be an absence of EEG abnormalities suggestive of epilepsy, and the sleep disturbance should not be better explained by any other sleep disorder, medical, mental or neurological condition, medication, or substance use. PSG is essential to establishing the diagnosis. In fact, RBD is the only parasomnia for which a sleep study is required for confirmation.

Three clinical subtypes of RBD have been described: (1) subclinical RBD, characterized by PSG findings consistent with RDB in the absence of a clinical history of dream enactment; (2) parasomnia overlap disorder, comprising RBD combined with a disorder of arousal (sleepwalking, sleep talking); and (3) status dissociatus, characterized by a state dissociation without clear sleep stages but with REM-related behaviors resembling RBD.

The pathophysiology of REM sleep behavior disorder in humans is based on the cat model (Figure 36.2). Bilateral pontine tegmental lesions result in permanent loss of REM atonia associated with prominent motor activity during REM sleep. The condition is frequently associated with neurodegenerative disorders, in particular the synucleinopathies such as Parkinson's disease, dementia with Lewy bodies, and multiple system atrophy. These disorders share a common pathologic lesion composed of abnormal aggregates of alpha-synuclein protein in specific nuclei of the brain. RBD may precede the diagnosis of the underlying neurodegenerative disorder by several decades and hence may serve as an indicator of an evolving synucleinopathy. Patients with neurologic lesions involving the REM generator centers in the brain due to stroke, multiple sclerosis, or neoplasm have also been reported to develop RBD. While the condition is more common in older men, its presence in younger patients should raise the possibility of narcolepsy. For reasons not understood, RBD is about 9 times more common in men than in women. Several medications have been implicated in exacerbating or even causing RBD. These include psychotropics, antidepressants such as selective serotonin reuptake inhibitors, serotonin-norepinephrine reuptake inhibitors, and tricyclic antidepressants. Alcohol and drug abuse or withdrawal and caffeine can also trigger RBD.

The differential diagnoses of RBD include NREM parasomnias, such as sleepwalking and sleep terrors, nocturnal seizures, obstructive sleep apnea, periodic limb movement disorder, nocturnal psychogenic dissociative disorders, and malingering.

Treatment with benzodiazepines is remarkably effective in treating RBD. Despite the lack of long-term trials, clonazepam is considered first-line therapy. Before therapy with benzodiazepines, patients must be evaluated for sleep apnea. Treatment of sleep related breathing disorders should be rendered prior to the use of benzodiazepines, as the severity of sleep apnea may be exacerbated by agents that suppress upper airway tone. Melatonin 3 to 12 mg at bedtime was found to be effective for RBD in one small case series, and it can also normalize EMG tone in patients with RBD. Alternative pharmacotherapy—such as dopamine agonists and precursors, newer antiepileptic agents, and propoxyphene—may be considered in patients who fail to respond to benzodiazepines or melatonin. Driving and home safety precautions should be recommended, particularly in patients with cognitive impairment.

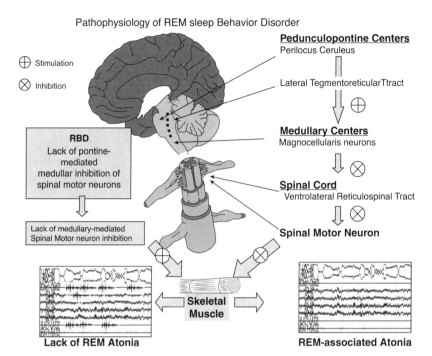

Pathophysiology of REM sleep Behavior Disorder

Stimulation

Inhibition

Pedunculopontine Centers
Perilocus Ceruleus

Lateral TegmentoreticularTtract

RBD
Lack of pontine-
mediated
medullar inhibition of
spinal motor neurons

Medullary Centers
Magnocellularis neurons

Spinal Cord
Ventrolateral Reticulospinal Tract

Lack of medullary-mediated
Spinal Motor neuron inhibition

Spinal Motor Neuron

Skeletal Muscle

Lack of REM Atonia

REM-associated Atonia

Figure 36.2 Muscle atonia characteristic of REM sleep results from pontine-mediated perilocus ceruleus inhibition of motor activity. This pontine activity exerts an excitatory influence on medullary centers (magnocellularis neurons) via the lateral tegmentoreticular tract. These neuronal groups, in turn, hyperpolarize the spinal motor neuron postsynaptic membranes via the ventrolateral reticulospinal tract. In REM sleep behavior disorder (RBD), the brainstem mechanisms generating muscle atonia in REM sleep are disrupted. In the experimental cat model of RBD, bilateral pontine lesions result in a persistent absence of REM atonia associated with prominent motor activity, similar to that observed in human RBD. The pathophysiology of RBD is thought to be related to reduction of striatal presynaptic dopamine transporters. Modified from Avidan, AY, Sleep Disorders in the Elderly, Primary Care: Clinics in Office Practice on Sleep Disorders. *Sleep Medicine* 2005;32(2):563–586. With permission from Elsevier.

Bibliography

Schenck CH, Mahowald MW. Long-term nightly benzodiazepine treatment of injurious parasomnias and other disorders of disrupted nocturnal sleep in 170 adults. *Am J Med.* 1996;100:548–554.

Schenck CH. REM sleep associated parasomnias. In Lee-Chiong TL, Sateia MJU, Carskadon MA, eds: *Sleep Medicine*. Philadelphia, Hanley& Belfus Inc., 2002, 215–223.

37

Peter and the Wolf

CARLOS RODRIGUEZ, MD

Case History

Peter was a 66-year-old retired attorney with disruptive behavior in sleep for the past 5 years. During a recent visit to his son and daughter-in-law, Peter began screaming in the middle of the night. Though his wife had witnessed this activity many times before, she had forgotten to tell his doctor. However, his son and daughter-in-law were quite concerned and managed to convince Peter to seek medical care. The attacks had variable manifestations, including screaming, swearing, arguing, gesturing, punching, and kicking. Once he fell out of bed during a spell, lacerating his scalp. These violent outbursts were uncharacteristic of Peter, who was described as a kind, gentle, and peaceful man. He generally had no memory of this activity and was shocked to hear the next morning what had transpired. About every other night, his wife would awaken predictably between 3:30 and 4 a.m. to find him in or near his bed, having an attack. Within 5 to 10 minutes, he was usually back to sound sleep. Peter and his wife described one particularly memorable night in which she was struck on the head but, fortunately, was uninjured. She shook him awake, and he recounted a dream in which he was attacked by a vicious wolf while making an argument in the court room. The wolf jumped on him, knocking him to the floor as he desperately attempted to defend himself by throwing a punch.

Peter denied a history of traumatic or violent experiences. He had snored for many years, but his wife had never observed breathing pauses in sleep. He denied waking up gasping for air or choking during sleep, although he generally woke up 2 to 3 times per night for no obvious reason. He would go to bed at 9:30 p.m. and wake at 7:30 a.m. every day. He denied daytime sleepiness (his Epworth Sleepiness Scale [ESS] score was 7), and he felt refreshed on awakening. His spells never resulted in tongue lacerations or incontinence, and he denied ever having a convulsion or loss of consciousness, balance problems, cognitive impairment, tremor, dizziness, or lightheadedness.

Peter had always enjoyed good health. He had diet-controlled hyperlipidemia, and he had a tonsillectomy and a hernia repair in childhood. He took no regular medications other than a daily aspirin. He smoked 1 cigar per month and had never used recreational drugs. He was a recovered alcoholic and had been abstinent for 15 years. His family history was negative for epilepsy, sleep apnea, parasomnias, and degenerative disorders.

Physical Examination

Peter was obese, with a body mass index of $33 \, kg/m^2$ and a neck circumference of $43 \, cm$. His upper airway exam was notable for a Grade III Friedman tongue position. There was no retrognathia, and his tonsils were surgically absent. There was no nasal congestion or nasal valve collapse. His general exam was otherwise unremarkable as was his neurological exam. Specifically, there was no masked facies, hypophonia, cogwheel rigidity or resting tremor. He exhibited normal arm swing and stride upon gait testing.

Evaluation

Peter was referred to the sleep lab to screen for sleep apnea and investigate his unusual night behaviors. A polysomnogram (PSG) with electroencephalography (EEG) and electromyography (EMG) recording from the upper and lower extremities was performed. He was found to have obstructive sleep apnea (OSA) moderate in severity but exacerbated to the severe degree when supine (his preferred sleep position). No epileptiform activity or unusual behavior was observed and EMG tone during REM sleep was normal (Figure 37.1, Table 37.1).

Diagnoses

Parasomnias due to medical condition.
Obstructive sleep apnea.
Obesity.

Outcome.

Peter was started on an acclimation CPAP setting of $5 \, cmH_2O$ and referred for a continuous positive airway pressure (CPAP) titration study. A pressure of

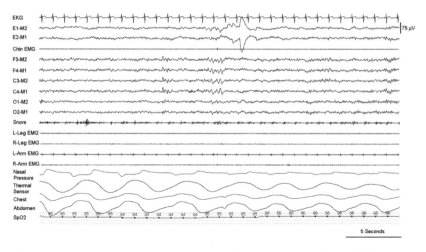

Figure 37.1 Polysomnogram tracing in REM sleep. This 30-second epoch demonstrates normal REM sleep. Rapid eye movements are present in the eye leads (E1-M2 and E2-M1) with low voltage desynchronized EEG, indicating REM sleep. There is no increased EMG tone present in the chin, legs, or arms as would be expected in REM sleep behavior disorder. Sensitivity scale: EEG leads 7 μV, EMG leads 50 μV.

12 cmH$_2$O normalized the apnea-hypopnea index (AHI), eliminated snoring and maintained the oxygen saturation above 90%. Peter and his wife were advised to implement safety measures, including removal of potentially dangerous objects from the vicinity of the bed. Since he had fallen out of bed in the past, placing the mattress on the floor or cushions on the floor around the bed was an additional consideration. His wife was informed that it was reasonable for her to sleep in the spare bedroom if she felt threatened by Peter's behavior, at least until the issue was corrected.

Following the initiation of therapeutic CPAP, Peter experienced a complete resolution of the dream-enacting behaviors when compliant with CPAP. Over the next year, his wife observed 5 to 10 recurrences, always on nights when Peter neglected to use his CPAP. Now, more than 3 years later, Peter remains healthy. He and his wife enjoy more peaceful nights of sleep without visits from the big bad wolf.

Discussion

Peter's case illustrates the co-existence of a parasomnia and OSA. Parasomnias are unpleasant or undesirable behavioral or experiential phenomena that occur predominately or exclusively during the sleep period.

The differential diagnosis of abnormal behaviors in sleep includes sleepwalking and sleep terrors given Peter's history of screaming, talking, agitation, and

Table 37.1 Polysomnogram data summary

Total sleep time: 328 min
Start time: 21:36:16
Stop time: 06:15:16
Sleep efficiency: 64.2%

Apnea-hypopnea index (AHI)	27.3
Supine AHI	42.3
Off-supine AHI	24.9
REM AHI	3.4
NREM AHI	30.2
Position time %	
Supine	13.4
Off-Supine	86.6
Oxygen saturation	
Mean Oxygen Saturation %	93.0
Lowest Oxygen Saturation %	87.0
Sleep stages %	
N1	32.0
N2	57.2
N3	0.0
REM	10.8
Limb movement data	
Periodic limb movement index (PLMI)	4.9
Periodic limb movement arousal index (PLMAI)	2.2

violent behavior in sleep. Sleepwalking and sleep terrors are disorders of arousal within the NREM parasomnia category. These disorders typically present in childhood and occur within 2 hours of sleep onset. Patients are usually difficult to awaken from events and appear confused afterwards. Dream recall, if any, is usually fragmentary and devoid of a coherent story. Sleepwalking and sleep terrors are often precipitated by sleep deprivation and stress.

Nocturnal seizures should be considered in the differential diagnosis given the history of altered consciousness and amnesia for the events. However, the lack of behavioral stereotypy, absence of epilepsy risk factors such as closed head injury, stroke, and CNS infection, normal neurological examination, and normal EEG made seizures less likely.

The lack of awareness and amnesia for the events excluded nocturnal panic attacks and sleep related hallucinations. There was no history of prior trauma suggestive of post traumatic stress disorder.

The primary consideration in Peters' case was REM sleep behavior disorder (RBD). The historical features that support this diagnosis include enactment of altered dreams at least 90 minutes after sleep onset with most events occurring in the second half of the night, when the majority of REM sleep normally is expected to occur. Peter demonstrated dream enactment with recall of unpleasant, violent, and disturbing dream content with a coherent story. In addition, his history illustrated an isomorphism, a phenomenon characteristic of RBD in which an observed sleep behavior corresponds with the dream action experienced by the patient. While Peter was dreaming of striking the wolf, he inadvertently delivered a blow to his wife. In order to make a diagnosis of RBD, a PSG demonstrating the presence of REM without atonia is required. Additional EMG of the upper and lower extremities should be monitored to fully assess muscle activity in REM sleep, as augmentation of EMG may be limited to one extremity or body part. While REM sleep time was limited in Peter's case, EMG activity was normal.

As a result, "pseudo-RBD" was the most likely diagnosis. This term describes cases of OSA presenting with abnormal behaviors in sleep, mimicking RBD. Patients with pseudo-RBD typically have severe OSA with significant oxygen desaturation, muscle atonia in REM on PSG, and clinical features including daytime sleepiness, unrefreshing sleep, witnessed apneas, and snoring, in addition to abnormal behaviors in sleep reminiscent of RBD. Pseudo-RBD is best classified as a parasomnia due to a medical condition—in this case, OSA. While Peter's history lacked many of the typical clinical features of OSA, he was found to have moderate to severe disease and muscle atonia in REM sleep on PSG. The diagnosis was confirmed by the resolution of the RBD-like behaviors with CPAP therapy and symptom relapse in the setting of CPAP noncompliance.

The differentiation of pseudo-RBD and RBD has important implications. The treatment of pseudo-RBD focuses on abolition of the breathing disturbance. In contrast, clonazepam, a benzodiazepine with myorelaxant properties, is the first-line therapy for RBD and can aggravate OSA by causing more frequent respiratory events, longer event duration, and/or more profound oxygen desaturation. From a prognostic standpoint, it is important to distinguish idiopathic RBD from pseudo-RBD, as the former is often associated with the subsequent emergence of a neurodegenerative disorder, such as Parkinson's disease, multiple system atrophy, or dementia with Lewy bodies, the risk of which would not be elevated in the OSA population.

Bibliography

Iranzo A, Santamaria J. Severe obstructive sleep apnea/hypopnea mimicking REM sleep behavior disorder. *SLEEP*. 2005;28(2):203–206.

Mahowald MW, Schenck CH. REM Sleep parasomnias. In: Kryger MH, Roth T, Dement CG, eds. *Principles and Practice of Sleep Medicine*. Philadelphia, PA: WB Saunders, 2005:897–910.

38

Why Can't John Go to a Slumber Party?

JENNIFER SCIUVA, MSN, PNP
JYOTI KRISHNA, MD

Case History

More than anything else, John wanted to sleep over at his friend's house when school let out in the summer. He hesitated when he opened the invitation, and a small tear ran down his face. His mother fully understood his predicament, as she had had the same problem when she was a child—John would have to decline because of his bed-wetting problem. He wet the bed every night and would be too embarrassed to wear pull-ups in the company of his friends. Most puzzling was the fact was that John had been dry at night by age 5, and now, at age 8, bed wetting was a big problem all over again. His mother was concerned not only for the embarrassment of bed wetting, but that John was snoring loudly, had breathing pauses, and could not get up for school in the morning. His grades were declining. John also had gained a lot of weight over the past year. His teacher had been sending home notes relating John's sleepiness and inability to focus on schoolwork. While his mother always made sure he had adequate sleep at night for his age, she realized it was time to make a visit to the sleep disorders clinic.

Overall, John was a healthy child. He lived with his mother and younger sister. He was in the third grade and was an average student. Past medical history included gastro-esophageal reflux disease, obesity, and speech delay. He had gained 28 pounds in the past year. He had been seen previously at the sleep center for sleepwalking and sleep terrors. At that time, a polysomnogram (PSG) with expanded EEG testing showed no snoring or significant sleep-disordered breathing. However, it did show a sudden arousal from slow-wave sleep consistent with parasomnias. He was diagnosed with a NREM parasomnia, specifically confusional arousals and sleepwalking, which he subsequently grew out of. No other EEG abnormalities had been observed.

Physical Examination

On examination, John was obese, with a body mass index (BMI) of $30.5\,kg/m^2$. His upper airway exam revealed minimal inferior turbinate hypertrophy and a Friedman tongue position of Grade III; tonsil size was Grade III as well, and there was no retrognathia. The rest of his examination was normal.

Evaluation

Urinalysis was negative, and serum electrolytes were normal. Due to his current sleep issues, a PSG was repeated. It showed moderate obstructive sleep apnea (OSA) worsening in REM sleep. The overall apnea hypopnea index (AHI) was 8.5; REM AHI was 11.4. The mean O_2 saturation was 96%, with a nadir of 89%. The capnogram was normal. Unlike the previous PSG, this time there were no arousals from slow-wave sleep suspicious for parasomnias. His bed was dry on the night of PSG.

Diagnoses

Obstructive sleep apnea.
Sleep enuresis (secondary type).
Obesity.

Outcome

Because of the OSA, John was referred to a pediatric ENT surgeon for evaluation of his upper airway, and he was advised to undergo an adenotonsillectomy. No pharmaceutical treatment was recommended for the nocturnal enuresis. The surgery went well, with no postoperative complications.

A follow-up PSG done 3 months postoperatively showed improved OSA with an overall AHI of 2.5. John's mother reported decreased, but persistent, symptoms of snoring and a distinct reduction in nocturnal enuresis (now less than twice weekly). His focus on schoolwork improved as well.

A referral to a nutritionist was suggested, with the expectation that further reduction in residual OSA would likely result from weight loss. A follow-up visit was planned for 6 months.

Discussion

According to the International Classification of Sleep Disorders, enuresis should occur with a frequency of more than twice a week to be considered clinically problematic, and it is generally not a consideration in children younger than 5 years of age. The distinction between primary and secondary types lies in the historical presentation. Whereas the former presents with a history of involuntary voiding during sleep since infancy, the latter, by definition, requires a recurrence of bedwetting after a clear period of dryness lasting for 6 months or more. Causes and associations for secondary sleep enuresis are many and include urinary infections, diabetes mellitus, diabetes insipidus, use of diuretics including caffeine, urinary tract malformations, neurological diseases, chronic constipation, OSA, and psychosocial stress, to name a few. A thorough physical exam and simple laboratory testing, including serum electrolytes and urinalysis, in otherwise healthy children usually suffices to guide clinical management in the majority of instances.

The prevalence of OSA in children ranges from 1%–3%, with most cases affecting children between ages 2 and 8. The prevalence of nocturnal enuresis ranges from 5%–15% in children between the ages of 5 and 10 years, with the prevalence declining with increasing age. The correlation between sleep related breathing disorder and nocturnal enuresis has been documented by various researchers. Reports from Turkey show increased nighttime symptoms such as bed wetting among snorers, and fully one-third of a sample of children undergoing adenotonsillectomy for presumed upper airway obstruction had nocturnal enuresis. In another study, from the United States, children between ages 4 and 17 with a polysomnographically measured respiratory disturbance index (RDI) greater than 1 had a higher prevalence of enuresis (47%) than those with an RDI less than 1 (17%) or literature controls, even after adjusting for age. No relationship was found between BMI and the prevalence of enuresis.

Several hypotheses have been proposed to explain why children with OSA may have a higher prevalence of sleep enuresis. These include insufficient arousal response (secondary to sleep fragmentation), impaired nighttime urodynamics (increased bladder pressure resulting from obstructed airway), and insufficient vasopressin levels during sleep. Atrial natriuretic peptide release (from increased right atrial pressure) also has been proposed to play a role. Reversal of some of these factors has been shown in treatment studies of sleep apnea subjects. Further, treatment of OSA via adenotonsillectomy, continuous positive airway pressure therapy, or dental devices has been reported to reduce or eliminate enuresis in children. Finally, it has been suggested that OSA should be considered in overweight children with enuresis.

Thus, even if an existing history of nocturnal enuresis were presumably to have introduced a selection bias in the population referred for upper airway obstruction in some of the above studies, the physiological plausibility for the mechanistic relationships between enuresis and OSA is strong. Our clinical experience certainly is in keeping with this notion (see also Chapter 17). Having said that, it is clear that additional research and educational awareness are needed to address the problem of nocturnal enuresis in patients with OSA, to establish treatment thresholds, and to assess outcomes with more rigorous study design.

Bibliography

Barone JG, Hanson C, DaJusta DG, et al. Nocturnal enuresis and overweight are associated with sleep apnea. *Pediatrics*. 2009;124:e53–59.

Basha S, Bialowas C, Ende K, Szeremeta W. Effectiveness of adenotonsillectomy in the resolution of nocturnal enuresis secondary to obstructive sleep apnea. *Laryngoscope*. 2005;115:1101–1103.

Brooks LJ, Topol HI. Enuresis in children with sleep apnea. *J Pediatr*. 2003;142: 515–518.

Cinar U, Vural C, Cakir B, et al. Nocturnal enuresis and upper airway obstruction. Int *J Pediatr Otolaryngol*. 2001;59:115–118.

39

Not Tonight, Dear

CRAIG BROOKER, MD
NANCY FOLDVARY-SCHAEFER, DO

Case History

Ben was a 28-year-old man who presented to the sleep center reporting embarrassing behaviors in sleep. Over the previous few years, he had begun to make advances toward his wife in sleep, talking and touching that was sexual in nature and for which he was completely amnestic. This activity contributed to their marital discord, ultimately leading to a divorce. On other occasions, he had vague recollection of thrusting his hips in the prone position during sleep, and he was surprised to find soiled bed linen in the morning. His current girlfriend reported equally disturbing behaviors. On one occasion, he was more forceful, grabbing both of her arms to initiate sex, but he stopped when she vehemently objected and repeatedly shouted "No!!!" In an attempt to lessen unanticipated advances, Ben and his girlfriend frequently engaged in sexual activity just prior to going to bed, however, this proved unsuccessful.

While he denied seizures, incontinence, and oral trauma in sleep, Ben had a history of sleepwalking from the ages of 4 to 10. His parents often locked him in his room at night for fear he would wander out and fall down the stairs. He came from a long line of sleepwalkers, and his mother had shared a bedroom with 2 younger sisters who "he described as meandering around the house" as zombies in the night. Ben also had nightmares as a child. Recently, he woke up abruptly from a dream swinging his arms in the air, sweating, and feeling as if his heart was pounding a mile a minute, and he recalled dream content in which something bad had happened to his girlfriend. None of his night behaviors ever resulted in physical injury to himself or his partner.

Ben generally went to bed at midnight and woke up at 6 a.m., often not feeling refreshed. Weekends allowed for 10 refreshing hours of sleep. He generally fell asleep within 10 minutes and usually did not wake up at night. But once or twice a week, he found himself lamenting financial concerns (he had lost 3 jobs in the past 4 years), his father's sudden death 4 years prior from cancer, and his recent divorce. He found himself tossing and turning and watching the clock until he finally fell asleep. His most offensive sleep related behaviors occurred after repeated nights of poor sleep. Additionally, bed partners complained of snoring, which was generally relieved by sleeping on his side. He was a mouth breather, which he attributed to allergies. On several occasions in the recent past, he woke up abruptly while sleeping on his back with a sensation of gasping for air, although bed partners never raised concern for apnea. He did not usually nap, though he complained of excessive daytime sleepiness (EDS) and had an Epworth Sleepiness Scale (ESS) score of 12. He drank 6 cups of coffee through-out the day, sometimes more, to stay awake, and had several beers on Friday and Saturday nights out. He denied sleep paralysis, cataplexy, and hypnagogic hallucinations.

Physical Examination

Ben weighed 191 lbs (86.6 Kg) and was 6 ft (183 cm) tall, resulting in a body mass index of 25.9 kg/m^2. His neck circumference was 16.5 inches (41.9 cm). He had nasal congestion with a midline septum, Grade II tonsils and a Grade I Friedman tongue position. There were no cranio-facial abnormalities. His heart and lung examinations, as well as a complete neurological exam, were normal.

Evaluation

Ben was referred to the sleep laboratory for a polysomnogram (PSG) with expanded EEG montage to screen for obstructive sleep apnea (OSA) and better characterize his abnormal sleep related behavior. The study revealed heavy snoring with an apnea-hypopnea index (AHI) of 14 that included 74 hypopneas and 13 apneas (9 obstructive and 4 central). Nearly all events occurred in the supine position (Table 39.1). The arousal index was 14 and oxygen saturation

Table 39.1 Polysomnography respiratory event data

	REM time (min)	REM AHI	NREM time (min)	NREM AHI	Total time (min)	Total AHI
Supine	16	23	84	49	100	45
Off-supine	41	7	230	2	271	3
Total	57	12	314	15	371	14

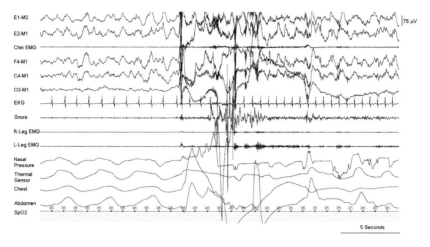

Figure 39.1 30-second epoch showing 1 of several arousals from N3 supportive of a NREM parasomnia.

was maintained above 90% for the entire recording. Frequent periodic limb movements (PLMS) were observed, resulting in a PLM-index of 20. The majority of these did not cause arousal. The EMG tone during REM sleep was at the lowest level of the entire night. Several unexplained abrupt arousals from stage N3, which constituted 17% of total sleep time, were observed (Figure 39.1). None were associated with unusual behavior. The EEG was normal without epileptiform discharges.

Diagnoses

Confusional arousal (sexsomnia variant).
Obstructive sleep apnea syndrome (OSAS).
Psychophysiological insomnia.

Outcome

Ben was offered treatment for all of his sleep problems and informed that his abnormal night behavior might improve with treatment of the OSA and insomnia. A trial of continuous positive airway pressure (CPAP) therapy was recommended to test just this. Yet despite the gravity of his sleep problem and the impact it had on his relationships, Ben was resistant to the idea. Since his OSA occurred predominately in the supine position, he preferred trying positional therapy. He was instructed on the importance of good sleep hygiene practices, including avoidance of sleep deprivation during the week and alcohol within

4 hours of bedtime, and the use of cognitive behavior strategies to clear his mind at night. While he was able to comply with sleeping on his side, he still felt sleepy, and his unpleasant night behaviors continued. While benzodiazepines were considered an option to control his parasomnia, due to concerns that they might negatively affect his OSA he was prescribed a trial of nortriptyline in the hope of reducing the frequency of episodes. However, this proved unsuccessful despite upward titration of the drug Unfortunately, his current relationship, too, ended, largely due to his sleep disorder.

Ben returned to the sleep center 2 years later, after starting a new relationship. Sexual advances in sleep continued, but this did not offend his new partner. He had gained 20 lbs since his first PSG and felt his sleep quality was worse. His girlfriend reported loud, disruptive snoring, and Ben reported occasionally waking from sleep suddenly gasping for air. He was counseled on the importance of diet and exercise, and he agreed to undergo another PSG, this time with CPAP titration, since oral appliance therapy and upper airway surgery were not felt to be better options. The study demonstrated abolition of respiratory events, oxygen desaturations, and snoring at a pressure of $10\,cmH_2O$. At his follow-up 3 months later, he reported better sleep quality, improved daytime alertness, and elimination of his abnormal nighttime behaviors. He was using CPAP virtually all night 7 nights per week and working on diet and exercise.

Discussion

Parasomnias are undesirable events that occur during sleep-wake transitions or during sleep. While PSG is not required for the diagnosis of the NREM parasomnias (in contrast to REM Behavior Disorder [RBD]), unexplained arousals from Stage N3 often preceded by a build-up of hypersynchronous, rhythmic delta or theta activity are supportive features of these disorders. The ICSD-2 recognizes sexsomnia as a variant of confusional arousals and sleepwalking. Confusional arousals are episodes of mental confusion or confusional behavior occurring during an arousal or awakening from nocturnal sleep or a daytime nap.

Sexsomnia constitutes a multitude of sexual behaviors occurring out of sleep that represent a subtype of the parasomnias. A recent review article by Schenck et al. (SLEEP 2007) on the topic revealed that sexual behaviors occurring during sleep most often represent parasomnias (31 cases) or sleep related seizures (7 cases). Parasomnias were further classified as confusional arousals with or without co-morbid OSA (26 cases), sleepwalking (2 cases), or RBD (3 cases). The parasomnia group exhibited behaviors including sexual fondling, intercourse, masturbation, sexual vocalization, and assault. All subjects reported amnesia for their behaviors and more than 90% also had confusional arousals, sleepwalking, sleep eating, or sleep driving. Roughly 80% were male, with onset usually in early adulthood. In about half the cases, sexsomnia was an isolated occurrence. In the others, recurrent episodes encompassing a range of behaviors were reported. Nearly 10% of patients had co-morbid OSA; in one case, treatment with CPAP abolished both the respiratory disturbance and the disturbing behaviors. Sexual behaviors were recorded during PSG in 4 cases. More than one-third of cases resulted in legal ramifications due to the disorder.

While most reports of sexsomnia are not recalled by the patients themselves, they are often very troubling for bed partners and family members and create significant relationship problems, often contributing to divorce. Even more disturbing are cases in which the affected individual makes advances toward others with whom he/she would not normally have sex. Several reports involve non-consenting adults and minors, including the children of the affected individual. The legal system has attempted to cope with cases of sexsomnia and apparent sexsomnia. Some courts have attempted to use sleepwalking cases (and the crimes committed apparently during sleepwalking) as a guide. Unfortunately, there is little consistency as to the use of the defense, when it should be applied, and which individuals should be ruled innocent or guilty. This is in part due to divergent language and interpretation of laws from state to state.

In the United States and Canada, sexsomnia rulings have generally fallen under the auspices of automatism, which the courts define as "…the existence in any person of behavior of which he is unaware and over which he has no conscious control. Automatism is behavior performed in a state of mental unconsciousness apparently occurring without will, purpose, or reasoned intention. Automatism connotes the state of a person who, though capable of action, is not conscious of what he is doing. Automatism manifests itself in a range of conduct, including somnambulism, hypnotic states, fugues, metabolic disorders, and epilepsy and other convulsions or reflexes" (*Schlatter vs. Indiana*). While automatism seems a reasonable classification, attempting to determine if any given act represented sexsomnia has been further challenging. To date, legal cases involving apparent sexsomnia continue to have inconsistent rulings, ranging from not guilty to guilty with prison time, in line with a rape conviction. If the range of outcomes is not troubling enough, some courts have even had a difficult time handling the suggestion that someone having sex might be sleeping.

Ben's history was highly suggestive of sexsomnia. After the onset of his abnormal night behaviors, he developed symptoms of OSA confirmed by PSG. While some patients with OSA have confusional arousals following apneic events, sexual behavior occurring exclusively in relation to respiratory events is unusual. Sexsomnia is the most common diagnosis in patients with sleep related sexual behaviors, although other disorders must be considered. Sexual vocalizations, masturbation, genital arousal, ictal orgasm, sexual automatisms, and assaultive sexual behavior are rare manifestations of partial seizures. While sexual hypermotoric pelvic or truncal movements have been reported in frontal lobe epilepsy, genital automatisms—like fondling and grabbing the genitals—are more likely to occur in seizures evolving from the temporal lobe. Sleep related sexual seizures were excluded in Ben's case by the absence of a history of seizures or risk factors for epilepsy and lack of epileptiform activity on EEG. Other less likely differential diagnoses excluded by his history and PSG include restless legs syndrome, RBD, narcolepsy, and Kleine-Levin syndrome.

At present, therapeutic options for the treatment of this parasomnia are the same as those applied to patients with other types of parasomnias. No clinical trials have been performed. Co-morbid sleep disorders should be treated, and known precipitants—such as stress, sleep deprivation, and alcohol and drugs—should be avoided or minimized. Benzodiazepines such as clonazepam may be effective but carry the potential for worsening OSA. Second-line agents include antidepressants such as sertraline as well as GABAergic agents such as valproate and lamotrigine. Psychiatric therapy, including cognitive behavioral therapy and psychotherapy, is recommended in select cases.

Bibliography

Leutmezer F, et al. Genital automatisms in complex partial seizures. *Neurology*. 1999;52(6):1188–1191.

Schenck CH, Arnulf I, Mahowalk MW. Sleep and sex: What can go wrong? A review of the literature on sleep related disorders and abnormal sexual behaviors and experiences. *SLEEP*. 2007;30:683–702.

Schlatter vs. Indiana, 891 N.E. 2d 1139, 1142.(Cir 2008).

Shapiro CM, Trajanovic NN, Fedoroff JP. Sexsomnia—A new parasomnia? *Can J Psychiatry*. 2003;48:311–317.

40

The Midnight Raider

STELLA BACCARAY, RN
NANCY FOLDVARY-SCHAEFER, DO

Case History

Jill was a 31-year-old woman who complained of binge eating at night for nearly 10 years. These episodes initially occurred only in times of extreme stress, but they increased dramatically in the past year after she was promoted at work to host a morning radio talk show. She made excursions to the kitchen 3 to 4 times per week, often multiple times in the night, typically during the first half of the sleep period. She usually ate high-carbohydrate foods, such as chocolates, cakes, cereal, pastries, muffins, and cookies. One morning she found a half-eaten plate of baked ziti in the microwave. In the refrigerator, she found a pie pan with only crumbs and a dirty spoon remaining, and once a nearly empty box of oatmeal crème pies with the individual wrappers strewn on the floor, which had been meant to go in her son's Spiderman lunchbox. In the morning, she would find crumbs and chocolate smears on her fingers and face, on the bed, or on the doorknob; frosting in her hair; and peanut butter in pockets of her robe. Finally, on a trip to New York City with her best friend, she awoke one morning to find she had raided the mini-bar and devoured the Godiva chocolate. After she spent the next day distraught, visiting 7-Elevens searching for the exact candy in order to avoid being charged the $5, she broke down and decided to speak with her doctor about the problem. She had no recall of her nighttime foraging and sloppy frenzies; she only saw the disturbing evidence left behind. During such episodes, she was difficult to arouse by her husband or friends and appeared confused upon awakening. She put a gate by the kitchen door and childproof locks on the cabinets, to no avail. Too often, her kids lost out on dessert as a result of her unplanned food fests. Jill expressed feelings of intense shame and embarrassment, which had prevented her from seeking medical attention in the past. She wondered how she could succumb to such a dramatic loss of control.

Jill typically went to bed at 11 p.m. and woke up between 6 and 7 a.m., generally not feeling refreshed. It took up to 30 minutes to fall asleep most nights, as she would lie in bed with her mind racing as she reviewed the line-up for the next morning's talk show. She had no appetite in the morning and never ate excessively during the day, to compensate for all of the calories ingested at night. Yet, she had gained 20 lbs in the past 6 months. She felt a bit sleepy and fatigued most days and had an Epworth Sleepiness Scale score of 9. Her husband told her she snored most nights and occasionally stopped breathing in sleep. She had a history of sleepwalking and nightmares in childhood, both of which remitted in her teen years, and denied sleep related injuries and dream enactment. Her father was a sleepwalker in childhood, as well. She denied symptoms of restless legs, narcolepsy, and psychiatric and eating disorders. Her Patent Health Questionnaire-9 score was 10, suggesting mild depression.

Jill's medical history was noteworthy for antiphospholipid antibody syndrome resulting in multiple miscarriages, gestational diabetes, and gastritis. She had developed depression and anxiety following a miscarriage several years prior and was briefly treated with alprazolam. She denied alcohol and tobacco use and took no regular medication.

Physical Examination

Jill was 5'6" tall and weighed 185 lbs, resulting in a body mass index of 29.9 kg/m². Her upper airway examination revealed a Grade II Friedman tongue position with normal nasal breathing and no retrognathia. The lungs were clear to auscultation. The heart rate and rhythm were normal without murmur. No edema was present in her extremities. Her neurological examination was normal.

Evaluation

Jill underwent a polysomnogram (PSG) to screen for sleep apnea, given her history of snoring, witnessed apnea, and recent weight gain. She was instructed to bring her favorite snacks, in hopes of recording an eating episode. The study revealed no sleep apnea (AHI was 3.2), periodic limb movements, or abnormal behaviors. However, spontaneous arousals from slow-wave sleep were observed.

Diagnoses

Sleep related eating disorder (SRED).
Psychophysiological insomnia.

Outcome

As a first-line course of treatment, Jill was started on a trial of bupropion (Wellbutrin XL) 150 mg per day to treat both her nighttime eating and her mild depressive symptoms. In addition, she was provided with good sleep hygiene tips and a session in progressive muscle relaxation to address her sleep-onset insomnia. She returned to the sleep clinic after 1 month of therapy reporting feeling more alert during the day but with the same frequency of night-eating episodes. Bupropion was increased to 300 mg per day, but she experienced only a modest improvement and continued to eat unknowingly 2 to 3 nights per week. As a result, Jill started treatment with topiramate 25 mg at bedtime and increased to 50 mg after 2 weeks. She experienced extreme nausea when she first increased to 50 mg but it subsided after 2 days. Night eating stopped briefly, only to resurface 2 weeks later. The dose was increased to 75 mg, which was well tolerated with full control of her eating frenzies. She stopped skipping breakfast and began eating balanced meals during the day. She reported a boost of energy and self-esteem. She joined a health club and began exercising 3 times per week. At her last follow-up visit, 8 months after she was diagnosed, her night eating remained controlled, save for rare nights of poor sleep due to extreme stress, and she proudly reported that she had lost 20 lbs.

Discussion

SRED is characterized by compulsive ingestion of food or drink occurring during recurrent partial arousals from sleep in which consciousness is only partially achieved (Table 40.1). Many patients have some recollection in the morning of their night behaviors, while others have none at all. Later on, when clues of their behavior become evident in the morning, they often feel ashamed and guilty, and they may develop self-hatred. Nocturnal eating episodes can occur nightly, often multiple times a night. SRED patients describe eating in an out-of-control manner and often consume unusual or inedible substances, such as raw meets, cleaning agents, cat food, coffee grounds and cigarettes. High-caloric foods are generally consumed. Females comprise more than two-thirds of cases, with a mean age of onset in the third decade of life.

Table 40.1 ICSD-2 diagnostic criteria for sleep related eating disorder

A. Recurrent episodes of involuntary eating and drinking occur during the main sleep period.

B. One or more of the following must be present with the recurrent episodes of involuntary eating and drinking:
   i. Consumption of peculiar forms or combinations of food or inedible or toxic substances.
   ii. Insomnia related to sleep disruption from repeated episodes of eating, with a complaint of nonrestorative sleep, daytime fatigue, or somnolence.
   iii. Sleep related injury.
   iv. Dangerous behaviors performed while in pursuit of food or while cooking food.
   v. Morning anorexia.
   vi. Adverse health consequences from recurrent binge eating of high-caloric foods.

C. The disturbance is not better explained by another sleep disorder, medical, or neurological disorder, mental disorder, medication use, or substance use disorder.

SRED patients have an increased risk of injuries, such as lacerations from food preparation, choking on thick foods, drinking excessively hot liquids, ingesting poisonous substances, and consuming foods to which they are allergic. Poor dentition may ensue, as feedings are not typically followed by dental hygiene practices, and because many will sleep with an oral bolus of food. These, combined with circadian decline in salivary flow, promote the development of caries.

SRED can be idiopathic, drug-induced, or linked to other sleep disorders. It has been proposed that if internally generated stimuli, such as periodic limb movements or sleep apnea, could trigger partial awakenings during NREM periods in predisposed patients, phenomena like sleep related eating may ensue. In the majority of SRED cases, a co-morbid primary sleep disorder or medication is thought to be a contributing or provoking factor. A history of sleepwalking is most common. SRED can be medication-induced with zolpidem or other psychotropic agents. SRED can also be associated with daytime eating disorders and with sleep related dissociative disorder. PSG reveals multiple confusional arousals arising from slow-wave sleep (Stage N3), light NREM sleep, and, rarely, REM sleep, with or without eating.

The differential diagnosis of SRED includes night eating syndrome (NES), other eating disorders, and psychiatric disorders. NES is characterized by overeating between the evening meal and nocturnal sleep onset and after awakenings from sleep with full recall. Daytime eating binges and the presence of purging or misuse of laxatives and diuretics raise concern for bulimia, although some SRED patients, Jill included, avoid eating during the day to counter the effects of the binging. Medical conditions that can cause recurrent sleep related eating include hypoglycemia, gastrointestinal disorders such as ulcers and gastroesophageal reflux disease, Kleine-Levin syndrome, and Klüver-Bucy syndrome.

Many consider the presence of impaired consciousness and subsequent amnesia for the eating episodes to be the major differentiating feature of SRED and NES. However, some SRED patients have eating episodes during EEG-defined wakefulness and clear recall for their behaviors. As a result, impaired level of consciousness cannot be the sole feature distinguishing SRED from NES. Rather than being 2 distinct disorders, SRED and NES may reflect opposite ends of a continuum of impairment of consciousness during nocturnal eating. Further support for this theory is provided by similarities in their clinical manifestations and long-term course. Both SRED and NES patients are at risk for weight gain, which may precipitate or aggravate pre-existing diabetes mellitus, hyperlipidemia, hypertension, cardiovascular disease, sleep disruption, and depression. Both experience morning anorexia that can interfere with nutrition.

Patients with NES are unable to initiate sleep without eating and have recurrent awakenings from sleep associated with an inability to fall back asleep without eating. They are not driven by true hunger—the urge to eat is an abnormal need. They have full awareness and recall the next day. NES is believed to represent a conditioned, conscious behavior that starts when an infant is given food in the middle of the night to appease him. NES also has been described as a circadian delay of food intake with normal circadian timing of sleep onset (or circadian delay in timing of feeding relative to sleeping). Foods eaten are similar to those eaten during the daytime. While eating, affected individuals feel tense, anxious, and guilty. Current NES criteria include the consumption of 50% or more of daily calories after the evening meal (evening hyperphagia), eating after waking from sleep (conscious night eating), and morning anorexia of at least 3 months duration. NES is often associated with an underlying mood disorder, such as depression, and not with a primary sleep disorder. NES has been effectively treated with selective serotonin reuptake inhibitors (SSRIs), which act through direct serotonergic effect in the hypothalamus, which controls circadian rhythms and feeding behavior. It has been suggested that high-carbohydrate food typically consumed by night eaters facilitates the availability of tryptophan, which is then converted into CNS serotonin, which promotes initiation of sleep and reversal of sleep disruption.

Treatment for SRED should be aimed at controlling co-morbid sleep disorders and eliminating provocative agents. Antiepileptic drugs (AED) have been effective in treating SRED. Topiramate, a second-generation AED, is a GABA agonist and glutamatergic antagonist. Sleep enhancement and appetite suppression are properties of topiramate, but the exact mechanism by which it improves SRED is unclear. Dopaminergic agents, such as pramipexole, also have been effective in treating SRED with therapy geared towards decreasing motor activity during sleep, thus decreasing arousals. Recurring chewing and swallowing movements and PLMS, present in the majority of SRED patients throughout all sleep stages, suggests a dysfunction of the dopaminergic system. In addition, dopaminergic dysfunction at the mesolimbic level plays a role in compulsive behaviors, including food-seeking behavior. Bupropion, unlike other antidepressants, has its major effect is on dopamine, and it has also been used to treat SRED, with some success.

When managing patients with SRED, video PSG with expanded EEG is helpful to better characterize the disorder and to identify other sleep disorders that may trigger arousals. Stress and anxiety management, counseling, and reducing alcohol and caffeine intake may be beneficial interventions in conjunction with pharmacotherapy. Sedatives should be avoided as they can increase confusion. Randomized placebo-controlled studies are needed to better isolate effective pharmacological agents.

Bibliography

Schenck C, Hurwitz T, Bundlie S, Mahowald M. Sleep-related eating disorder: polysomnographic correlates of a heterogeneous syndrome distinct from daytime eating disorders. *SLEEP*. 1991;14:419–431.

Vetrugno R, Manconi M, Ferini-Strambi L, Provini F, Plazzi G, Montagna P. Nocturnal eating: Sleep-related eating disorder or night eating syndrome? A videopolysomnographic study. *SLEEP*. 2006;29:949–954.

Winkelman J. Clinical and polysomnographic features of sleep-related eating disorder. *J Clin Psychiatry*. 1998;59:14–19.

41

The Case of the Sick Coyote

MADELEINE GRIGG-DAMBERGER, MD
NANCY FOLDVARY-SCHAEFER, DO

Case History

Diego was a 14-year-old boy who was brought by his mother to the sleep medicine clinic for "incredibly loud groaning and moaning like a sick coyote" when sleeping. This problem began at 8 years of age and had gotten louder and deeper since his voice changed. Periods of moaning and groaning recurred several times every night for periods lasting 30 to 60 minutes. He went to bed at 9:30 p.m. on school days, fell sleep within 10 to 20 minutes, and slept soundly, awakening to an alarm at 6:30 a.m. On weekends he went to bed nearer to 11 p.m., sleeping without awakening until 10 to 11 a.m. His mother denied snoring, breathing pauses in sleep, gasping/choking, excessive sweating, respiratory distress of any sort, leg movements in sleep, sleepwalking, sleep terrors, or seizures. Diego felt his sleep was refreshing and he denied shortness of breath, restless legs, daytime sleepiness, or awareness of the sounds he made when sleeping. He had mild exercise-induced (not nocturnal) asthma when younger, but this had resolved. He had a normal birth and developmental history, and his immunizations were up-to-date. He was a B student in the ninth grade. He had no allergies, took no medications, and did not drink caffeinated beverages or use tobacco or illicit drugs. His Epworth Sleepiness Scale Score was 3 of 24. His mother hoped his groaning could be treated so that everyone else in the house could sleep.

Physical Examination

On examination, Diego appeared to be a healthy adolescent in no apparent distress. His vital signs were normal, and his body mass index was 18 kg/m².

His general and neurologic examinations were normal. He had no dysmorphic features, a normal chin size and location, a Friedman tongue position Grade I, and no tonsillar tissue.

Evaluation

A polysomnogram (PSG) with video, expanded electroencephalography (EEG), and additional electrodes placed on the upper extremities was performed to rule out sleep apnea, seizures, and parasomnias. Sleep onset was in 5 minutes after lights out. REM sleep was first seen 149 minutes after sleep onset. Sleep efficiency was 96%. During the 432 minutes of sleep, 24% was NREM 1, 45% NREM 2, 17% NREM 3, and 14% REM sleep. Eighteen minutes of wake after sleep onset were observed. A mean of 44 arousals and 3 awakenings per hour of sleep was noted, the majority related to respiratory events. Four episodes of repeated prolonged expiratory groaning and moaning were observed during NREM sleep ranging from 4 to 36 minutes in duration. During groaning episodes, the respiratory rate fell to 4 breaths per minute and the heart rate fell into the low 40s; the end-tidal CO_2 rose slightly, from 38 to 40 torr to 42 to 44 torr, while the SpO_2 was maintained at 94%–96% (Figure 41.1 and see video 1). A mean of 13 central apneas per hour of sleep was observed, which typically lasted 14 to 15 seconds, rarely as long as 21 seconds, almost all occurring in NREM sleep during or just before the onset of a groaning cluster. Central apneas usually did not cause oxygen desaturation. Between groaning clusters, the SpO_2 averaged 96% awake, 93% during NREM, and 94%–96%

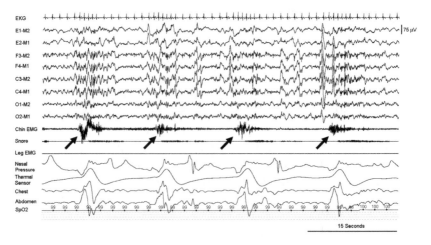

Figure 41.1 Thirty-second epoch from the overnight polysomnogram representative of the patient's sleep related behavior. Note the repeated EMG artifact in the chin and snore channels coinciding with groaning (arrows).

during REM sleep. The nadir SpO$_2$ was 91%. The obstructive apnea-hypopnea index was 6, the majority of which occurred during sleep-state transitions and were associated with noisy breathing only. Sleep related bruxism was noted both during and in between groaning episodes. Continuous positive airway pressure (CPAP) was tried toward the end of the study and increased to 8 cmH$_2$O with suppression of groaning and obstructive events. No epileptiform activity was observed on EEG.

Given the presence of central apneas, a brain MRI was performed that showed no brainstem abnormalities.

Diagnoses

Sleep related expiratory groaning (catathrenia).
Obstructive sleep apnea-hypopnea syndrome.
Sleep related bruxism.

Outcome

Diego's PSG demonstrated a repetitive pattern of prolonged expiratory groaning that emerged from NREM sleep. Vocalizations began following a spontaneous arousal from NREM 2 or 3 sleep with an abrupt deep breath followed by a prolonged expiratory groan that usually was accompanied by a central apnea or a hypopnea without snoring. These findings are characteristic of sleep related expiratory groaning, also called catathrenia. CPAP was effective in suppressing mild obstructive sleep apnea (OSA) and catathrenia, delighting his family, who could now sleep in peace.

Discussion

Catathrenia was first reported in 1983 in a young man with expiratory groaning during REM sleep. In 2001, 4 more cases were reported, with symptom onset between 5 and 16 years of age. These patients experienced groaning beginning 2 to 6 hours after sleep onset, usually from REM sleep and less commonly from Stage N2. Expiratory groans lasted 2 to 20 seconds and recurred in clusters lasting for up to 1 hour multiple times per night. Like Diego, these patients denied respiratory distress and had no awareness of their groaning. The authors coined the term catathrenia, from the Greek words "kata," below or under, and "threnia," to lament, for this strange sleep related behavior.

A recent review article detailed the clinical and polysomnographic characteristics of 21 cases of catathrenia. Most were young adults who had symptoms for more than a decade prior to presentation. There was a slight male predominance. Three patients had a family history of catathrenia; in 2 of these, an autosomal dominant mode of inheritance was suggested. In nearly 40% of cases, other parasomnias—including bruxism, somnambulism, somniloquy, and sleep terrors—were reported in family members. Polysomnography was performed in 16 cases, and catathrenia was documented in 12. The expiratory groan was characterized as a loud, monotonous noise that was stereotyped within a given subject but varied in quality among subjects. Episodes were isolated and brief (about 10 seconds) in some patients, and recurred in sequences (lasting up to 4 minutes) in others. Nearly 90% of catathrenia episodes occurred during REM sleep. Intercostal EMG was not increased during episodes, and there was no relationship between episodes and body position. None of the patients had sleep apnea, significant periodic limb movements, or oxygen desaturations, although daytime sleepiness was observed in one-third of cases. The disorder was chronic in all cases. Attempts to treat catathrenia with clonazepam, gabapentin, pramipexole, carbamazepine, trazodone, paroxetine, and dosulepine were either ineffective or produced short-term benefit only.

The differential diagnosis for catathrenia includes somniloquy, sleep related laryngospasm, stridor, nocturnal asthma, and vocalization associated with epileptic seizures. Snoring is easily distinguished from catathrenia, since it is a supraglottic sound occurring primarily during inspiration. The prolonged expiratory noise of catathrenia can be differentiated from other sleep related sounds—such as snoring, stridor, and wheezing due to asthma—with PSG and video analysis. Snoring occurs during inspiration, and stridor will not appear sporadically in clusters. Central sleep apnea is differentiated by the lack of vocalization associated with breathing. Seizures can be characterized by a variety of types of vocalizations and speech, but they typically produce motor manifestations in sleep and are associated with EEG abnormalities, features not observed in Diego's case.

The pathophysiology of catathrenia remains uncertain. A variety of hypotheses have been proposed, including a vestigial sleep related respiratory pattern due to an abnormality in brainstem respiratory centers, functional occlusion of the vocal cords with forced expiration, breathholding concurrent with closure of the glottis, or unmasking of a primitive brainstem central pattern generator. Even the classification of catathrenia as a parasomnia is debated, some suggesting it may represent a form of sleep-disordered breathing. CPAP seemingly suppressed the groaning and OSA in Diego. Others have reported similar findings. A trial of CPAP assessing its effect upon the catathrenia, arousals, and sleep apnea is warranted in view of these anecdotal successes. We need to learn more about this rare chronic sleep disorder, which begins in childhood, appears to be lifelong, and so disrupts the sleep of others it forces the patient to sleep alone.

Bibliography

De Roek J, Van Hoof E, Cluydts R. Sleep-related expiratory groaning. A case report. *Sleep Res.* 1983;12:237.

Guilleminault C, Hagen CC, Khaja AM. Catathrenia: parasomnia or uncommon feature of sleep disordered breathing? *SLEEP.* 2008;31(1):132–139.

Marder E, Bucher D. Central pattern generators and the control of rhythmic movements. *Current Biology.* 2001;11:R986–R996.

Oldani A, Manconi M, Zucconi M, Castronovo V, Ferini-Strambi L. Nocturnal groaning: Just a sound or parasomnia? *J Sleep Res.* 2005;14:305–310.

Vetrugno R, Provini F, Plazzi G, Vignatelli L, Lugaresi E, Montagna P. Catathrenia (nocturnal groaning): A new type of parasomnia. *Neurology.* 2001;56: 681–683.

42

When More Is Less

JOYCE LEE-IANNOTTI, MD

CHARLES BAE, MD

Case History

Gene was a 77-year-old retired physician who presented to the sleep disorders clinic for evaluation of fatigue and involuntary leg movements during sleep. In his late 60s he developed unrefreshing sleep and unexplained night awakenings. His primary care physician ordered a polysomnogram (PSG) that showed frequent periodic leg movements in sleep (PLMS) and in wakefulness (PLMW) but no evidence of sleep apnea (Figure 42.1). He was started on clonazepam to treat the PLMS though his symptoms persisted. He started napping during the day and was unable to play with his grandchildren for extended periods of time. More than 20 years prior, he began to experience an urge to move his legs at night that he described as "irritating—as if bugs were crawling all over my legs." This initially was a no more than a nuisance, but it had become much more intense in the recent past. Stretching his legs or pacing in the bedroom would transiently alleviate this sensation, only to return once he got back into bed. He recalled that his mother had had a similar problem with her legs at night beginning in her late 40s. He denied tingling, numbness, weakness, or leg pain during the day.

Gene's physician switched him to pramipexole, gradually titrated to 0.5 mg per night, without significant improvement. Pramipexole was then switched to ropinirole, which significantly reduced his night awakenings, PLMS, and fatigue. He did well for nearly 6 years, but then his symptoms recurred and his uncomfortable leg sensations began to occur during the day whenever he was sedentary. Ropinirole was increased to a total daily dosage of 3.5 mg, divided in as many as 7 doses, which he took when his legs bothered him. With this adjustment,

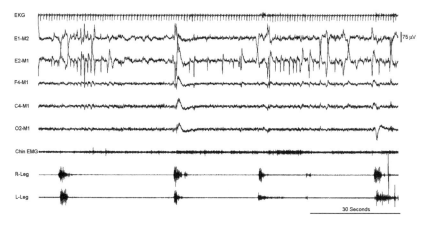

Figure 42.1 Two-minute PSG tracing during wake. Note the periodic limb movements (arrows) occurring at 25- to 30-second intervals. Periodic limb movements and intermittent elevations in EMG tone during wake are a characteristic feature of patients with RLS.

his symptoms became more tolerable, but only for a few months. He began to adjust the timing and dosage of ropinirole to control daytime leg sensations, ultimately taking 0.75 mg 8 times daily (total daily dosage of 6 mg), but this only made matters worse. He was then started on a rotigotine transdermal patch increased steadily to 6 mg daily, but he began to feel "drugged," with morning headaches, necessitating dose reduction to 4 mg.

At the time of presentation, Gene reported an average sleep duration of 6 to 7 hours per night. He would go to bed at 10 p.m. and wake up at 5:30 a.m. every day, never feeling refreshed. It typically took 30 to 60 minutes to fall asleep, depending on how intensely his legs disturbed him. He reported frequent awakenings throughout the night and would have trouble falling back to sleep due to leg discomfort. He would take one or two 30-minute naps per day and reported 2 near-accidents in the last year due to feeling drowsy behind the wheel. His leg symptoms were present virtually around the clock, with the exception of a few hours in the morning after awakening, when he was able to sit and read the newspaper without distraction until about 10 a.m. He scored a 22 (severe range) on the International Restless Legs Syndrome Study Group (IRLSSG) rating scale (see Appendix). He denied snoring, witnessed apnea, cataplexy, sleep paralysis, and parasomnia symptoms.

Gene's medical history was notable for atrial fibrillation and hypertension. He was married for 42 years with 3 grown children. He did not use caffeine, tobacco, or alcohol. He was an avid woodworker but had recently given up his favorite hobby due to safety concerns related to the use of power tools while sleepy. His medications included rotigotine 4 mg transdermal patch daily, ropinirole 6 mg per day divided into 8 doses, warfarin, atorvastatin, amlodipine besylate, flecainide, and a multivitamin.

Physical Examination

Gene was a mildly overweight Caucasian man with a body mass index of 28 kg/m² and a neck circumference of 16 inches. His upper airway exam revealed a Grade II Friedman tongue position, patent nares, and no retrognathia. On neurological exam, his mental status, language, and cranial nerves were intact. His motor examination revealed normal tone, bulk, and strength bilaterally. Deep tendon reflexes were 2+ and symmetric and his plantar responses were flexor. There were no signs of cerebellar dysfunction. The sensory examination was normal to light touch, pinprick, vibration, and proprioception in the upper and lower extremities bilaterally. Peripheral pulses were intact. His gait examination was normal. He was able to tandem walk and assume the Romberg position.

Evaluation

A complete metabolic panel, thyroid stimulating hormone, complete blood count, total iron binding capacity, serum iron level, and serum ferritin (98 ng/mL) were normal.

Diagnoses

Restless legs syndrome.
Augmentation due to dopaminergic medication.

Outcome

Gene was diagnosed with RLS complicated by augmentation related to the use of 2 dopamine agonists, ropinirole and rotigotine, prescribed simultaneously. He was started on gabapentin 300 mg 3 to 4 hours before bedtime and 300 mg at bedtime. Over the course of a 2-month period, the dopamine agonists were slowly withdrawn and the gabapentin titrated to a dose of 1500 mg a day (1200 mg at 6 p.m., since his symptoms usually intensified at around 7:30 to 8 p.m., and 300 mg between 10 and 11 p.m., before bedtime).

Gene experienced a 75% reduction in symptom severity on this regimen (IRLSSG rating scale score decreased from 22 to 7). His total sleep time increased from 6 to 8 hours per night, and his daytime sleepiness and fatigue improved

(Epworth Sleepiness Scale score decreased from 10 to 4 and Fatigue Severity Scale score dropped from 53 to 39). His sleep was more consolidated, and he was able to resume activities he had put on hold due to the disabling nature of his RLS. Now, 2 years after dopaminergic agent withdrawal, he remains virtually free of troubling RLS symptoms.

Discussion

Gene's case is fairly typical of primary RLS complicated by augmentation due to the use of dopamine agonists. One of the earliest accounts of RLS was made in the 17th century by Sir Thomas Willis, who described patients who couldn't fall asleep because of "leaping and contractions" of the arms and legs. In 1944, Karl Ekbom coined the term "restless legs syndrome," sometimes referred to as Ekbom's disease. RLS has since been described as "the most common disorder no one has ever heard of." While people of all ages and races are affected, older women have a slightly higher rate of RLS, and the prevalence and severity of the disorder increases with age. RLS affects approximately 10% of the population over 65 years of age. The hallmarks of RLS include an urge to move the legs, usually accompanied or caused by uncomfortable or unpleasant leg sensations that begin or worsen during periods of rest or inactivity, are partially or totally relieved by movement, and are worse or occur solely in the evening or night (Table 42.1).

The majority of RLS cases are classified as primary or idiopathic. A positive family history is present in more than 50% of patients with primary RLS. Onset before 45 years of age is more likely to be associated with an autosomal dominant inheritance pattern. Secondary causes, including iron deficiency,

---

Table 42.1 ICSD-2 diagnostic criteria for restless legs syndrome

A. The patient reports an urge to move the legs, usually accompanied or caused by uncomfortable and unpleasant sensations in the legs.
B. The urge to move or the unpleasant sensations begin or worsen during periods of rest or inactivity, such as lying or sitting.
C. The urge to move or the unpleasant sensations are partially or totally relieved by movement, such as walking or stretching, at least as long as the activity continues.
D. The urge to move or the unpleasant sensations are worse, or only occur, in the evening or night.
E. The condition is not better explained by another current sleep disorder, medical or neurological disorder, mental disorder, medication use, or substance use disorder.

peripheral neuropathy, renal disease, and medications (antihistamines, dopamine receptor antagonists, antidepressants) should be ruled out in all patients presenting with RLS.

Therapy for primary RLS consists of nonpharmacologic strategies and pharmacologic agents. Nonpharmacologic strategies include counter-stimulation (rubbing the legs, heating pads) and distraction activities, such as video games and crossword puzzles. Pharmacologic agents are classified primarily into four groups: (1) dopaminergic agents (dopamine agonists, levodopa); (2) benzodiazepines; (3) anticonvulsants (gabapentin, pregabalin, carbamazepine); and (4) opioids. Medical therapy is generally quite effective, alleviating symptoms in over 70% of cases. However, treatment with dopaminergic agents can be complicated by a peculiar phenomenon called augmentation.

Augmentation was first described in 1996 by Allen and Earley as the change in symptom severity, timing, and distribution with prolonged use of dopaminergic agents. Patients with augmentation report more severe symptoms, earlier

Table 42.2 NIH criteria for augmentation

RLS augmentation can be diagnosed if either of the following two criteria are met:

A. Criterion 1
RLS symptoms occur at least 2 hours earlier than was typical during the initial course of beneficial stable treatment.

B. Criterion 2
Two or more of the following key features of RLS augmentation are present:
- An increased overall intensity of the urge to move or sensations is temporally related to an increase in the daily medication dosage, or a decreased overall intensity of the urge to move or sensations is temporally related to a decrease in the daily medication dosage.
- The latency to RLS symptoms at rest is shorter than the latency either during initial therapeutic response or before treatment was instituted.
- The urge to move or sensations are extended to previously unaffected limbs or body parts.
- The duration of treatment effect is shorter than the duration during initial therapeutic response
- Periodic limb movements while awake occur for the first time or are worse than either during initial therapeutic response or before treatment was instituted.

C. In addition to meeting 1 of these 2 criteria, the diagnosis requires both of the following:
Augmented symptoms meeting these criteria present for at least 1 week for a minimum of 5 days, and
No other medical, psychiatric, behavior, or pharmacological factors explain the exacerbation of the patient's RLS and the augmented symptoms meeting these criteria.

Table 42.3 Differentiating rebound and augmentation

Early morning rebound	Augmentation
Early morning symptoms (between midnight and 10 a.m.)	Afternoon or evening symptoms
	Anticipation of time of onset
Delayed onset of symptoms	Followed by usual course of symptoms
Followed by symptom-free interval	Additional features (expansion to other body
No additional features	parts, shorter latency to symptoms at rest,
	increased intensity of symptoms)

symptom onset at night, emergence of daytime symptoms, shorter latency to symptom recurrence after discontinuing movement, and involvement of other parts of their body, such as the upper limbs and trunk (Table 42.2). Patients may also report a shorter duration of medication effect as in Gene's case. Augmentation is most common in patients taking levodopa, for whom it has been estimated to occur in 27%–82% of cases, but is also associated with the use of dopamine receptor agonists. Augmentation must be distinguished from rebound, which also occurs with the use of dopaminergic agents. Rebound manifests in patients who initially report benefit from dopaminergic agents but experience symptom recurrence 2 to 6 hours later, necessitating additional

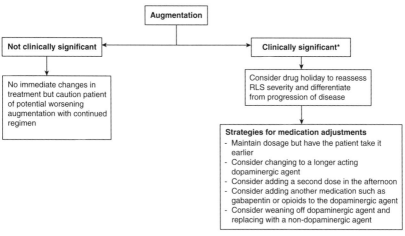

Adapted from Garcia-Borreguero D, Allen R et al. Augmentation as a treatment complication of restless legs syndrome: concept and management. Movement Disorders. 2007; 22:476–484.

*Leads to 1) change in daily activities and/or behavior; 2) negative impact on quality of life; 3) need to change the treatment dose or the patient needs to take the dose earlier in the day (e.g. dividing the dose); 4) adjustments in concomitant medication are made to compensate for augmented RLS symptoms (e.g. and increased intake of analgesics or hypnotics to cover an increase in symptom intensity).

Figure 42.2 Treatment algorithm for augmentation. Adapted from Garcia-Borreguero D, Allen R, et al. Augmentation as a treatment complication of restless legs syndrome: concept and management. *Movement Disorders.* 2007;22:476–484.

medication in the early morning hours. In contrast to early morning rebound, augmentation is characterized by an increase in symptom severity beyond baseline (Table 42.3).

Prior to adjusting dopaminergic medications in the setting of augmentation, one should verify that the patient is on the lowest effective dose and determine whether other explanations for RLS progression are present. Not uncommonly, these may include offending medications, caffeine and alcohol use, or iron deficiency. In the absence of such causes, the dose of the dopaminergic agent should be either reduced or divided into multiple doses over the course of the day. If augmentation persists, the dopaminergic agent should be discontinued and replaced temporarily with a non-dopaminergic medication (Figure 42.2). As illustrated by Gene's case, augmentation can be more disabling than the RLS itself and difficult to recognize in patients with severe RLS. However, prompt diagnosis and treatment, usually requiring frequent, sometimes aggressive, medication adjustments and careful clinical monitoring. can lead to marked symptom relief and rapid improvement in sleep quality.

Bibliography

Allen RP, Picchietti D, Hening W, Trenkwalder C, Walters A, Montiplasir J. Restless legs syndrome: Diagnostic criteria, special considerations, and epidemiology. A report from the Restless Legs Syndrome Diagnosis and Epidemiology Workshop at the National Institutes of Health. *Sleep Med.* 2003;4:101–119.

Garcia-Borreguero D, Allen R, Benes H, Earley C, Happe S, Hogl B, Kohnen R, Paulus W, Rye D, Winkelmann, J. Augmentation as a treatment complication of restless legs syndrome: concept and management. *Movement Disorders.* 2007; 22: 476–484.

Walters AS, LeBrocg C, Char A, Hening W, Rosen R, Allen RP, Trenkwalder C. International Restless Legs Syndrome Study Group. Validation of the International Restless Legs Syndrome Study Group rating scale for restless legs syndrome. *Sleep Med.* 2003(Mar);4(2):121–132.

43

They Call Me "Twinkle Toes"

AI PING CHUA, MD
LI LING LIM, MBBS, MRCP, MPH
NANCY FOLDVARY-SCHAEFER, DO

Case History

Julie was a 63-year-old Mary Kay cosmetic sales representative from Ohio who presented to the sleep center complaining that her legs had "gone wild" for the past 6 months. When she settled down in the evenings, either on her couch or in bed, she would experience intense, almost unbearable, aching cramps in her legs. Rubbing, shaking, or stretching her legs or walking around the house would quickly calm them. She denied upper extremity involvement. The annoying sensations would keep her awake until 1 to 2 a.m., and she would wake up at 7 a.m. to start her day feeling unrefreshed and tired. Julie recalled occasional nights with similar sensations in her legs over the past few years, but these never prevented her from getting a good night's sleep. In his later years, her husband had given her the nickname "Twinkle Toes" after the constant movements he observed during her sleep. During the day, her legs didn't bother her as long as she was on her feet. However, things flared up when she had to sit still for longer than 15 or 20 minutes. On a recent road trip with colleagues to Florida, she had to pull over every few rest stops to "shake out" her legs. Julie admitted to feeling sleepy at times, and typically drank 2 to 3 cups of coffee per day to stay awake. She had an Epworth Sleepiness Scale (ESS) score of 6 and a Fatigue Severity Scale (FSS) score of 36. She denied snoring, gasping, or choking in sleep and abnormal sleep related behaviors. Despite the recent loss of her husband, she felt her mood was good and denied symptoms of depression or anxiety.

Julie's medical history was notable for diet-controlled hyperlipidemia, fibromyalgia, irritable bowel syndrome, esophageal reflux, and allergic rhinitis.

She reported past renal calculi, for which she had undergone laser lithotripsy and laparoscopic pyeloplasty. She had a history of left lower limb deep vein thrombosis after blunt trauma to the leg. She reported diffuse myalgias and joint pain, for which she had been on steroids for several years, although a workup for rheumatological disorders was negative. She denied abdominal pain, nausea, vomiting, hematemesis, melena, hematochezia, hemoptysis, and easy skin bruisability. She had a hysterectomy 10 years prior that had corrected abnormal vaginal bleeding. She had not had hematuria since treatment for renal stones 4 years prior. There was no history of peripheral neuropathy. Julie's medications included prednisolone, escitalopram, trazodone, pantoprazole, potassium citrate, coumadin, fluticasone, a multivitamin, calcium, and vitamin D supplements. She had been keeping herself busy with work after her husband passed away. There was no exposure to tobacco and she consumed alcohol rarely. She was enrolled in a preventive cardiology and rehabilitation program and had recently started a regular exercise regimen. She was not a vegetarian but rarely consumed red meat. There was no family history of restless legs syndrome (RLS) or thalassemia.

Physical Examination

Julie was a well-groomed lady who looked mildly cushingoid. Her body mass index was $26\,kg/m^2$. Her upper airway exam revealed normal nares, a Grade I Friedman tongue position and no retrognathia. There were no skin changes in the lower extremities and all peripheral pulses were palpable. Her motor exam revealed normal tone, bulk, and strength bilaterally. She had intact pinprick, temperature, and vibratory sensation in the upper and lower extremities. The rest of her general and neurological examinations were normal.

Evaluation

Julie scored 20 on the International Restless Legs Syndrome study group (IRLSSG) rating scale, indicating RLS of moderate severity. Laboratory testing included complete blood count (CBC), serum iron panel, urea, creatinine, glucose, and calcium. Serum ferritin was $16.5\,ng/mL$ (normal: 18–300). The remaining tests were normal. Stool was negative for occult blood.

Diagnosis

Restless legs syndrome (secondary to iron deficiency).

Outcome

Julie was started on ferrous sulfate SR 325 mg (65 mg elemental iron) with vitamin C (ascorbic acid) 500 mg, 3 times per day. Four months later, the ferrous sulfate was reduced to twice daily as she reported that her leg symptoms, daytime sleepiness, and fatigue were markedly improved. After 6 months of treatment, serum ferritin was 97 ng/mL and her RLS symptoms had virtually vanished. She was scheduling more Mary Kay parties farther from home as she was able to drive longer distances comfortably. In fact, she had recently returned from a family reunion with her sister and 90-year-old father in Georgia and reported an uneventful car ride.

Discussion

RLS is characterized by an irresistible urge to move the legs, often accompanied by paresthesias, typically in the evening or at night, precipitated and/or aggravated by rest or inactivity and temporarily relieved by movement. The disorder is classified as primary (idiopathic or hereditary) or secondary to an identifiable cause. Some of the more common secondary forms of RLS are shown in Table 43.1.

Given the unique clinical features, a thorough sleep history is usually all it takes to diagnose RLS and differentiate it from other disorders associated with sensorimotor disturbances of the lower extremities. These include akathisia and

Table 43.1 Secondary causes and conditions associated with RLS

A. Iron or folate deficiency
B. End stage renal failure
C. Pregnancy
D. Peripheral neuropathy
E. Others: Parkinson's disease, depression, diabetes, rheumatoid arthritis, fibromyalgia, hypothyroidism
F. Drugs:
   i. Antidepressants (selective serotonin reuptake inhibitors, tricyclic antidepressants, mirtazapine)
   ii. Neuroleptics (typical and atypical antipsychotic agents such as risperidone, olanzapine)
   iii. Lithium
   iv. Anticonvulsants (phenytoin, zonisamide, methsuximide)
   v. Anti-emetics (metoclopramide, chlorpromazine, prochlorperazine)
   vi. Others: H1-antihistamines, beta-blockers, ethanol, caffeine, opiate withdrawal

habitual foot tapping; "sleep starts," also known as hypnic jerks; myoclonus of various etiologies; and leg discomfort or pain due to nocturnal leg cramps, vascular insufficiency, painful neuropathy, and arthritis.

Once RLS is diagnosed, secondary causes and aggravating factors should be excluded, as symptoms typically improve or resolve completely with treatment of the underlying disorder. The initial evaluation should include a CBC to screen for anemia and hypochromic microcytosis, blood urea nitrogen and creatinine for uremia and renal dysfunction, and calcium and glucose for hypocalcaemia and hyperglycemia/diabetes mellitus respectively, both of which can cause peripheral neuropathy. A serum ferritin level should be obtained, even in the absence of anemia, as correction with iron therapy has been shown to relieve symptoms. Further tests may be necessary to investigate the cause of anemia associated with iron deficiency and exclude bleeding, including occult blood loss from the gastrointestinal tract. Measures of thyroid function, vitamin B12, and an oral glucose tolerance test are performed if peripheral nerve disease is present. Nerve conduction studies and electromyography (EMG) including small fiber studies are indicated in cases of suspected peripheral neuropathy. The diagnosis of RLS is established based on clinical criteria and polysomnography (PSG) is not routinely required. However PSG should be performed if another primary sleep disorder, such as obstructive sleep apnea (OSA), is suspected. Characteristic PSG findings include periodic limb movements in sleep (PLMS) with or without arousal, and augmentation of leg EMG tone and PLMS in wake (PLMW) prior to sleep onset when symptoms are present (see videos 1 and 2).

Patients with frequent or disturbing symptoms, insomnia, daytime sleepiness, and fatigue should receive treatment. Management of secondary RLS involves addressing the underlying etiology and removing any associated triggers, such as repleting iron and folate stores. Symptoms dramatically improve or resolve entirely in patients with renal failure following renal transplant and in pregnant women after delivery. Patients with coexisting depression may require a change in therapy as selective serotonin reuptake inhibitors (SSRIs) and tricyclic antidepressants (TCAs) can trigger or exacerbate symptoms. Patients with seemingly intractable RLS may improve quickly after withdrawal of offending agents. Drugs that exacerbate RLS should generally be avoided. Treatment should be individualized with consideration of cognitive behavioral therapy in select cases. Drug therapies similar to those used for primary RLS are reserved for patients with persistent symptoms following correction of the underlying cause (Table 43.2). Dopaminergic agents improve the symptoms of RLS and anti-dopaminergic drugs exacerbate them. Effective treatments include the dopaminergic agents (carbidopa-levodopa, pramipexole, and ropinirole), anticonvulsants, benzodiazepines, and opioids. Dopaminergic drugs and opioids are more effective at suppressing PLMS than are benzodiazepines and anticonvulsants. Anticonvulsants are often preferred in cases associated with painful neuropathy.

Table 43.2 Pharmacotherapy of RLS

Drug	Dose range (mg/day)	Timing before sleep (h)	Half life (h)	Metabolism/elimination	Adverse effects
L-dopa/carbidopa	50–200	1.5–2.0	0.75–1.5	Hepatic, gastrointestinal	Rebound, augmentation, orthostatic
Pramipexole	0.125–1.5	2	8–10	Negligible, 90% unchanged in urine	hypotension, nausea, vomiting, hallucinations,
Ropinirole	0.25–3.0	1–2	6	Hepatic	nasal congestion, constipation, leg edema
Gabapentin	300–3600	1	5–7	Eliminated unchanged in urine	Sedation, dizziness, peripheral edema, ataxia,
Pregabalin	150–600	1	6	Negligible, 90% unchanged in urine	behavior change, weight gain
Carbamazepine	200–600	1–2	Variable	Hepatic	Nausea, dizziness, rash, blood dyscrasis, sedation
Clonazepam	0.125–4	1–2	19–39	Hepatic	Sedation, tolerance, dependence, bradypnea
Propoxyphene	100–600	2–2.5	6–12	Hepatic	Sedation, nausea, vomiting, constipation, dry
Tramadol	50–300	1.5–2	6–8		mouth, pruritis, respiratory depression, tolerance,
Codeine	30–180	0.5–1	2.5–3.5		dependence
Oxycodone	5–30	0.25–0.5	2–3		
Methadone	2.5–20	0.5–1	8–59		

* Opioids are presented in order of increasing potency

Iron Deficiency

Iron deficiency with or without anemia is common among RLS patients. Secondary RLS has been noted in pregnant, anemic, and dialysis patients with low iron status. Iron is a cofactor for tyrosine hydroxylase, a rate-limiting enzyme in the biosynthesis of dopamine, and it is the ferritin molecule that carries iron across the blood–brain barrier. Thus, the prevailing "iron hypothesis" is that RLS results from low levels of iron in the brain, interfering with dopamine synthesis. Compared to controls, patients with RLS have lower cerebrospinal fluid levels of ferritin and higher levels of transferrin, reflective of iron-deficient states, although the differences are not statistically significant. On brain magnetic resonance imaging, RLS patients have significantly lower iron content in the substantia nigra and putamen compared to age-matched healthy controls; disease severity correlates with the extent of nigrostriatal iron depletion. Iron is involved in the physiological regulation of dopamine-2 (D2) receptor binding sites. Single photon emission computed tomography (SPECT) and positron emission tomography (PET) studies of human and animal models have reported a diminution in D2 receptor binding and dopamine transporter activity in the striatum and putamen that normalizes after iron supplementation in subjects with RLS. Why iron deficiency specifically affects D2 receptors and not adrenergic, muscarinic cholinergic, serotoninergic or dopamine-1 receptors is unclear. It may be that iron is part of the receptor site, as many dopamine agonists and antagonists are iron chelators. Alternatively, iron may be important in the conformation of the receptor or the formation of the D2 receptor protein. Studies of neuromelanin cells in autopsied RLS brains have demonstrated decreased iron regulatory protein-1 (IRP-1) activity responsible for the post-transcriptional regulation of transferrin receptors and under-expression of these transferrin receptors, suggesting a defective response to the iron-deficient state. Lesions of A11, a hypothalamic nucleus from which the only descending dopaminergic pathway to the spinal cord arises, result in behavioral changes in rats not unlike those seen in RLS patients. These behaviors further increase when an iron-deprived state is induced and decrease with administration of the dopamine agonists pramipexole and ropinirole. The expression of Thy-1 protein, a T-cell protein responsible for the structural integrity of synaptic membranes of the dopaminergic system, is decreased in RLS autopsy tissue and animal models of iron-deficiency.

Iron deficiency should be assessed in patients with RLS, bearing in mind that serum iron is highly variable and transferrin and ferritin are not specific to iron metabolism. It is important to note that ferritin is an acute phase reactant that will rise during an acute illness, and therefore its level should not be sampled during or shortly following an acute illness. Low serum ferritin (50 ng/mL), even with normal hemoglobin and iron levels, has been reported in RLS patients and correlate with more severe RLS symptoms, PLM arousals, and decreased sleep efficiency. Iron supplementation reduces symptom severity and is generally recommended when serum ferritin is less than 45 to 50 ng/mL. Importantly, iron may be beneficial in RLS patients with serum ferritin above this level. Oral iron is effective in repleting body iron stores, and it is safe and inexpensive. It is often administered as iron sulfate 2 or 3 times daily. Iron should be taken on an empty stomach with vitamin C to facilitate absorption. Antacids can block iron absorption by chelating with iron and should be taken at least 2 to 4 hours apart.

Pregnancy

RLS occurs in nearly 25% of pregnant women and is more prevalent during the third trimester. Patients with primary RLS can experience worsening of their symptoms during pregnancy. The pathophysiology underlying this association is uncertain, but hormonal shifts have been implicated. Low serum ferritin, folate deficiency, and depression that arise during pregnancy may actually be the triggers, rather than pregnancy itself. Deficiencies of serum ferritin and folate have been found in pregnant women with RLS, and the resolution of RLS appears to correlate with normalization of folate and iron levels postpartum. The prevalence of RLS in women receiving folate supplementation throughout pregnancy is lower than in untreated women. Symptoms are mild in most cases and resolve promptly postpartum. However RLS during pregnancy may predict future recurrence of chronic disease. A conservative approach in this group of RLS patients is advocated, including education and reassurance on the benign and transient nature of the disease, encouraging a folate- and iron-rich diet, and folate supplementation. The recommended daily intake of folate is 600 to 800 mcg to prevent fetal neural tube defects and maintain normal metabolism during a time when red blood cells are increasing by 30%. Except for the most refractory of cases, the pregnant patient with RLS rarely requires additional therapy. Iron, folate, and vitamin B12 are the only Category A drugs proven to be safe and beneficial in pregnancy. Oxycodone, methadone, and magnesium are Category B drugs that are not shown to cause harm in controlled studies. Levodopa, clonazepam, codeine, propoxyphene, clonidine, and the anticonvulsants are Category C drugs that are demonstrated to be toxic in animal studies (although they may be used if the benefits of therapy outweigh the risks). Temazepam is a Category D drug proven to be teratogenic in humans.

Folate Deficiency

Folate deficiency has been implicated in RLS and several other neurological diseases as well as in pregnancy. Generally, serum folate measurements are preferred to red cell folate. Although red cell folate more accurately reflects tissue folate stores, the red cell folate assay is technically more challenging, resulting in poorer precision and reliability. It is also expensive, is not readily accessible, and lacks specificity and sensitivity. Furthermore serum folate has been shown to correlate well with red cell folate. Serum folate levels should be obtained in pregnant patients with RLS, especially in the absence of adequate folate supplementation, and in those presenting with peripheral neuropathy or intractable RLS symptoms not responding to conventional therapy. RLS symptoms improve with folate replacement. Unlike ferritin, it is uncertain what constitutes a healthy serum folate concentration in pregnant or neuropathic patients with RLS. Most pregnant women are already on folate replacement and have seemingly normal range serum concentrations. Further investigation in this area is required.

Uremia

RLS is common in patients with end stage renal failure, with a reported incidence of up to 60%. Severe RLS is associated with lower quality of life due to neuropsychiatric and cognitive dysfunction resulting from chronic insomnia and sleep fragmentation. Recent data has linked RLS symptoms with increased mortality in renal failure patients. Symptom severity may be a marker for underdialysis, inflammation, sleep fragmentation, and coexisting diabetes mellitus, which are all associated with increased cardiovascular morbidity and mortality. Likewise, the urge to move may hinder hemodialysis, leading to premature termination of dialysis and urea clearance, which in turn further exacerbates the disorder. Iron deficiency and peripheral neuropathy, common in patients with renal failure, can cause RLS and should be excluded. Hemodialysis improves RLS symptoms temporarily. Intravenous iron dextran infusion is effective in relieving symptoms in renal patients but is not widely utilized due to the lack of established long-term safety, efficacy, and availability. Dose reduction is required when administering drugs like opioids, gabapentin, and pregabalin that depend primarily on renal clearance. Similarly, higher doses for dialyzable drugs such as gabapentin are required in renal dialysis patients.

Peripheral Neuropathy

RLS has been linked to many peripheral nerve disorders. Nerve conduction studies and EMG are not part of the routine workup for RLS, but they should be considered in patients manifesting signs of peripheral neuropathy, such as sensorimotor deficits, and those with underlying metabolic disorders, including diabetes mellitus, hypo- or hyperthyroidism, vitamin B12 deficiency, and vasculitis. RLS patients with peripheral neuropathy should be screened for impaired glucose tolerance, electrolyte abnormalities, thyroid dysfunction, and B12 deficiency. RLS symptoms normally respond to treatment of the underlying cause of the neuropathy. Gabapentin and pregabalin are effective treatments for patients with neuropathic or painful RLS.

Depression

Depression is associated with RLS in up to 40% of patients. While the pathophysiology of this relationship has not been fully elucidated, many drugs used in the treatment of depression can precipitate or aggravate RLS symptoms. These include SSRIs and TCAs. Bupropion and trazodone which have both dopaminergic activity and antidepressant effects—are the drugs of choice.

Bibliography

Allen RP, et al. Restless legs syndrome: diagnostic criteria, special considerations, and epidemiology. A report from the Restless Legs Syndrome Diagnosis and Epidemiology Eorkshop at the National Institutes of Health. *Sleep Med.* 2003(Mar);4(2):101–119.

Connor JR. Pathophysiology of restless legs syndrome: evidence for iron involvement. *Curr Neurol Neurosci Rep.* 2008(Mar);8(2):162–166.

44

A 52-Year-Old Man with Flying Legs at Night

FAHD ZARROUF, MD

KUMAR BUDUR, MD, MS

Case History

Michael was a 52-year-old man who presented with difficulty staying asleep, excessive daytime sleepiness, and fatigue for the past 2 to 3 years. He reported having had a regular sleep-wake schedule for many years and never had any problem with falling or staying asleep in the past. However, in the recent years, he started waking up 4 to 5 times during the night for no apparent reason, though he was able to fall back to sleep in 5 to 10 minutes. He went to bed at around 10 p.m. and was able to fall asleep within 10 minutes, usually while watching TV. He denied restless, uncomfortable, or painful sensations in his legs in the evening or at bedtime. His wife reported that sometimes Michael appeared restless, moved around in the bed, and "legs appear to fly sometimes." No dream enactment, snoring, or witnessed apneas were reported.

Michael woke up most mornings feeling still slightly sleepy, but he felt much worse in the afternoon, especially after lunch. He frequently dozed off sitting in front of the TV, reading or watching a movie, but denied driving accidents or near-miss incidents because of excessive sleepiness during the day. He scored 17/24 on the Epworth Sleepiness Scale (ESS).

Michael saw his primary care physician 1 year prior to presentation and was prescribed trazodone 50 mg at bedtime. The medication did not reduce the number of nighttime awakenings, but it did allow him to get back to sleep faster. However, his wife felt that he was more sleepy during the day. He was subsequently prescribed eszopiclone 2 mg followed by zolpidem 10 mg at bedtime, without obvious benefits at night but worsening of daytime sleepiness.

He denied depressed mood; anhedonia; feelings of hopelessness or guilt; anxiety; and psychosocial stressors.

Michael had had a polysomnogram (PSG) 2 years prior at another facility, and he was told he had mild sleep apnea. He was prescribed continuous positive airway pressure (CPAP) but did not return for the CPAP titration study. He felt his sleep actually worsened and discontinued CPAP use.

His past medical history was significant for hypertension, coronary artery disease, hypothyroidism, and peptic ulcer disease. His medications included amlodipine, hydrochlorothiazide, levothyroxine, lovastatin, aspirin, and famotidine. He had no family history of insomnia, sleep apnea, restless legs syndrome, or Parkinson's disease. He denied use of caffeine, tobacco, alcohol or illicit drugs.

Physical Examination

Physical examination showed a well-built man in no apparent distress, with upper airway examination showing a Grade III Friedman tongue position. Cardio-Respiratory exam was within the normal limits, without wheezes or murmurs. His neurological exam showed an awake and alert man, fully oriented, with no abnormal movements. Deep tendon reflexes were within normal limits bilaterally.

Evaluation

A PSG was performed to re-evaluate his sleep apnea and assess for possible periodic limb movements. The study showed an overall AHI of 9.9 and REM AHI of 1.9. The arousal index was 102, sleep latency of 13 minutes, total sleep time of 240 minutes, and sleep efficiency of 73%. The minimum oxygen saturation was 90%. There were 744 periodic limb movements during sleep (PLMS), resulting in a periodic limb movement index (PLMI) of 186 and a PLM arousal index (PLMAI) of 84 (Figure 44.1). The serum ferritin was normal.

Michael had a CPAP titration study. At a CPAP setting of 8 cmH$_2$O, the AHI was reduced to 0.2. During this study the periodic limb movement indices remained elevated, with a PLMI of 115 and PLMAI of 76 (see video 1).

Diagnoses

Periodic limb movement disorder.
Obstructive sleep apnea syndrome.

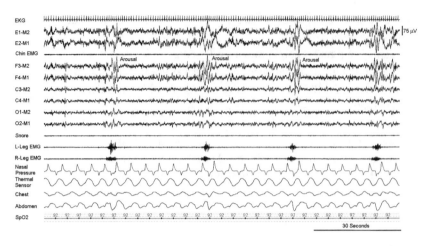

Figure 44.1 A 2-minute epoch of the polysomnogram showing frequent periodic limb movements with arousals.

Outcome

Michael wanted to try CPAP again. Since he did not think the leg movements were waking him at night, he declined treatment with a dopamine agonist at that time. At his follow-up appointment 8 weeks later, he continued to report daytime sleepiness and multiple awakenings, despite using CPAP all night every night. His wife again confirmed that he seemed restless at night, with leg jerks. She had become more aware of the leg movements after the findings on the sleep study. At this stage, Michael was started on ropinirole 0.25 mg at bed time and the dose was titrated up every 3 days to a total of 1 mg at night. At this dose, he reported consolidated sleep with only 1 to 2 awakenings at night. He also felt refreshed in the morning and did not report any daytime sleepiness. His wife also reported that Michael was no longer restless at night and that she had not observed any leg movements during sleep. His ESS score dropped from 17 to 7. He and his wife both were satisfied with the outcome.

Discussion

Michael's sleep complaints included multiple spontaneous awakenings at night with daytime sleepiness and fatigue.

Sleep disordered breathing was a diagnostic consideration, since he had had a previous sleep study that had showed mild sleep apnea. The repeat PSG showed an AHI of 9.9. However, this was unlikely to account for all of his symptoms and the exceptionally high ESS score of 17. Furthermore, his symptoms did not improve with CPAP at an appropriate pressure.

During the CPAP titration study, PLMI and PLMAI were markedly elevated. Limb movements are a common finding in patients with OSA, and the majority of the times these are secondary to respiratory events, resolving with adequate CPAP therapy. Therefore, Michael's PLMS could not be attributed to sleep apnea in isolation.

Apart from PSG (see Table 44.1), no further evaluation is needed in most PLMD patients. It is to be noted about 70% of patients with RLS have PLMS. This patient denied RLS symptoms.

The first step in managing patients with PLMD is to carefully evaluate other medications that may play role in causing or worsening of PLMS, such as selective serotonin reuptake inhibitors (SSRIs), tricyclic antidepressants, lithium, anxiolytics, or antiemetics. Serum ferritin may be useful although, unlike the

---

Table 44.1 ICSD-2 criteria for periodic limb movement disorder

A. Polysomnography demonstrates repetitive highly stereotyped limb movements that are:
  i. 0.5 to 5 seconds in duration.
  ii. Of amplitude greater than or equal to 25% of toe dorsiflexion during calibration.
  iii. In a sequence of 4 or more movements.
  iv. Separated by an interval of > 5 seconds (from limb movement onset to limb movement onset) and < 90 seconds.
B. The PLMS index exceeds 5 per hour in children and 15 per hour in most adults. Note the PLMS index must be interpreted in the context of a patient's sleep related complaint. In adults, normative values higher than the previously accepted value of 5 per hour have been found in studies that did not exclude respiratory events-related arousals (using sensitive respiratory monitoring) and other causes for PLMS. New data suggest a partial overlap of PLMS Index values between symptomatic and asymptomatic individuals, emphasizing the importance of clinical context over an absolute cutoff value.
C. There is clinical sleep disturbance or a complaint of daytime fatigue. If PLMS are present without clinical sleep disturbance, the PLMS can be noted as a polysomnographic finding, but criteria are not met for a diagnosis of PLMD.
D. The PLMS are not better explained by another current sleep disorder, medical or neurological disorder, mental disorder, medication use, or substance use disorder (i.e., PLMS at the termination of cyclically occurring apneas should not be counted as true PLMS or PLMD).

case with RLS, there is no established cut-off below which iron therapy is recommended. A PSG is recommended not only to confirm the diagnosis of PLMD, but also to rule out other conditions that can cause PLMS, such as sleep apnea. Caffeine can worsen leg movements during sleep and should be avoided.

Several medications have been reported to be helpful in PLMD, but none of these have been specifically studied or approved by the U.S. Food and Drug Administration (FDA) for this disorder. Benzodiazepines (mainly clonazepam and temazepam) are useful in some patients by improving the subjective measures of sleep quality, but they may worsen the PLMI in other patients. Dopamine agonists such as pramipexole and ropinirole have shown to decrease PLMS in RLS patients, but their efficacy in PLMD is not well established. Other medications that have been found to be helpful include opioids, gabapentin, and melatonin.

Bibliography

Baran AS, Richert AC, Douglass AB, May W, Ansarin K. Change in periodic limb movement index during treatment of obstructive sleep apnea with continuous positive airway pressure. *SLEEP.* 2003(Sep);26(6):717–720.

Hening W. The clinical neurophysiology of the restless legs syndrome and periodic limb movements. Part I: diagnosis, assessment, and characterization. *Clin Neurophysiol.* 2004(Sep);115(9):1965–1974.

Kunz D, Bes F. Exogenous melatonin in periodic limb movement disorder: an open clinical trial and a hypothesis. *SLEEP.* 2001(Mar 15);24(2):183–187.

45

The Woman Who Moved Her Feet with a Beat

SALLY IBRAHIM, MD
ROXANNE VALENTINO, MD

Case History

Janice was a 53-year-old Caucasian woman who presented to the sleep clinic with complaints of difficulty sleeping through the night. She reported going to sleep at approximately 10 p.m. on weekdays and 11 p.m. on weekends. On most nights, it took no more than 15 to 20 minutes to fall asleep. She would wake up once or twice per night, but it typically took an hour or 2 to fall back to sleep. During this time, she would feel discomfort in her legs and an irritating need to reposition them that was relieved by getting out of bed and walking. About 1 night per week, these symptoms occurred just before going to sleep at night. This problem first developed 30 years prior, during her first pregnancy, though it had increased in recent years. Involuntary leg movements would jolt her awake at night and her bed partner complained of leg jerks and kicking that disrupted his sleep. In addition, almost every night she experienced uncontrollable leg movements prior to going to sleep that were not necessarily bothersome to her but that annoyed her bed partner.

In the last few years, Janice developed low back pain after gaining 30 lbs. She took Tylenol PM most nights, without improvement in night awakenings. She felt sleepy and fatigued during the day and had an Epworth Sleepiness Scale score of 13 and a Fatigue Severity Scale score of 42. She drank three 8-oz cups of coffee daily to stay awake. She snored, which bothered her bed partner, but denied apneic episodes in sleep.

Janice's medical history was positive for hypertension, asthma, and a total hysterectomy 4 years prior to presentation. Her regular medications included diltiazem, hydrochlorothiazide, losartan, fluticasone-salmeterol, aspirin, and calcium.

She worked first shift as a registered nurse. She smoked a couple of cigarettes per week and drank alcohol at social functions. Both of her sisters had sleep problems; one had restless legs syndrome (RLS) and obstructive sleep apnea (OSA) and the other had insomnia.

Physical Examination

Janice was morbidly obese with a body mass index (BMI) of $45.3\,kg/m^2$ and a neck circumference of 46 cm. Her oropharyngeal examination showed a Grade III Friedman tongue position. Her neurological examination, including motor and sensory testing of the lower extremities, was normal. Her general examination was unrevealing.

Evaluation

Janice underwent a polysomnogram (PSG) due to concerns about OSA given her history of snoring, night awakenings, daytime sleepiness, and obesity. The study revealed a sleep efficiency of 77%, a sleep latency of 11 minutes, and increased wake time after sleep onset, corresponding to her reported sleep pattern at home. Her sleep stage percentages were normal with the exception of a reduced amount of N3 sleep (7%) and slightly increased N1. The arousal index was elevated at 33. One obstructive apnea and 74 hypopneas were observed, resulting in an apnea-hypopnea index (AHI) of 14. The mean oxygen saturation during sleep was 93%, periodically dropping following respiratory events with a nadir of 83%. There were 386 periodic limb movements during sleep (PLMS), resulting in a PLM index of 73 and a PLM arousal index of 16. During the initial wake period, rhythmic leg EMG elevations were noted in trains of 5 to 60 seconds with a frequency of 0.5 to 1.5 Hz (Figure 45.1). Some of these leg movements alternated between legs (Figure 45.2, video 1).

Laboratory testing revealed a normal complete blood count, BUN, creatinine, electrolytes, fasting glucose, and thyroid stimulating hormone. Serum ferritin was low (20 ng/mL).

Diagnoses

Obstructive sleep apnea (OSA).
Restless leg syndrome (RLS), secondary, due to iron deficiency.
Hypnagogic foot tremor (HFT) and alternating leg muscle activation (ALMA).

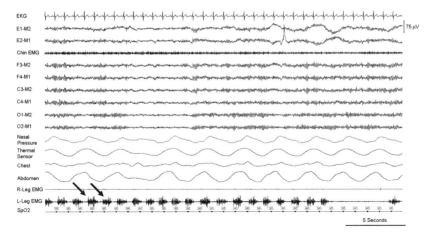

Figure 45.1 Hypnagogic foot tremor. Note the repetitive leg movements (arrows) during wake before sleep onset having a frequency of about 1 Hz.

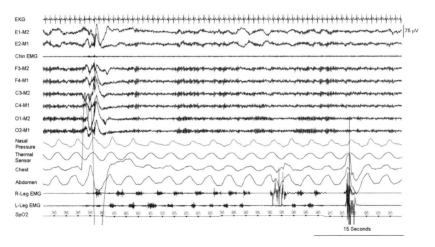

Figure 45.2 Alternating leg muscle activation. Note the leg movements in this 60-second epoch alternating between the left and right legs.

Outcome

Janice was first treated for OSA and RLS. She underwent treatment with continuous positive airway pressure (CPAP) therapy. Her night awakenings resolved and she felt more refreshed in the morning. She was placed on ferrous sulfate 325 mg 3 times per day for treatment of secondary RLS due to iron deficiency, with plans to check a serum ferritin level in 3 to 6 months to determine if ongoing supplementation was required. Her RLS symptoms improved significantly after a few months of treatment, and her bed partner reported that leg kicking in sleep had virtually stopped. However, she continued to have leg movements prior to going to sleep. These were more bothersome to her bed partner than they were to her. The couple was counseled regarding HFT and ALMA discovered on the PSG with appropriate reassurance given which alleviated their concerns.

Discussion

Although Janice was successfully treated for OSA and RLS, this case focuses on the incidental polysomnographic findings of HFT and ALMA on PSG (Table 45.1). HFT is a benign condition in which the feet or toes move rhythmically during the transition from wake to sleep or during stages 1 and 2 of NREM (see video 2). In fact, patients may not complain about these movements, but bed partners may bring them to the attention of the patient, as in Janice's case. There can be voluntary control over these movements. ALMA is an alternating pattern involving brief activations of the anterior tibialis muscle in one leg alternating with the other leg. ALMA usually occurs during sleep or arousals from sleep. Like most cases of HFT and ALMA, Janice had other sleep

---

Table 45.1 ICSD-2 diagnostic criteria for hypnagogic foot tremor (HFT) and alternating leg muscle activation (ALMA)

A. The patient reports foot movements that occur at the transition between wake and sleep or during light sleep (HFT only).
B. PSG demonstrates characteristic pattern
  i. For HFT:
- Recurrent EMG potentials or foot movements typically at 1-2Hz (range 0.5–3Hz) in one or both feet.
- Burst potentials longer than the myoclonic range (greater than 250 milliseconds) and usually less than 1 second.
- Trains lasting 10 or more seconds.
  ii. For ALMA:
- Pattern of brief, repeated activation of the anterior tibialis in 1 leg alternating with similar activation in the other leg.
- At least 4 discrete and alternating muscle activations occur with less than 2 seconds between activations.
- Individual activations last between 0.1 and 0.5 seconds and occur at a frequency of 0.5–3Hz (usually 1–2Hz).
- Sequences of alternating activations last between 1–30 seconds that may recur periodically (e.g. 1–4 times per minute).
C. The disorder is not better explained by another sleep, medical or neurological disorder, mental disorder, medication use, or substance use disorder (for HFT).

---

disorders (RLS and OSA), but these conditions did not explain the rhythmic leg movements.

HFT and ALMA are discussed together because the conditions are related and may represent variations of the same phenomenon. The etiology is unknown, although a large number of patients with ALMA have been reported to take antidepressant medications. HFT and ALMA are not known to be associated with other pathology. Up to 8% of adults referred for PSG are found to have these movements. While the movements can lead to sleep disruption, most affected patients are asymptomatic. Rhythmic foot movements while falling asleep usually present in children and may persist in adulthood.

The differential diagnosis of HFT and ALMA includes myoclonus, PLMS in patients with periodic limb movement disorder and RLS, painful legs and moving toes syndrome, and hypnic jerks. Myoclonic jerks are typically of shorter duration, lack an oscillating rhythmic pattern, and cannot be voluntarily suppressed like HFT and ALMA. PLMS have a duration of EMG bursts similar to HFT and ALMA, but have longer intervals between movements (at least 4 seconds). Additionally, PLMS predominate in NREM sleep, whereas HFT and ALMA typically occur in wake-sleep transitions, NREM sleep, and after arousals from NREM/REM sleep. In painful legs and moving toes syndrome, patients complain of pain or burning in the lower extremities that does not meet criteria for RLS. It is usually associated with spinal cord pathology or neuropathy. Hypnic jerks are differentiated from HFT by their sudden and brief nature, as well as the tendency to involve the upper extremities.

There is no specific treatment for HFT and ALMA. Although treatment is often not required, identifying the movements can help to counsel patients and their bed partners about their benign nature. However, patients with rhythmic foot movements should be treated for concomitant sleep disorders. In Janice's case, HFT and ALMA persisted after successful treatment of OSA and RLS, although the movements did not adversely affect her sleep quality.

Bibliography

Chervin RD, Consens FB, Kutluay E. Alternating leg muscle activation during sleep and arousals: A new sleep-related motor phenomenon? *Movement Disorders*. 2003;18:551–559.

Walters, AS. Clinical Identification of the simple sleep-related movement disorders. *Chest*. 2007;131:1260–1266.

Wichniak A, Tracik F, Geisler P, Ebersbach G, Morrissey SP, Zulley J. Rhythmic feet movements while falling asleep. *Movement Disorders*. 2001;16(6):1164–1170.

46

Sleepless in Kalamazoo

SILVIA NEME-MERCANTE, MD
NANCY FOLDVARY-SCHAEFER, DO

Case History

Meg was a 49-year-old, left-handed woman referred to the Cleveland Clinic by her neurologist in Kalamazoo, Michigan for evaluation of abnormal behaviors in sleep. She had croup at 9 months of age and 1 month later had 2 or 3 episodes of transient reduction in awareness without motor features. She was evaluated by her pediatrician, but the etiology of these events was unclear, and she was not treated. In her early elementary school years, she developed spells during her sleep similar to her current spells that would occur no more than once or twice per year. She had a normal electroencephalogram (EEG) and head computerized topography (CT) and was started on phenytoin without improvement.

When she reached her early 20s, the frequency of nighttime spells increased. Over time, they became more distressing to Meg and her husband, and the resultant sleep fragmentation affected her ability to function during the day. Spells almost always occurred between the hours of 1 and 4 a.m. and were characterized by a sudden arousal from sleep associated with a feeling of anxiety, after which she would roll over and grab the headboard or wall involuntarily. At times, this would evolve to shaking of both arms and legs. She would laugh softly or sigh afterwards and then return to sleep. She was fully aware during spells but would not speak, claiming that intense concentration could lessen their intensity and/or duration. In recent years, more severe spells were associated with urinary incontinence, though she never experienced oral trauma and her husband did not describe convulsive activity. Episodes would last 20 to 40 seconds and occur at least 2 to 3 nights per week, sometimes repeatedly during the night and worse surrounding menses. While the nighttime episodes scared her, the daytime sleepiness, fatigue, and difficulty with concentration, attention, and cognitive processing the next day were her primary complaint. After nights of repetitive spells, she had difficulty functioning at her job as a loan officer. In fact, her supervisor had recently suggested she consider resigning; otherwise, Meg would face a performance improvement plan at her next annual evaluation. Most nights she had trouble falling asleep and would wake up repeatedly during the night for fear of having a spell. Once awake, she worried incessantly about what she would do if she lost her job and health benefits. She snored lightly but denied witnessed apnea, restless legs symptoms, sleepwalking, and dream enactment behaviors. Her husband was distressed by Meg's spells. Fearing she might die in her sleep, he spent hours awake every night watching her and was experiencing daytime sleepiness, fatigue, and moodiness as a result of sleep loss.

Meg's birth and development were normal and she had no significant medical, psychiatric, or surgical history. She had a paternal cousin with seizures that remitted in childhood. She denied a history of closed head injury, central nervous system infection, or febrile seizures. She had had numerous brain magnetic resonance imaging (MRI) studies and EEGs over the years that were normal. Despite this, she had been treated with numerous antiepileptic drugs (AEDs)—including phenobarbital, valproic acid, topiramate, clonazepam, tiagabine, and acetazolamide—that were ineffective. She was taking levetiracetam, carbamazepine, and lamotrigine at the time of presentation. One year prior, she underwent a 5-day video EEG (VEEG) evaluation during which several typical spells were recorded without EEG change. She was diagnosed with psychogenic seizures and referred to a psychiatrist, who in turn told her she had no psychiatric diagnosis. She had discontinued her medications several times over the years and found that the frequency of spells was no different on or off AED therapy.

Physical Examination

Meg had normal vital signs and a body mass index of $22.8\,\text{kg/m}^2$. Her general examination was normal. On neurological exam, she had a normal mental status with intact fund of knowledge, memory, and processing speed. Her speech was fluent and comprehension, naming, and repetition were intact. Examination of the cranial nerves was intact. Her motor exam revealed normal tone, bulk, and strength bilaterally with no involuntary movements. Coordination and sensory examinations including pinprick, vibration, and proprioception were intact. The deep tendon reflexes were 2/4 and symmetric, and plantar stimulation was flexor. The gait was normal.

Evaluation

Due to concerns that Meg likely had medically refractory epilepsy, she underwent VEEG using the 10–20 electrode system placements with additional anterior temporal, frontal, and sphenoidal electrodes. Her AEDs were discontinued and she was asked to comply with sleep deprivation in order to record spells. Despite the extensive scalp montage, the interictal EEG showed no epileptiform discharges, although she had generalized intermittent slow activity. Eleven events were recorded with nearly identical clinical manifestations (see video 1). The clinical onset was characterized by abrupt arousal from Stage 2 sleep, accompanied by a sense of fear. This was followed by a vocalization ("unhum") after which she turned onto the prone position and grabbed the bed rail. Her heart rate increased from a baseline of 72 to 102 bpm and she was observed by staff to hyperventilate and have facial flushing. She was able to repeat and follow commands. Postictally, she responded immediately, was able to remember the word given to her during the seizure, and stated that she was clenching the bed rail because she felt dizzy and was afraid she might fall. The ictal EEG showed no clear ictal pattern (Figure 46.1). She had an ictal single photon emission computed tomography (SPECT) study during the evaluation but the injection was approximately 40 seconds after clinical onset, and therefore was not felt to reliably predict the area of seizure onset. The study showed an area of hyperperfusion in the left mesial frontal lobe. A positron emission tomography (PET) scan showed hypometabolism in the bilateral anterior mesial temporal regions (5–10%) and less than 5% in the left frontal region with no predominant focus.

Additional testing included a 3-Tesla MRI and neuropsychological testing. The MRI demonstrated subtle findings suspicious for a transmantle malformation of cortical development in the right frontal lobe (Figure 46.2). The neuropsychological evaluation revealed difficulty with verbal fluency and mental flexibility as well as occasional word-finding problems. Her performance on measures of other cognitive functions—including measures of verbal and visual intellectual reasoning, verbal and visual memory, simple attention, and verbal and nonverbal working memory—was within normal range.

Based on the character and stereotypy of spells, EEG manifestations, and imaging findings, Meg was diagnosed with nocturnal frontal lobe epilepsy, likely arising from the right frontal lobe. Since her seizures failed to respond to numerous AED trials, she was offered an intracranial EEG evaluation to precisely localize the onset of seizures. Prior to electrode implantation, she underwent a functional MRI for language lateralization. The study demonstrated Broca's area activation in the left hemisphere while receptive speech was represented bilaterally with greater activation in the right hemisphere.

The intracranial VEEG evaluation was performed with subdural grids overlying the right fronto-parietal convexity (A plate), mesial frontal (B plate), orbitofrontal (C plate), and mesial fronto-parietal regions (D plate), and

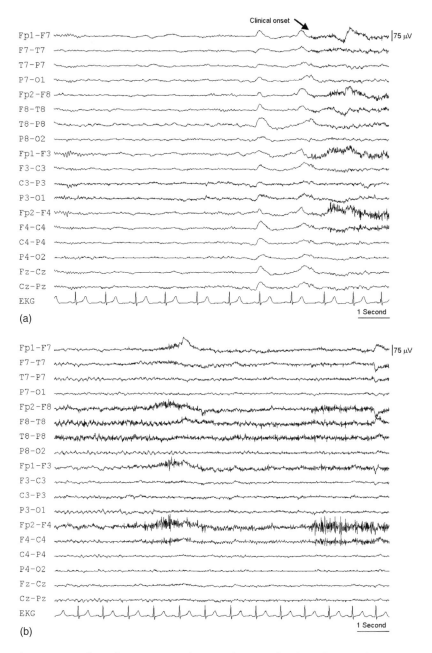

Figure 46.1 Scalp ictal EEG tracing of a typical event. The clinical onset (a) was an arousal from sleep (arrow) without any clear change in the EEG seen in the ensuing 10 to 15 seconds (b).

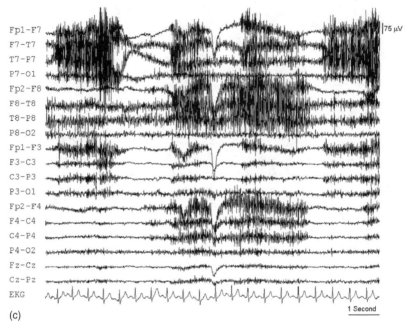

Fp1-F7
F7-T7
T7-P7
P7-O1
Fp2-F8
F8-T8
T8-P8
P8-O2
Fp1-F3
F3-C3
C3-P3
P3-O1
Fp2-F4
F4-C4
C4-P4
P4-O2
Fz-Cz
Cz-Pz
EKG

|75 µV

1 Second

(c)

Figure 46.1 Cont'd. Twelve to 15 seconds later. (c), there is an abrupt onset of movement artifact and tachycardia with a heart rate increase from a baseline heart rate of 72 to 102 beats per minute as seen in the EKG channel.

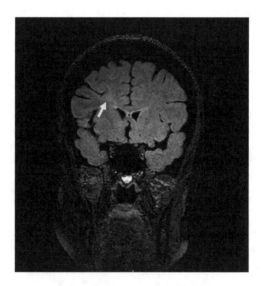

Figure 46.2 Coronal FLAIR MRI of the brain in a patient with frontal lobe epilepsy. Note the area of hyperintensity in the right frontal lobe (arrow) suspicious for a transmantle malformation of cortical development.

temporo-parietal convexity (E plate). An electrode was placed near the suspected malformation in the depths of the superior frontal sulcus (Figure 46.3). Interictal spikes were recorded from the right lateral, mesial and orbitofrontal regions and the inferior parietal lobule (Figure 46.3). Three seizures, clinically identical to those observed in the scalp evaluation, were recorded (see video 2). The ictal EEG was characterized by low-voltage activity followed by rhythmic spikes involving the depth electrode near the lesion, evolving to the B and E plates. Once seizures were captured, her AEDs were restarted and electrical stimulation was performed to delineate motor and language areas (Figure 46.3).

Diagnoses

Nocturnal frontal lobe epilepsy due to a malformation of cortical development. Insomnia due to medical condition (epilepsy).

Outcome

Based on the invasive EEG evaluation, Meg underwent a right premotor frontal resection involving the superior and middle frontal gyri, sparing the inferior frontal lobe (which was not part of the ictal onset zone or MRI lesion). The pathology demonstrated marked architectural disorganization and neuronal cytomegaly consistent with a malformation of cortical development. She developed transient left-sided neglect that resolved gradually over 2 to 3 months. She became entirely seizure free, and at 18 months postoperatively her AED regimen was reduced to monotherapy. A postoperative neuropsycological assessment showed a significant improvement on a variety of measures including problem solving, complex visuomotor sequencing and phonemic fluency.

Since surgery, both Meg and her husband were sleeping better at night. Over time, as she became less worried about seizures, her insomnia resolved. Without the frequent interruptions in sleep due to seizures and medication reduction, she no longer experienced daytime sleepiness or fatigue. She began to volunteer at the local library and decided to return to school in pursuit of a degree in social work. Her husband, now more at ease that Meg's seizures were a thing of the past, was sleeping better, too.

Discussion

In 1981, Lugaresi described a series of patients with stereotyped movements in sleep, including asymmetric tonic or dystonic posturing and bizarre behaviors having choreoathetoid or ballistic features lasting 20 to 30 seconds without

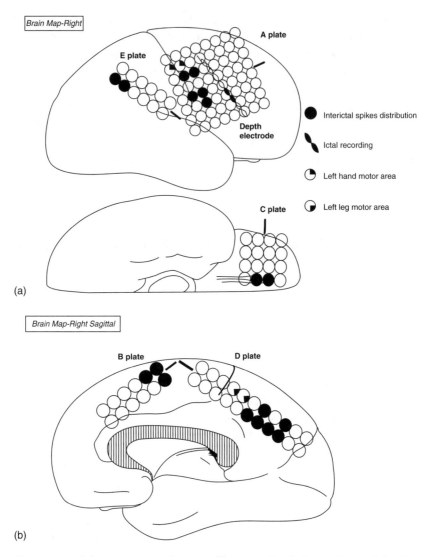

Figures 46.3 Invasive EEG maps showing placement of right hemisphere subdural grids and depth electrode on the lateral and inferior (3a) and mesial (3b) surfaces. The evaluation included fronto-parietal convexity (A plate), mesial frontal (B plate), orbitofrontal (C plate), and mesial fronto-parietal regions (D plate), and temporo-parietal convexity (E plate) coverage, and a single depth electrode placed in the superior frontal sulcus in the lesion. The location of interictal discharges, seizure onset and motor functions are shown.

associated EEG abnormalities. He questioned whether this—initially called hypnogenic paroxysmal dystonia, and later nocturnal paroxysmal dystonia (NPD)—represented a previously unrecognized form of epilepsy. Subsequently, detailed analyses of seizures arising from the orbitofrontal and mesial frontal regions confirmed that the semiology of Lugaresi's cases overlapped with that of frontal lobe epilepsy (FLE). The epileptic nature of NPD was confirmed by intracranial EEG recordings and the term nocturnal frontal lobe epilepsy (NFLE) was coined.

NFLE is a heterogeneous disease. Familial, sporadic, idiopathic, cryptogenic, and symptomatic forms have been observed. The familial form, known as autosomal dominant nocturnal frontal lobe epilepsy (ADNFLE), constitutes as many as 25% of cases. Linkage studies have localized genes for ADNFLE to chromosomes 20q13 and 15q24 with mutations in the transmembrane region of the neuronal nicotinic acetylcholine receptor (nAChR) alpha4-subunit (CHRNA4), beta2-subunit (CHRNB2), and alpha2-subunit (CHRNA2). The nAChRs are ion channels distributed widely on neuronal and glial membranes in cortical and subcortical regions of the brain. These channels regulate the release of acetylcholine, gamma-hydroxybutyric acid and glutamate and have a modulatory effect on arousals at the cortical and thalamic levels. It is hypothesized that these receptor mutations cause changes in neuronal excitability preferentially affecting the mesial prefrontal area and regulate microarousals thereby destabilizing sleep.

Seizures in patients with NFLE occur exclusively or predominately during sleep and can be of virtually any type. Asymmetric tonic posturing, dystonic, dyskinetic, and hypermotor activity as well as agitated wandering that can be difficult to differentiate from sleepwalking are observed. Most attacks are brief and repetitive, with sudden onset and offset and accompanied by marked autonomic activation, as illustrated by Meg's case. Consciousness is usually preserved, and motor features are stereotyped. The age at onset typically ranges from infancy to adolescence, and there is a slight male predominance. A personal or family history of parasomnia is present in more than one-third of cases. In nearly half of affected individuals, the EEG (ictal and interictal) fail to disclose epileptiform activity. Carbamazepine is effective in reducing or abolishing seizures in the majority of patients, although approximately 30% are resistant to medical therapy.

Many patients with epilepsy experience insomnia related to fears of having a seizure in sleep, fears of dying in sleep, or the psychosocial limitations imposed by a chronic neurological disorder. Patients with epilepsy are faced with a variety of challenges that adversely affect quality of life, including unemployment and underemployment, driving restrictions, financial stressors, and the stigma associated with epilepsy. Meg's nocturnal seizure pattern led to difficulty falling asleep and maintaining sleep, largely due to fears of having seizures. In turn, her husband developed insomnia due to his own fears that she might die in her sleep from a seizure. Her and her husband's insomnia resolved once her seizure disorder was controlled, supporting the diagnosis of insomnia due to her medical condition.

The differential diagnosis of NFLE includes NREM arousal disorders (confusional arousals, sleep terrors, and sleepwalking), nocturnal panic attacks, movement disorders, and psychogenic disorders. Unlike nocturnal frontal lobe seizures, panic attacks, psychogenic seizures, and arousal disorders lack stereotypy; spells are variable in duration, usually much longer than in NFLE, and clinical manifestations are more variable. Movement disorders typically present during wakefulness and are associated with abnormalities on neurological examination. Differentiating NFLE from a parasomnia by EEG recording alone is often challenging. Only about a third of frontal lobe seizures are accompanied by clear ictal rhythms on scalp EEG. Another third are characterized by diffuse, nonlateralized EEG changes not unlike that of the NREM arousal disorders, while the remaining third are accompanied by no recognizable EEG changes other than those attributed to muscle artifact.

In patients with stereotyped spells strongly suggestive of NFLE, high resolution MRI, ictal SPECT, and PET studies can provide indirect evidence of epileptogenicity. In medically resistant cases, the use of intracranial EEG is typically required to localize the ictal onset zone and map eloquent brain functions so that resective surgery can be performed with minimal risk of neurological morbidity.

Bibliography

Provini F, Plazzi G, Tinuper P, Vandi S, Elio Lugaresi E, Montagna P. Nocturnal frontal lobe epilepsy: A clinical and polygraphic overview of 100 consecutive cases. *Brain*. 1999;122(6):1017–1031.

Marini C, Guerrini R. The role of the nicotinic acetylcholine receptors in sleep-related epilepsy. *Biochem Pharmacol*. 2007;74(8):1308–1314.

Oldani A, Zucconi M, Ferini-Strambi L, Bizzozero D, Smirne S. Autosomal dominant nocturnal frontal lobe epilepsy: electroclinical picture. *Epilepsia*. 1996;37: 964–976.

47

Seizures and Stimulators and Sleep, Oh My!

JOANNA FONG, MD

CHARLES BAE, MD

KWANG IK YANG, MD

NANCY FOLDVARY-SCHAEFER, DO

Case History

Gary was a 43-year-old, right-handed man with a history of Type I diabetes mellitus who developed seizures at 36 years of age. His birth and development were normal. There was no history of head trauma, central nervous system (CNS) infection, developmental delay, or febrile seizures. His daughter developed temporal lobe seizures in early childhood.

Gary's seizures were preceded by an aura of fear followed by unresponsiveness and oral and manual automatisms. At times, partial seizures evolved to secondary generalized tonic clonic seizures (GTCs). Prior to the onset of epilepsy, he worked as a substitute grade school teacher with hopes of being hired into a full-time position. Since developing epilepsy, he had become a stay-at-home father. He had also stopped driving since his first seizure. His seizures persisted despite trials of more than 10 antiepileptic drugs (AEDs) in monotherapy and various combinations. As a result, he underwent vagus nerve stimulation (VNS) implantation to improve his seizure control.

After VNS implantation, Gary's seizures decreased from 3 to 4 per week to 1 to 2 per week. However, he developed excessive daytime sleepiness (EDS) and fatigue. For the first time in their 10 years of marriage, his wife began to complain of his loud snoring and irregular breathing patterns during sleep. She likened the sounds he made to a "sputtering motor" with escalating snoring, interrupted by brief pauses in respiration that did not improve even when she nudged him to roll onto his side. Gary had not gained weight since college.

He slept for 7 to 8 hours per night, between midnight and 8 a.m. Since VNS implantation, his night awakenings increased from 1 to 2 to as many as 5 times per night. He had no idea what woke him up and denied a choking sensation or seizures in sleep. He felt sluggish in the morning and had begun taking naps most afternoons. He denied symptoms of restless legs syndrome or parasomnias. His regular medications included controlled-release carbamazepine and aspirin.

Several months prior to presentation, Gary underwent a polysomnogram (PSG) to evaluate for sleep apnea. The apnea-hypopnea index (AHI) was 28, and events were predominately obstructive in nature. He subsequently underwent titration with continuous positive airway pressure (CPAP), but the AHI remained in the range of 20 to 40 titrated to a maximally tolerated pressure of 14 cmH$_2$O. He was prescribed CPAP at home but did not use it for more than a few weeks since it did not seem to alter any of his sleep symptoms.

Physical Examination

Gary was 6 feet tall and weighed 189 lbs. His neck circumference was 16 inches. His upper airway exam was notable for a Grade III Friedman tongue position with patent nares and no retrognathia. The rest of the general examination was unremarkable, with the exception of a scar under the left clavicle under which the VNS generator was palpable. His neurological examination was normal other than mild horizontal nystagmus.

Evaluation

Failure of apneic events to improve with PAP therapy raised concern that Gary's sleep related breathing disturbance was secondary to the firing of his VNS. Initially, a PAP titration study was performed, with CPAP followed by bi-level PAP due to unacceptable mask leaks at CPAP pressures of 10 cmH$_2$O and higher despite interface adjustments. The AHI remained elevated in the range of 22 to 28 at a maximally tolerated bi-level PAP pressure of 20/16 cmH$_2$O. Virtually all events were hypopneas occurring at 1.8 - minute intervals coinciding precisely with activation of the VNS (Figure 47.1).

A second overnight PSG was performed. This was designed as a "split-night" study with the VNS device off for the first 2 hours and on for the remainder of the study (Figure 47.2, Table 47.1).

The initial portion of the study (VNS off) revealed a normal AHI with oxygen saturation at or above 92%. With the VNS activated, oxygen therapy followed by adaptive servo-ventilation (ASV) was administered to assess whether there was a central component to the respiratory events. The AHI remained in the moderate range of severity (22 to 28) despite both treatments.

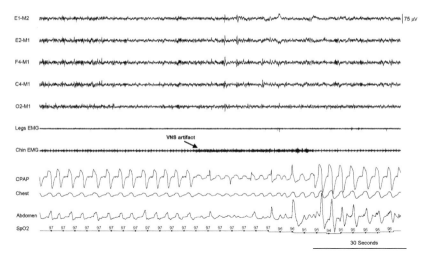

Figure 47.1 Two-minute PSG tracing showing a hypopnea coinciding with VNS activation recorded from the chin EMG electrode (arrow). The VNS activation (and hypopnea) lasts for 30 seconds after which respirations return to baseline.

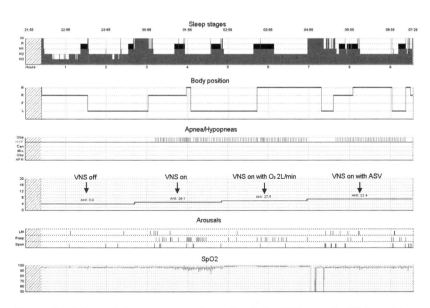

Figure 47.2 Split study hypnogram performed with the VNS turned off followed by oxygen therapy and ASV titration with the VNS turned on. Note the absence of respiratory events when the VNS was deactivated. Recurrent hypopneas coinciding with VNS activation persisted despite both treatments.

Table 47.1 Polysomnography findings based on VNS condition

Condition	TST min	REM TST min	REM TST sup%	Resp Events	Total AHI	Sup AHI	REM AHI	Arousal Index	SpO$_2$ min %	SpO$_2$ mean %
VNS off	131	18	0	0	0	0	0	2	92	96
VNS on	103	28	6	50	29	46	30	20	83	95
VNS on/O$_2$ 2 lpm	124	30	59	57	28	29	32	7	93	98
VNS on/ ASV	118	34	52	44	22	24	28	16	90	95

AHI, apnea-hypopnea index; ASV, adaptive servo-ventilation; Sup, supine; TST, total sleep time

Diagnoses

Obstructive sleep apnea syndrome.
Left temporal lobe epilepsy (TLE).
Status post vagus nerve stimulator implantation.

Outcome

After his second sleep study, which was recorded with the VNS on and off, it was clear that the pattern of Gary's respiratory events correlated with the firing of the VNS. The VNS was deactivated, and his sleep apnea resolved. His nighttime awakenings lessened and daytime sleepiness improved. However, without the VNS, his seizure frequency increased, and he decided to consider surgical treatment of his epilepsy.

Gary underwent a video electroencephalography (VEEG) evaluation with scalp and sphenoidal electrodes. The interictal EEG revealed frequent spikes and sharp waves in the left anteromesial temporal region maximal at the FT9 electrode (Figure 47.3). Several seizures were recorded, characterized by an aura of fear (during wake seizures) followed by oral and manual automatisms, staring and unresponsiveness (see video 1). Postictal testing revealed difficulty naming objects after recovery of consciousness supportive of a postictal aphasia. Seizures were associated with an evolution of rhythmic activity in the left temporal region on EEG (Figure 47.4). A high resolution magnetic resonance imaging (MRI) study showed mild volume loss in the left hippocampal formation without signal change. Neuropsychological testing and an intracarotid amytal test revealed intact verbal memory. Due to the risk of memory decline associated with a temporal lobe resection, an intracranial VEEG evaluation was performed with placement of subdural and depth electrodes to localize the onset of his seizures. Using this technique, seizures were found to arise from the left mesial

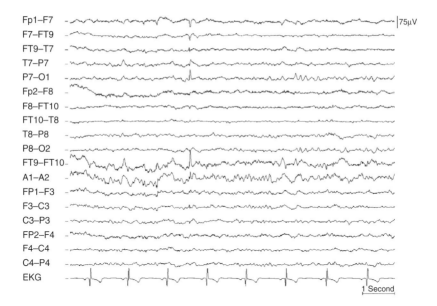

Figure 47.3 Ten-second EEG epoch showing a left anteromesial temporal sharp wave with a negative phase reversal at FT9.

basal temporal region. Thus, it was determined that resection of the hippocampal formation would be required to maximize his chance of a seizure-free outcome. After much thought, Gary decided to forego the temporal lobe surgery. Instead, he enrolled in an investigational device trial called the Responsive Neurostimulator System Study (NeuroPace, Inc.). This study involved implantation of intracranial electrodes (left mesial and anterior temporal, in Gary's case) in the suspected seizure onset zone that connected to an impulse generator placed under the scalp. The electrodes recorded electrical activity from the brain and delivered stimulation to suppress seizures. The device was programmed using a computer and a hand-held wand, much like the VNS. The VNS was removed before Gary entered the study.

At his 6-month follow-up visit, Gary reported a reduction in seizures from 8 to 3 episodes per month. Soon after the VNS was removed, his wife stopped complaining of snoring and breathing pauses in sleep, and he stopped waking up during the night. As a result, his daytime sleepiness improved considerably. He was able to run a 10K race, and a year later he completed a half-marathon, determined to not allow seizures to get the best of him.

Discussion

Temporal lobe epilepsy (TLE) constitutes nearly two-thirds of focal epilepsies that present during adolescence and adulthood. The syndrome of mesial temporal

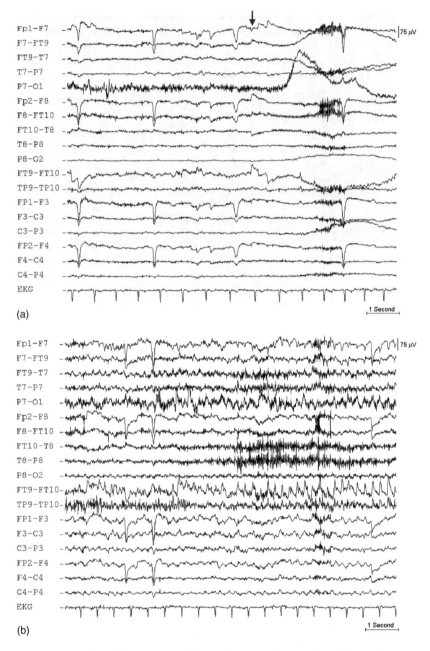

Figure 47.4 Ictal EEG during a typical partial seizure. The patient wakes up from sleep at the beginning of the first epoch (a) and begins to exhibit oral automatisms at the time of EEG seizure onset (arrow). In the next 10-second epoch (b),

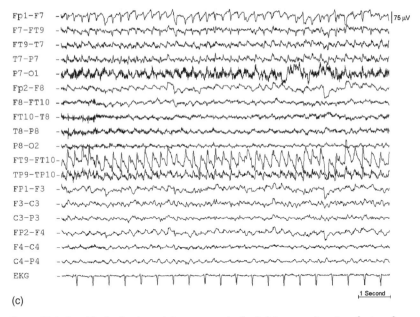

Fp1–F7		75 μV
F7–FT9		
FT9–T7		
T7–P7		
P7–O1		
Fp2–F8		
F8–FT10		
FT10–T8		
T8–P8		
P8–O2		
FT9–FT10		
TP9–TP10		
FP1–F3		
F3–C3		
C3–P3		
FP2–F4		
F4–C4		
C4–P4		
EKG		

(c)

⌐ 1 Second ⌐

Figure 47.4 Cont'd. rhythmic activity appears in the left temporal region that evolves into sustained 5 to 6 Hz theta activity 20 seconds after EEG seizure onset (c).

lobe epilepsy (MTLE)—in which seizures arise from the hippocampus, amygdala, and/or parahippocampal gyrus—represents the majority of cases. Patients with MTLE commonly have a history of childhood febrile seizures, CNS infection, head trauma, or a positive family history of epilepsy. Seizure onset ranges from the latter half of the first decade of life to early adulthood, typically beginning after a latency period following the presumed cerebral insult. Seizures commonly begin with an aura of fear or abdominal sensations and evolve to partial seizures with automatisms and alteration in awareness. The presence of postictal language disturbances is highly predictive of epilepsy arising from the dominant temporal lobe. Approximately 50% of patients also experience GTCs. Seizures usually occur during sleep and wakefulness, but they are exclusively nocturnal in a minority of cases. In general, nocturnal temporal lobe partial seizures are usually associated with less motor activity than frontal lobe seizures and, therefore, they are less likely to be confused with parasomnias. The EEG shows epileptic discharges localized to the anterior temporal or sphenoidal electrodes in more than 90% of cases. The ictal EEG is typically characterized by a gradual buildup of lateralized or localized rhythmic alpha or theta that may be preceded by diffuse or lateralized suppression or arrhythmic activity. Mesial temporal sclerosis is the most common pathologic substrate of MTLE, although neoplasms, vascular malformations, and malformations of development are also observed. At least 30–40% of patients continue to have seizures despite appropriate medical management. In treatment-resistant cases, resection of the anteromesial temporal lobe can produce a seizure free state in 70–90% of cases. While the procedure is usually associated with low morbidity, patients with left MTLE and intact verbal memory are at increased risk of verbal memory loss postoperatively.

Vagal nerve stimulation was approved by the FDA in 1997 as adjunctive therapy for partial epilepsy in patients over 12 years of age and, in 2005, for major depression in patients over 18 years of age. The device consists of a pulse generator, a spiral bipolar lead, a handheld magnet, and a programming wand with a handheld computer. The VNS pulse generator is encased in titanium and is the size of a silver dollar. This generator is implanted subcutaneously in the left infraclavicular region (Figure 47.5). The bipolar electrode lead is threaded under the skin to attach around the left vagus nerve in the neck. Because the left vagus nerve has fewer cardiac efferent fibers than the right, there tend to be less cardiac side effects using this approach. Although the exact mechanism is unknown, VNS reduces the frequency and severity of seizures by delivering small pulses of electrical stimulation (on-time) at preset regular intervals interrupted by periods of no stimulation (off-time). A hand-held magnet can be used

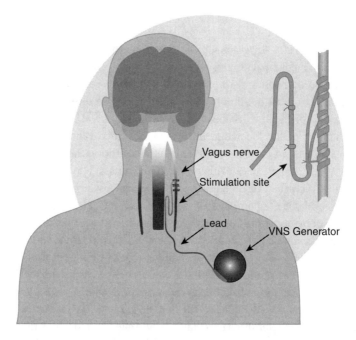

Figure 47.5 VNS generator with bipolar lead. The generator is implanted in the left chest wall and connected to a wire attached to the left vagus nerve through a lateral neck incision (modified with permission from Cyberonics, Inc).

to deliver an extra pulse of stimulation during a seizure to reduce the intensity or duration of the event.

The efficacy of VNS in the treatment of epilepsy was demonstrated in 5 clinical studies from 1988 to 1996. Overall, approximately one-third of subjects experienced a greater than 50% reduction in mean monthly seizure frequency, one-third experienced a less than 50% reduction in seizures, and one-third had no benefit. Only 5% of subjects achieved seizure freedom after VNS implantation. Common side effects include hoarseness, cough, throat pain, pharyngitis, dyspnea, paresthesias, and muscular pain.

Alterations in respiration have been reported in epilepsy patients treated with VNS. The first report detailed sleep related decreases in airflow and effort coinciding with VNS activation in four patients. In 2 cases, a reduction in VNS frequency ameliorated respiratory events. The mechanism by which VNS influences breathing during sleep is unclear, with both central and peripheral mechanisms proposed. Stimulation of vagal afferent fibers peripherally may activate motor efferents whose cell bodies originate in the dorsal motor nucleus of the vagus nerve and nucleus ambiguous. Activation of these efferents alters upper airway neurotransmission, thereby reducing airway patency. It is equally plausible that VNS might influence respiration through central projections to the pontine and medullary reticular formation to affect pontomedullary nuclei involved in the regulation of breathing and upper airway tone.

The emergence or worsening of apneas and hypopneas with VNS therapy has been reported in both adults and children with epilepsy. In one of the larger series, 16 adults with treatment resistant epilepsy underwent PSG before and 3 months after VNS implantation. At baseline, only 1 subject had OSA with an AHI of 5 or greater. Post implantation, the AHI increased in 14 of the 16 subjects, and all subjects had decreased airflow and diminished effort with or without tachypnea coinciding with device activation. Five subjects developed mild OSA. A recent pediatric series reported the emergence of sleep related breathing disturbances in 8 of 9 children following VNS implantation, including one who developed severe OSA (AHI = 37). Resolution of VNS-related apneas was observed after device deactivation. In contrast to Gary's case, CPAP therapy normalized the AHI in all subjects affording patients the opportunity to continue VNS treatment. As a result of these reports, the manufacturer of VNS added a warning statement to their product label stating that patients with OSA may have increased apneic events during stimulation. Treatment with VNS in patients with pre-existing OSA or patients with typical OSA risk factors (high BMI, large neck circumference, male gender, snoring, or witnessed apneas) should be pursued with caution. Lower stimulating frequencies or prolonging off-time may prevent OSA exacerbations. Polysomnography should be considered in all patients prior to VNS implantation, and careful follow-up thereafter is warranted.

Bibliography

FineSmith RB, Zampella E, Devinsky O. Vagal nerve stimulator: A new approach to medically refractory epilepsy. *NEJM.* 1999(Jun);96(6):37–40.

Hsieh T, Chen M, McAfee A, Kifle Y. Sleep-related breathing disorder in children with vagal nerve stimulators. *Pediatr Neurol.* 2008;38:99–103.

Malow BA, Edwards J, Marzec M, Sagher O, Fromes G. Effects of vagus nerve stimulation on respiration during sleep: A pilot study. *Neurology.* 2000;55:1450–1454.

Marzec M, Edwards J, Sagher O, Fromes G, Malow BA. Effects of vagus nerve stimulation on sleep-related breathing in epilepsy patients. *Epilepsia.* 2003;44(7): 930–935.

Rychlicki F, Zamponi N, Cesaroni E, Corpaci L, Trignani R, Ducati A, Seerrati M. Complications of vagal nerve stimulation for epilepsy in children. *Neurosurg Rev.* 2006;29:103–107.

48

The Boy Who Seized Every Time He Slept

TOBIAS LODDENKEMPER, MD
PRAKASH KOTAGAL, MD

Case History

Andrew was a 6-year-old boy who presented for evaluation of seizures. At the age of 4 years, his parents began waking in the middle of the night to the sound of gurgling noises from his bedroom and would find him in bed with his eyes open, mouth salivating, and face twitching. These episodes would last 1 to 2 minutes and were followed by 30 to 60 minutes of confusion. When Andrew woke up in the morning, he had no recollection of what had transpired. He underwent an EEG at a local hospital and was diagnosed with seizures. Medications were not initiated, as the episodes were exclusively nocturnal and occurred only once every few months.

At 5 years of age, Andrew developed daytime seizures. These were characterized by sudden jerking of the neck and left arm and upward deviation of the eyes, causing him to drop objects from his hands. His knees would buckle, and at times his limbs would jerk or he would stutter. These lasted no more than 5 seconds and occurred several times per week. Treatment with oxcarbazepine reduced them to a brief shiver or twitch of the upper body.

At 6 years of age, Andrew developed staring seizures, rarely associated with oral and manual automatisms. At around the same time, his seizures increased in frequency to several per day, often causing him to stumble. Both seizure types persisted despite maximum clinically tolerable doses of oxcarbazepine (41 mg/kg/d). Further antiepileptic drug (AED) trials including levetiracetam, valproic acid and clonazepam failed to improve seizure frequency.

Behavioral and school problems became apparent at 6 to 7 years of age. While no concerns were noted by his kindergarten teacher, Andrew had to repeat the first grade due to frequent seizures and medication side effects. Hearing and vision screens were normal. An individualized education plan was put in place.

Andrew was the product of a normal pregnancy and prolonged labor. Within his first 6 months of life, Andrew's parents noted reduced use of the left hand. As he grew older, his pediatrician found him to have a left hemiparesis and a spastic gait. Andrew's parents denied a history of febrile seizures, stroke, cerebral tumor, head trauma, or central nervous system infection. His parents also denied sleep disturbances, including snoring, witnessed apnea, and sleepwalking. Andrew had daytime sleepiness that was attributed to AED therapy, as it fluctuated with medication adjustments.

Physical Examination

Andrew's general examination was unremarkable. Specifically, he had no dysmorphic features and no neurocutaneous stigmata. Auscultation of the heart and lungs was within normal limits. There was no hepatosplenomegaly, and there were no orthopedic deformities or scoliosis. On neurological examination, his visual fields were intact. His left arm was held flexed at the elbow. Tone was increased in the left arm and leg. The strength in his leg arm showed a pyramidal distribution of weakness, while the strength in his left leg was nearly intact. He used the left hand as a helper hand only, although he was able to lift it against gravity. There were no fine finger movements of the left hand. Deep tendon reflexes were 4/4 on the left and 2/4 on the right. Plantar reflex was extensor on the left and flexor on the right. There was ankle clonus on the left.

Evaluation

Andrew underwent video EEG monitoring (VEEG) in the pediatric epilepsy monitoring unit. The interictal EEG showed a waking posterior background rhythm of 8 to 9 Hz with continuous slowing in the right centro-temporal region. Spike and sharp waves were present in the right temporal, fronto-central, and centro-parietal regions (60% maximum T8/P8, 30% maximum C4/P4, 10% maximum P4/P8) that were markedly activated in sleep. During light NREM sleep, normal sleep structures such as spindles and K-complexes were notably absent. Generalized electrographic status epilepticus consisting of diffuse spike wave complexes during NREM sleep was observed (Figure 48.1).

During the VEEG evaluation, seizures characterized by staring and unresponsiveness evolving to eye blinking and generalized body jerks were recorded (see video 1). In addition, more than 30 subclinical seizures (EEG seizures without clinical signs) were recorded. Clinical and subclinical seizures were

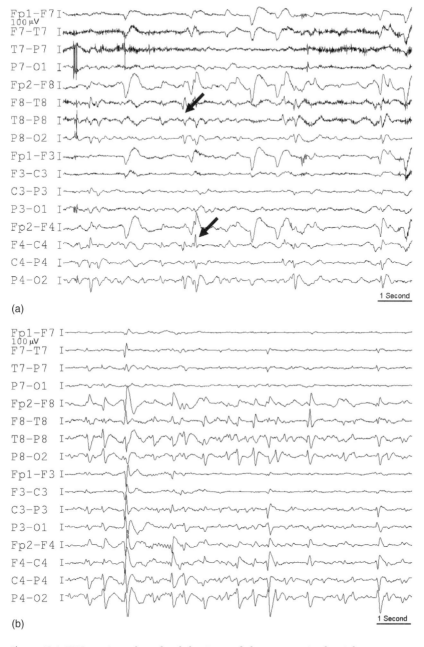

Figure 48.1 EEG tracings show focal slowing and sharp waves in the right centro-temporal region (arrows) during wakefulness (a). In Stage 2 NREM sleep, sharp waves occurred in long runs and sleep spindles, and K complexes were absent (b).

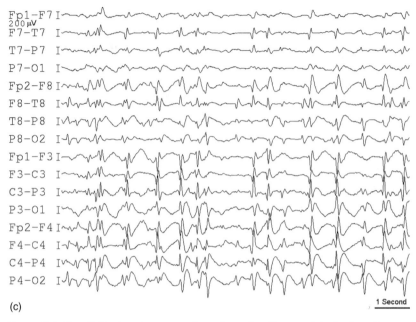

```
Fp1-F7 I
200μV
F7-T7  I
T7-P7  I
P7-O1  I
Fp2-F8 I
F8-T8  I
T8-P8  I
P8-O2  I
Fp1-F3 I
F3-C3  I
C3-P3  I
P3-O1  I
Fp2-F4 I
F4-C4  I
C4-P4  I
P4-O2  I
```

(c)   1 Second

Figure 48.1 Cont'd. During slow-wave sleep, the epileptiform activity had a wide-spread distribution over both hemispheres and occupied almost the entire epoch (c).

associated with a generalized EEG seizure pattern sometimes preceded by runs of right centro-temporal spikes (Figure 48.2). Late into the seizures, spike wave discharges became more lateralized to the right before becoming generalized again.

MRI of the brain revealed an extensive abnormality involving the right hemisphere sparing the occipital cortex and partially sparing the parietal cortex. Cortical thickening, shallow sulci, and serrated subcortical white matter were observed, most marked along the sylvian fissure. Diffuse gyral thickening and a paucity of sulci was seen in the right temporal region. Findings were consistent with diffuse right hemispheric polymicrogyria (Figure 48.3).

Diagnoses

Continuous spike waves during NREM sleep.
Right hemisphere malformation of cortical development.
Cognitive impairment.
Left spastic hemiparesis.

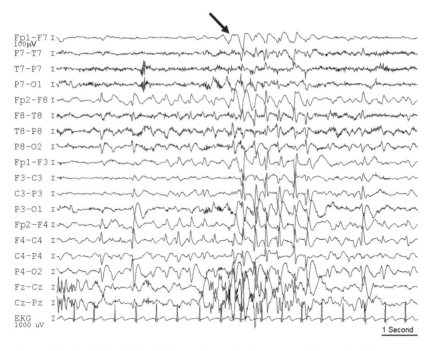

Figure 48.2 Ictal EEG of the child's axial myoclonic seizure while awake. The arrow denotes the clinical onset. Generalized spikes are observed that are preceded by epileptiform discharges in the right hemisphere.

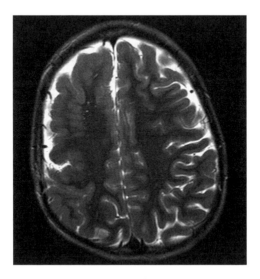

Figure 48.3 Axial T2-weighted brain MRI showing an extensive malformation of cortical development involving the anterior two-thirds of the right hemisphere (see text for detailed description).

Outcome

At 8 years of age, Andrew underwent a right functional hemispherectomy due to right hemispheric epilepsy in the setting of malformation of cortical development (Figure 48.4). The sleep related EEG abnormalities and seizures remitted postoperatively. His left hemiparesis remained unchanged. Now, 1 year after hemispherectomy, Andrew has remained seizure free. AED withdrawal was offered but his parents chose to continue medications for another 6 months. Academically, Andrew completed the second grade with As and Bs.

Discussion

Continuous Spike Waves during NREM Sleep (CSWS), previously known as electrical status epilepticus in sleep (ESES), is a rare epilepsy syndrome affecting 0.5%–1% of people with epilepsy. The diagnostic criteria for CSWS include (1) continuous generalized spike wave activity occupying at least 85% of NREM sleep, (2) seizures, and 3) neuropsychological impairment. Physiological REM sleep patterns are usually preserved, whereas NREM sleep stages are disrupted with occasional complete lack of normal sleep structures such as spindles, vertex waves, and K-complexes. REM sleep can be readily identified by the prominent decrease or complete resolution of CSWS. The ultradian organization of sleep is generally preserved.

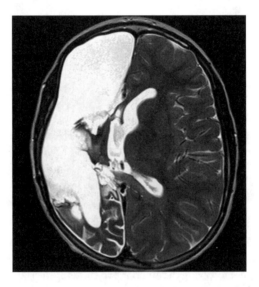

Figure 48.4 Postoperative T2-weighted axial MRI after right functional hemispherectomy.

CSWS occurs only in children and the course is age related. Seizures usually start between 2 months and 12 years of age, with a peak at around 5 years, as in Andrew's case. The typical EEG pattern may be detected between 3 and 14 years, usually a few years after the onset of seizures. The EEG pattern typically persists for 8 to 12 years and gradually normalizes in the late teenage years. Many affected children undergo developmental regression and present with deficits in language, socialization skills, memory, global intellect, and motor function, beginning 1 to 2 years after seizure onset, sometimes earlier. The loss of developmental milestones often correlates with the duration of CSWS. While the course of CSWS is usually self-limited, cognitive deficits frequently persist long after the EEG pattern resolves and are believed to be due to interference with memory formation during sleep. Other clinical features of CSWS, such as perinatal distress and abnormalities on neurological exam, such as congenital hemiparesis, are seen in up to 50% of cases.

The differential diagnosis of the clinical presentation of CSWS includes other epileptic encephalopathies, such as Landau-Kleffner syndrome (acquired epileptic aphasia preferentially affecting the temporal lobe) and atypical benign focal epilepsy of childhood. However, these disorders rarely present with hemiparesis, and seizures are generally characterized by more focal manifestations, such as unilateral right focal motor features. Other early, large structural lesions, frequently involving the thalamus, such as perinatal strokes, may present with a similar clinical presentation to Andrew.

There is no clear consensus on the optimal treatment of CSWS. Additionally, it is unclear if sleep-potentiated spiking on the EEG contributes to memory loss and cognitive deficits and, if so, whether pharmacological treatment for the electrical abnormalities alone is warranted. As neuropsychological regression seems to be related to CSWS and other interictal epileptiform discharges on EEG, AED therapy with agents such as valproic acid, ethosuximide, and high-dose diazepam is generally recommended in patients with seizures. Because of the self-limiting course of the illness in many cases, surgical treatment has been controversial. Nonetheless, surgical approaches including multiple subpial transections and focal resections have been performed in cases presenting with devastating developmental outcome and/or catastrophic epilepsy that fail to improve over time. Seizure and neuropsychological outcome following surgical therapy is not well studied.

Andrew did exceptionally well after a functional hemispherectomy. The procedure involved disconnection of the epileptogenic hemisphere from the rest of the brain with limited resection of tissue in order to prevent complications. In his case, epilepsy surgery was indicated for the treatment of frequent disabling seizures due to a large malformation of development in the right hemisphere. As Andrew's case illustrates, select children with unilateral brain lesions and seizures or neuropsychological impairment may benefit from surgery aimed at one hemisphere despite the generalized electrical abnormalities characteristic of CSWS.

Bibliography

Hirtum-Das M, Licht EA, Koh S, Wu JY, Shields WD, Sankar R. Children with ESES: Variability in the syndrome. *Epilepsy Res.* 2006;70 Sup1:S248–S258.

Loddenkemper T, Cosmo G, Kotagal P, Haut J, Klaas P, Gupta A, Lachhwani DK, Bingaman W, Wyllie E. Epilepsy surgery in children with electrical status epilepticus in sleep. *Neurosurgery.* 2009;64:328–337.

Tassinari CA, Bureau M, Dravet C, Dalla Bernadina B, Roger J. Epilepsy with continuous spikes and waves during slow sleep-otherwise described as ESES (epilepsy with electrical status epilepticus during slow sleep). In Roger J, Bureau M, Dravet C, Dreifuss FE, Perret A, Wolf P, eds. *Epileptic Syndromes in Infancy, Childhood and Adolescence.* London: John Libbey & Company; 1992:245–256.

49

The Case of the "Sleepy Stiff"

JESSICA VENSEL-RUNDO, MD
CARLOS RODRIGUEZ, MD

Case History

Brian was a 56-year-old man with Parkinson's disease who presented to the sleep center with recurrent awakenings from sleep for the past 7 years, unrefreshing sleep, and excessive daytime sleepiness (EDS). He was diagnosed with mild obstructive sleep apnea (OSA) 2 years prior after his primary care physician recommended a polysomnogram (PSG). The study revealed an apnea-hypopnea index (AHI) of 12, supine AHI of 16, and REM AHI of 14. Brian was started on continuous positive airway pressure (CPAP) therapy and underwent a second PSG, during which a CPAP setting of $7\,cmH_2O$ abolished the respiratory events. Neither study reported periodic limb movements (PLMS) or other unusual behaviors. Despite Brian's reported compliance with CPAP (using it 6 hours per night 7 days per week), his nonrestorative sleep, EDS, and frequent awakenings persisted. Treatment with zolpidem and, later, temazepam did not improve the situation. One year prior to his presentation to the Cleveland Clinic, Brian's neurologist prescribed modafinil 200 mg daily, which provided no relief from his extreme EDS. Further, his daytime sluggishness had contributed to a 10 lb weight gain since his last PSG.

Although he did not routinely take planned naps, Brian often fell asleep reading, watching TV, and working on his computer. On several occasions, he had even fallen asleep behind the wheel. He scored 15 on the Epworth Sleepiness Scale (ESS) and 40 on the Fatigue Severity Scale (FSS). Brian normally went to bed at 11 p.m. and woke up at 6 a.m., but he estimated a total sleep duration of no more than 5 hours per night on average. He woke up 5 to 7 times per night feeling stiff and uncomfortable and would find it difficult to reposition himself in bed. He denied cataplexy, hypnagogic hallucinations, sleep paralysis and symptoms of restless legs syndrome (RLS), but reported vivid dreams. For the past year, his wife had witnessed strange behaviors a few times per month, almost always in the early morning hours, in which Brian would yell and thrash in bed, once kicking her repeatedly. After she shook him awake, he recounted with horror dreaming that he was being chased by a pride of lions and falling to the ground as one descended upon him.

Brian was diagnosed with idiopathic Parkinson's disease 5 years prior and had a history of gastroesophageal reflux disease (GERD), hypercholesterolemia, and hypothyroidism. He took modafinil 200 mg daily, carbidopa/levodopa 25/100 mg 4 times daily, levothyroxine 125 mcg daily and pravastatin 20 mg daily. He was a lifetime nonsmoker and drank alcohol only on special occasions. He worked as a supervisor for a medical equipment distributor. In the past year, his co-workers had noticed he was becoming forgetful and called this to the attention of Brian and his wife.

Physical Examination

Brian was mildly overweight with a body mass index (BMI) of $27 \, kg/m^2$. His nares were patent with a midline nasal septum. He had Grade I tonsils and had a Friedman tongue position Grade III. He had mild hypophonia, a mask-like facial expression, and decreased blink rate. The motor examination was notable for cogwheel rigidity and a low-frequency rest tremor of the right upper extremity, and reduced arm swing bilaterally. His gait was slow and shuffling. His mental status and language were intact.

Evaluation

Due to Brian's severe and persistent EDS, frequent awakenings, and recent weight gain, a CPAP titration study was performed to verify that his CPAP pressure setting was adequate. Frequent respiratory events were observed on his home CPAP setting of $7 \, cmH_2O$. However, at a CPAP setting of $10 \, cmH_2O$ the AHI and the arousal index were normalized, snoring was eliminated, and the oxygen saturation was maintained above 90%. During REM sleep, excessive muscle activity was recorded from EMG electrodes on the arms and legs consistent with REM sleep without atonia (Figure 49.1). No PLMS or other abnormal movements or behaviors were observed. Thyroid stimulating hormone, complete blood count, and complete metabolic panel were normal.

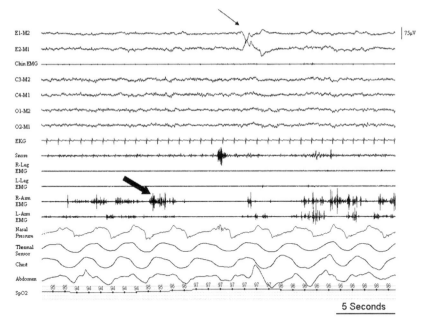

Figure 49.1 PSG tracing demonstrating REM sleep without atonia in REM behavior disorder. Rapid eye movements are present in the eye leads (line arrow) with low voltage desynchronized EEG indicating REM sleep. There is, however, increased muscle tone in both left and right arm leads (block arrow), which would normally be absent during REM sleep. EMG activity in the submental (chin) and leg EMG channels is low, underscoring the importance of recording from multiple muscle groups when RBD is suspected.

Diagnoses

Insomnia due to medical condition (Parkinson's disease).
REM sleep behavior disorder (RBD).
Obstructive sleep apnea.

Outcome

Brian was diagnosed with insomnia related to Parkinson's disease (Table 49.1) and RBD in addition to OSA and underwent a series of sleep interventions over time (Table 49.2). Despite an increase in CPAP pressure to $10\,cmH_2O$, his EDS did not improve, and he continued to have frequent awakenings at night due to body stiffness and discomfort. Carbidopa/levodopa 50/200 mg controlled release (CR) at bedtime produced a dramatic improvement in his

Table 49.1 ICSD-2 diagnostic criteria for insomnia due to medical condition

A. The patient's symptoms meet the criteria for insomnia.
B. The insomnia is present for at least 1 month.
C. The patient has a coexisting medical or physiologic condition known to disrupt sleep.
D. Insomnia is clearly associated with the medical or physiologic condition. The insomnia began near the time of onset or with significant progression of the medical or physiologic condition and waxes and wanes with fluctuations in the severity of this condition.
E. The sleep disturbance is not better explained by another sleep disorder, mental disorder, medication use, or substance use disorder.

Table 49.2 Brian's sleep interventions and outcomes

Intervention	Sleep symptoms	Epworth Sleepiness Score
Baseline	Sleep maintenance insomnia, EDS, nighttime motor symptoms	16
CPAP 7 cmH$_2$O, modafinil 200 mg	Sleep maintenance insomnia, EDS, nighttime motor symptoms	15
CPAP 10 cmH$_2$O, modafinil 200 mg	Sleep maintenance insomnia, EDS, frequent night awakenings, nighttime motor symptoms	15
Carbidopa/levodopa CR 50/200 mg, modafinil discontinued	Resolution of insomnia, EDS and nighttime motor symptoms	9
After 3 years of PD progression, multiple antiparkinson agents, modafinil 400 mg	Recurrence of sleep maintenance insomnia, EDS, nighttime motor symptoms	14
DBS, modafinil discontinued	Resolution of insomnia, EDS and nighttime motor symptoms	8

EDS, excessive daytime sleepiness; DBS, deep brain stimulation

stiffness, allowing him to move around more freely in bed. He slept longer (7 to 8 hours) and more deeply through the night. He felt that his EDS virtually resolved and his ESS score dropped to 9. He was able to watch movies with his wife again without falling asleep, and he got back to reading suspense novels on Saturday afternoons. However, Brian's wife remained troubled by his violent dreams and had grown tired of being kicked at night—now as often as 2 to 3 times per week—fearing someday she might be seriously injured. To treat the RBD, clonazepam 0.5 mg at bedtime was prescribed. Within a few weeks, the bad dreams and acting out completely resolved.

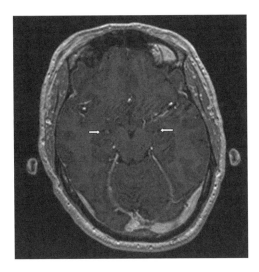

Figure 49.2 Axial T1-weighted brain MRI with gadolinium at the level of the midbrain showing bilateral subthalamic nuclei deep brain stimulation electrodes. (hypointense circumscribed signal intensities at the tips of the arrows)

Over the ensuing 3 years, the Parkinson's symptoms progressed and Brian's night awakenings and EDS returned, forcing him to take early retirement and stop driving. The severity of his motor fluctuations required treatment with escalating doses of carbidopa/levodopa followed by a variety of other anti-Parkinsonian agents, including apomorphine, ropirinole, pramipexole, and entacapone. Modafinil was resumed and titrated to 400 mg for treatment of EDS, although his ESS remained elevated at 14. Despite these measures, his motor impairment led to progressive disability prompting treatment with bilateral subthalamic nucleus deep brain stimulation implantation (DBS, Figure 49.2). At his 2-month postoperative assessment, Brian had significant improvement in his motor symptoms, and his night awakenings had essentially resolved. His ESS was reduced to 8, and he was able to discontinue modafinil and return to driving short distances.

Discussion

Parkinson's disease is a neurodegenerative disorder characterized by bradykinesia, tremor, and rigidity due to loss of dopaminergic neurons in the nigrostriatal and mesocorticolimbic systems of the brain. Up to 90% of patients with Parkinson's disease have sleep disturbances. Brian's case illustrates the spectrum of sleep disorders observed in patients with Parkinson's disease.

His presenting complaint of daytime sleepiness and recurrent night awakenings has a variety of potential causes.

Insomnia is the most frequent sleep disturbance in Parkinson's disease patients, with an incidence of 27%, as compared to 9% in the general population. Sleep maintenance insomnia is often due to movement disturbances, including tremor, bradykinesia, rigidity, dyskinesias, and dystonias that pose difficulty repositioning in bed. In addition, patients with Parkinson's disease experience treatment-related nocturnal disturbances, such as nightmares and hallucinations, and psychiatric symptoms that interfere with sleep, including depression, anxiety, and panic attacks. Parkinson's disease patients are also at risk for primary sleep problems that contribute to the recurrent awakenings at night, including OSA, RBD, and RLS with PLMS. Treatment of the underlying cause of the insomnia is required, sometimes combined with the use of nonbenzodiazepine hypnotic agents.

Brian had a known history of OSA which was suboptimally treated, so a diagnosis of hypersomnia due to OSA was considered. Parkinson's disease patients are predisposed to develop OSA due to abnormal upper airway tone and dyskinetic movements of respiratory muscles. Despite lower BMIs when compared to controls, more than 40% of Parkinson's patients have OSA. Standard treatments for OSA, most commonly with PAP therapy, are recommended. In Brian's case, the EDS appeared to be out of proportion or excessive for the severity of his OSA. Furthermore, his daytime sleepiness did not improve with therapeutic CPAP, supporting the suspicion that other causes were operative. Anti-Parkinsonian agents, including levodopa and dopamine agonists, are known to cause or exacerbate EDS in patients with Parkinson's disease. Sleep attacks occur in up to 9% of Parkinson's disease patients who take dopamine agonists. Therefore, the diagnosis of hypersomnia due to drug or substance should be considered. However, Brian's EDS began prior to treatment with dopaminergic agents. While his medical therapy may have worsened the EDS, was not the initial or sole cause.

Hypersomnia due to medical condition and narcolepsy due to medical condition are diagnostic considerations in patients with Parkinson's disease and EDS. These diagnoses are most often suspected in the setting of severe daytime sleepiness despite adequate sleep at night. However, Brian's sleep duration had become significantly curtailed over time due to difficulty falling asleep and recurrent night awakenings. As a result, treatment of the factors contributing to poor sleep quality and reduced duration was planned with reconsideration of these disorders if the EDS persisted.

Insomnia due to medical condition (Parkinson's disease) was the most likely diagnosis in Brian's case. Brian reported typical sleep duration of only 5 hours per night, the primary cause of which was thought to be suboptimal control of his neurodegenerative disorder. A deficiency in dopaminergic tone during the night produced motor fluctuations impeding his ability to make postural adjustments during sleep, in turn leading to recurrent awakenings, inability to fall back to sleep and EDS. The addition of carbidopa/levodopa 50/200 mg CR eliminated the motor fluctuations and prevented the nocturnal akinesia which were responsible for Brian's immobility at night. Alternative approaches included the use of a long acting dopamine agonist or the addition of a catechol-O-methyltransferase (COMT) inhibitor to his evening dose of carbidopa/levodopa.

Finally, Brian also experienced vivid dreams, and his wife reported dream enactment in the second half of the sleep period, features highly suggestive of REM sleep behavior disorder. RBD is a parasomnia characterized by injurious, potentially injurious, or disruptive behaviors during sleep associated with sustained or intermittent elevation of submental EMG tone or excessive phasic, submental, or extremity EMG twitching during REM sleep on PSG. RBD is associated with the synucleinopathies, neurodegenerative disorders including Parkinson's disease, dementia with Lewy bodies, and multiple system atrophy. The common pathologic feature of this group of disorders is accumulation of the insoluble alpha synuclein protein in vulnerable groups of neurons and glial cells. Approximately 65% of patients with idiopathic RBD are subsequently diagnosed with Parkinsonism and/or dementia. Clonazepam is the most common treatment for RBD, effective in approximately 90% of cases. Benzodiazepine hypnotics, such as clonazepam, can affect nocturnal breathing by reducing upper airway pharyngeal dilator muscle activity and increasing the arousal threshold. Therefore, caution should be taken when prescribing these medications in patients with sleep apnea. Safety precautions,—such as removal of dangerous objects from around the bed, securing windows and doors, and padding the floor next to the bed—should also be taken.

Although the exact mechanism of DBS is unclear, high frequency (130 Hz) stimulation of the subthalamic nucleus acts to inhibit its function, ultimately resulting in increased activation of the motor cortex in the brain. In addition to the primary effect on the motor system, DBS of the subthalamic nucleus has been shown to reduce sleep disturbances in patients with Parkinson's disease. Improved mobility during sleep, increased total sleep time, increased slow-wave sleep, and decreased wakefulness after sleep onset have been reported.

Most patients with Parkinson's disease and other neurodegenerative disorders have sleep complaints that are often overlooked as concerns regarding mobility and cognition take center stage. A smaller percentage of patients are diagnosed with and treated for their sleep disorders. Untreated sleep disorders not only result in medical co-morbidities (hypertension in OSA, for example), but negatively impact on quality of life, preventing patients from participating in the activities they most enjoy. Thus, routine assessment of sleep and wake disturbances should be part of the comprehensive evaluation and treatment of all patients with neurodegenerative disorders.

Bibliography

Cicolin A, Lopiano L, Zibetti M, Torre E, Tavella A, Guastamacchia G, Terreni A, Makrydakis G, Fattori E, Lanotte MM, Bergamasco B, Mutani R. Effects of deep brain stimulation of the subthalamic nucleus on sleep architecture in Parkinsonian patients. *Sleep Med*. 2004;5(2):207–210.

Diedrich NJ, et al. Sleep apnea syndrome in Parkinson's disease. A case control study in 49 patients. *Movement Disorders*. 2005;20:1413–1418.

Friedman JH, Millman RP. Sleep disturbances and Parkinson's disease. *CNS Spectrums*. 2008;13(3 Sup4):12–17.

Oerlemans SGH, de Weerd AW. The prevalence of sleep disorders in patients with Parkinson's disease. A self-reported, community-based survey. *Sleep Med*. 2002;3: 147–149.

Verbaan D, van Rooden SM, Visser M, Marinus J, van Hilten JJ. Nighttime sleep problems and daytime sleepiness in Parkinson's disease. *Movement Disorders*. 2008;2:35–41.

50

It's Never Too Late, or Is It?

WILLIAM NOVAK, MD

Case History

Fred was an 88-year-old gentleman with a known history of mild to moderate cognitive impairment following a fall resulting in a closed head injury 6 months prior. Initially, Fred's family noticed that he started forgetting appointments and would misplace things around the house. Fred also was aware of his cognitive decline, and although he was living independently, he was worried about the risk his cognitive decline presented to him. As a result, he sold his car and arranged his own placement in an assisted living facility.

Prior to his moving into assisted living, Fred reported a history of hypertension (well-controlled on medications) and nocturia (2 to 3 times nightly). He never used tobacco and drank only an occasional alcoholic beverage on holidays. He was taking an acetylcholine-esterase inhibitor as prescribed by his primary care physician.

Approximately 3 months after his move, Fred presented to the Sleep Center accompanied by his son with complaints of significantly worsening cognitive function and nocturnal hallucinations. Fred's son reported that his father's cognitive function appeared to be stable until 1 month after he moved. He seemed to be more confused in his new surroundings.

When asked about his new living conditions, Fred stated that it was taking more time to get used to things than he had expected. He was not making new acquaintances and was spending most of his time within his apartment, often with the blinds closed. In addition, he noticed that he began falling asleep later and later. While previously he had been able to fall asleep around 10 p.m., now it was often well past midnight before he was getting into bed. He denied racing thoughts, worries, and feeling depressed. His sleep duration remained unchanged (approximately 7 hours nightly), but instead of waking between 7 and 8 a.m., he was now sleeping until 10 a.m. Whenever his son visited him during morning hours, Fred appeared tired and would often fall asleep in the middle of conversations.

Fred also began to have nocturnal visual hallucinations that included seeing family members (both deceased and living), children unknown to him, and animals. His son recalled that one night Fred called reporting there was a dog, a bird, and cats in his apartment. The people and animals in his hallucinations were very real to Fred, and only with strong and repeated encouragement of family could he be convinced they were not real. As time passed, Fred's nocturnal hallucinations began to present a risk to both himself and others in the community.

One night alone in his apartment around 2 a.m., Fred began having visions of children calling out for help. He somehow managed to exit the facility and gain access to a neighbor's vehicle. He drove to his son's home and at approximately 3 a.m. began to bang frantically on his son's door, screaming "We have to save the children!" He pointed to a van parked on the street and said that children were trapped inside. Furthermore, he believed the van was filling with water. He began to strike the vehicle's windows, repeating screaming, "We have to save them… I hope we're not too late." Eventually, Fred's son was able to coax him into his home where he returned to baseline in approximately 30 minutes, but he had little memory of the event.

Physical Examination

Fred's workup included a head CT, chest X-ray, urinalysis with culture, and blood tests (vitamin B12, rapid plasma reagin, antinuclear antibody test, sedimentation rate, complete metabolic panel, complete blood count, and thyroid stimulating hormone), all of which were normal.

Evaluation

Fred's general and neurological exams were unremarkable except for an abnormal score on the Folstein Mini Mental Status Exam (MMSE). During the MMSE, the patient was found to have poor orientation to time; not being able to correctly state the date, day, month or season. He was unable to recall the Thanksgiving holiday which was less than one week prior. He also was unable to recall all three objects following five-minute interval. His MMSE score was 20/30, which indicated moderate dementia. Fred had difficulties providing basic directions from his house to popular neighborhood places and recalling Presidents in reverse chronological order: "Bush, Clinton … I have no idea … Nixon?"

Diagnoses

Circadian rhythm sleep disorder, delayed deep phase type (with "sundowning").
Dementia.
History of closed head injury.

Outcome

Significant changes in Fred's life included his moving to a new home, increase in social isolation, and difficulties falling asleep before midnight. The focus of initial therapy was the delay in Fred's sleep schedule - a delay in both sleep onset and waking. The goal of treatment was to advance his sleep onset and wake times to what they were prior to his moving to assisted living. Thus, he was initiated on 3 mg of synthetic melatonin 5 hours before his sleep time. He was also advised to wake up 1 hour early and try to advance sleep and wake time by an hour every week. He was encouraged to increase his daytime light exposure, starting from the time of his waking, at 9 a.m and to minimize exposure to light and mental/physical stimulating activities late in the evening and at night. He was advised to avoid naps during the day, even when he felt sleepy. In addition, Fred's son arranged for him to take part in planned social activities throughout the day. Caretakers at the assisted living facility were instructed on how to help Fred adhere to the treatment plan.

Within 3 weeks of initiating treatment, Fred began to fall asleep regularly at 10 to 11 p.m., and waking at 7 to 8 a.m., spontaneously. He found himself to be more alert in the mornings. He began to interact more with others at the assisted living facility and would even volunteer for odd jobs throughout the day. He was able to go to sleep at his preferred bedtime and no longer felt lonely or bored at night. More important, the visual hallucinations had resolved, and he attributed this to his ability to sleep well at night. Fred returned to the sleep clinic 4 weeks later. At that time, his general and neurological exams remained unchanged. He was advised to continue to follow the same recommendations (i.e., melatonin, exposure to light in the morning, no naps, minimize stimulation at night, and regular sleep-wake schedule.) Now, almost 2 years later, Fred's condition (including cognitive function) remains stable.

Discussion

Elderly people with cognitive impairment or dementia often experience abnormal behaviors in the evening or during the night known as "sundowning". A person who is experiencing sundowning may become abnormally demanding, suspicious, upset, or disoriented. In addition, they may have visual or auditory hallucinations, appear irritable or agitated, or wander, posing a risk for accidents and injuries. These abnormal behaviors are commonly observed in patients with moderate to severe dementia of the Alzheimer's type. Fred exhibited several features consistent with sundowning.

Fred's history, although rare for this age group, was consistent for a circadian rhythm abnormality, of the delayed sleep phase type. Based on the International Classification of Sleep Disorders criteria, the patient had a complaint of an inability to fall asleep at a desired clock time, an inability to spontaneously awaken at a desired awakening time, phase delay of major sleep episode in relation to desired sleep time, and his symptoms were present for greater than 1 month.

It is not uncommon for elderly patients with dementia to have cognitive decline accompanied by disturbances of mood, behavior, sleep, and activities of daily living. The triggers for change in sleep patterns remains uncertain. Degenerative changes in the suprachiasmatic nucleus, the master biological clock, have been proposed. In addition, people with dementia have been shown to have greater percentages of total daily motor activity at night, less strict circadian motor activity rhythms, and later acrophase (peak) of both motor activity and temperature rhythms, all of which are consistent with a delayed sleep phase type circadian abnormality.

While Fred's underlying dementia may have played a role in his circadian abnormality and associated sundowning, the most likely cause was a life adjustment, in this case, a new place of residence. This life change resulted in Fred becoming socially isolated. Additionally, by having limited exposure to daylight, he essentially removed critical photic cues that allowed for the entrainment of his sleep-wake cycle.

The correction of his circadian abnormality necessitated strict changes in his life habits as well as the use of melatonin. The rationale for such a treatment plan was based on a series of reports on the ability of physiological levels of melatonin to advance the circadian phase and sleep onset. Happily, Fred not only advanced his circadian phase, but had an overall improvement in his cognitive function.

Bibliography

Riemersma-van der Lek R, Swaab DF. Effect of bright light and melatonin on cognitive and concognitive function in elderly residents of group care facilities: Randomized control trial. *JAMA*. 2008;299(22):2642–2655.

Volicer L, Harper DG, Manning BC, et al. Sundowning and circadian rhythms in Alzheimer's disease. *Am J Psych*. 2001;158:704–711.

51

"Mom, I Have a Bad Headache, I'm Tired, and I Can't Go to School"

DAVID ROTHNER, MD

Case History

Jonathan, a 15-year-old young man, was evaluated for chronic headaches. He was the product of a normal pregnancy, labor, and delivery. His growth and development were normal. His past medical history was negative for significant medical problems. His academic function was above average until 18 months ago, when his headaches began.

Jonathan's headaches began without apparent precipitating cause. At first they were occasional, nondescript, and of moderate severity. Over the subsequent 2 months, they evolved into daily headaches and then became 24/7. They were bifrontal in location, graded 5-6/10, and described as squeezing. They were worsened by activity. They were not associated with nausea, vomiting, phonophobia, photophobia, or neurological features. He had never had a typical migraine.

For the last 1.5 to 2 years or so, his parents noted that he had increasing difficulty with falling asleep, remaining awake until 2 to 3 a.m., and habitual delay in rise times on weekends. This sleep pattern began even before his headaches became constant. They reported that his difficulty with earlier bedtimes was not always due to headaches. He also had multiple nocturnal awakenings and increasing difficulty with getting up in the morning for school. No loud snoring, apnea, or abnormal leg movements were noted. The development of these sleep complaints worsened his headache and aggravated school issues. At school he was noted to have deteriorating grades and he frequently fell asleep in class. At the time of the office visit, he had missed 31 days of school. He consumed 3 to 4 caffeinated sodas daily, but almost never in the evening.

Evaluations by his primary care physician and neurologist had previously been undertaken. Laboratory testing—including thyroid studies, dilated eye exam and electroencephalogram, as well as computerized tomogram and magnetic resonance imaging (MRI) scans of the brain—were all negative. No Chiari malformation was noted. Lumbar puncture showed normal opening and closing pressures and normal protein, sugar, and cells on cerebrospinal fluid analysis.

Prior unsuccessful treatments included gabapentin, topiramate, acetazolamide, and trigger point injections. He drank caffeinated soda to excess and used Fioricet and Vicodin several times daily.

Family history revealed significant marital discord and paternal alcoholism. His older siblings were healthy and in college. There was no significant family history of headache.

Physical Examination

On examination, Jonathan was obese with a body mass index of $32\,kg/m^2$. He stated that his headache was a 7 on a scale of 10, but he did not appear to be in distress. A detailed general examination and neurological examination were normal.

Diagnoses

Insomnia due to medical condition—chronic daily headache (CDH).
Possible delayed sleep phase syndrome (DSPS).
Possible medication overuse headache (caffeine overuse).
Somatoform disorder.

Outcome

Jonathan was admitted to the inpatient adolescent pain program. Discontinuation of all medications and caffeine, daily psychological counseling and group therapy, a rigorous physical rehabilitation program, occupational and physical therapy, adequate hydration, and a balanced diet were implemented. Regular sleep routines were enforced. For headaches, amitriptyline was initiated at 5 mg before bedtime. Due to the possibility of delayed sleep phase, melatonin at a dose of 3 mg was also added at 7 p.m.

Within 10 days, noticeable changes in function and attitude were noted. At the end of 3 weeks, sleep quality was significantly improved and headaches, though still daily, were less severe. He reported a bedtime of 10 p.m. and was generally asleep by 10:30 p.m. He woke up at 6:30 a.m. on school days and no later than 8 a.m. on weekends. He denied need for naps and felt more energetic during the day. Outpatient follow up visits, continued counseling, lifestyle changes, melatonin and amitriptyline therapy, avoidance of analgesics, and mandatory school attendance were emphasized.

Discussion

"The stupid looking lazy child who frequently suffers from headaches in school, breathes through his mouth instead of his nose, snores and is restless at night and wakes with a dry mouth in the morning, is well worthy of the solicitous attention of the school medical officer."

Since Hill made this observation in 1889 the relationship of sleep to head-ache has fascinated both physicians dealing with headache as well as those with primary interest in sleep disorders. Bille, in his classic monograph (1962), which initiated the modern era of the study of headache in children, noted that sleep disturbances were present in 47% of children with migraines. Additional mile-stones highlighting the sleep-headache relationship include Guilleminault's description of sleep apnea in children (1976), Barabas's observation (1986) that children with migraine had a higher incidence of somnambulism, and Bruni's study (1997) that showed children with migraine and those with ten-sion-type headaches had less sleep and longer sleep latencies than controls. More recently, Luc reported (2006) that children with headache have a higher prevalence of excessive daytime somnolence, narcolepsy, and insomnia.

The most common forms of headache seen in pre-adolescents include migraine followed by CDH. Seventy to 85% of migraine patients have migraine without aura; 15–30% have migraine with aura. CDH implies more than 15 days of headache per month. Tension-type headaches are experienced on the majority of days, whereas migraines are noted on half or fewer days.

The statistics are reversed in adolescents, where the majority of patients have CDH and fewer have migraine alone. Associated co-morbidities include school absences, medication overuse, family strife, sleep irregularity, and academic deterioration; obesity and psychological stress additionally make the problem more difficult to treat. A multidisciplinary approach is therefore needed.

Sleep related headaches are infrequent in children and teens, according to the International Classification of Sleep Disorders (ICSD-2). Cluster headaches and hypnic headache are rare in children and adolescents. Migraine on occa-sion will begin during sleep, but this does not occur frequently. If a child or teen has increasing frequency and severity of headache, and the headache awakens the patient from sleep, a space-occupying mass must be considered.

The spectrum of sleep disorders seen in youngsters with headaches varies depending on the type of headache (migraine vs. TTH) and the patient's age.

Younger children with headache have a high incidence of sleep disorders. These include sleeping too little (42%), co-sleeping with parents (25%), and snoring (23%). Those with migraine were also noted to have sleep anxiety, parasomnia, and sleep resistance.

Adolescents with headaches (both migraine and TTH) also have a higher frequency of sleep disorders. These include insufficient total sleep (66%), daytime sleepiness (23%), difficulty falling asleep (41%), and nocturnal awakenings (38%). Although not mentioned, DSPS is frequently encountered in adolescents with CDH.

DSPS results in difficulty with falling asleep and awakening at the proper time (see also Chapters 30 and 31). The predisposing factors are multifactoral and may include genetic, environmental, physical, and psychological precipitants. It can result in significant sleep deprivation and impaired daytime function. It can cause deterioration in academic function and change in disposition. Treatment is multifaceted, and may include psychological counseling, pharmacotherapy, chronotherapy, controlled light/dark exposure, and early-evening melatonin. Lack of compliance, overt or covert, on the part of the patient and family can make treatment difficult.

It has been noted that sleep disorders are more frequent in children and adolescents with headache than in the general childhood population. Successful treatment of "difficult" headache disorders requires a number of lifestyle changes, especially restoration of a normal sleep pattern.

When evaluating a refractory headache patient, and when alteration of the normal sleep-wake cycle or sleep related symptoms are noted, a sleep specialist consultation and/or evaluation in a sleep laboratory can be quite helpful. Expert advice in diagnosis and treatment leading to improved restorative sleep is a major component of successful headache treatment.

Our patient had refractory CDH, which is also known as chronic nonprogressive headache, tension-type headache, muscle contraction headache, mixed headache, chronic migraine, transformed migraine, and comorbid headache. The episodic variety occurs fewer than 10 to 15 days per month, and children or adolescents with episodic TTH are seldom seen in consultation. If, however, the headaches occur more than 10 to 15 days per month, interfere with normal school and family functions, or are associated with medication overuse or excessive school absences, then the patient needs to be evaluated. These headaches are not associated with symptoms of increased intracranial pressure or progressive neurologic disease. They often combine features of tension-type and migraine. Examinations of patients are mostly normal both during the headache and between headaches. Laboratory studies, including MRI, are generally nonrevealing. These headaches, although not life threatening, are among the most refractory to treatment. They are often associated with psychological factors, lifestyle issues, overuse of medications, excessive school absences, low socioeconomic status, and sleep disorders such as insomnia, excessive daytime sleepiness, sleep apnea, and DSPS.

Less well-recognized and less well-studied is the headache frequency in children and adolescents with sleep disorders. In a preliminary study of 34 patients from a headache clinic and 23 from a sleep laboratory, the headache group had an increased frequency of a wide variety of sleep disorders (30/34) and the sleep laboratory group had an increased frequency of headache (18/23), including migraine and CDH.

The importance of the relationship between headaches and sleep in adults is underscored by the inclusion of *Sleep related headaches* as a diagnostic category under the broader listing of *Sleep disorders classifiable elsewhere* in the ICSD-2. The classification acknowledges that cluster headaches, migraines, and chronic paroxysmal hemicrania are generally daytime phenomena, but it cautions that these may also occur in sleep. Migraines, for instance, tend to occur most commonly between 4 and 9 a.m. in older adolescents and adults, and many of the headache types may arise out of REM sleep. Hypnic headaches are peculiar to sleep but do not occur in children and adolescents. Patients are generally elderly and likely to awaken from REM sleep with a headache that may last from several minutes to a couple of hours with no associated autonomic features.

Other sleep related associations of headaches include disorders of insomnia, hypersomnia, and sleep apnea. In a retrospective analysis of 80 consecutive adult patients from Cleveland Clinic, 60% reported headaches in the prior year and 48% reported awakening headaches (AH). The AH were more common in patients who were diagnosed with obstructive sleep apnea (OSA) as compared to a set of controls diagnosed with periodic limb movement disorder. Further, the AH generally lasted less than 30 minutes, and were worse in those with more severe OSA. Treatment of OSA improved headache symptoms in those specifically reporting AH rather than those with other headache types.

In summary, the relationship between headache and sleep is bidirectional with added influence from many organic and psychiatric conditions. Further study of both groups is needed. Data concerning polysomnography in patients with headache is sparse and additional data is needed. The known clinical, anatomical, and physiological relationships between headache and sleep make this group of disorders worthy of investigation.

Bibliography

Barabas G, Ferrari M, Matthews WS. Childhood migraine and somnambulism. *Neurology*. 1986;33:948–1048.

Bille BS. Migraine in school children. *Acta Paediart Scand*. 1962;51(Sup136):1.

Bruni O, Fabrizi P, Ottaviano S, Cortesi F, Giannotti F, Guidetti V. Prevalence of sleep disorders in children and adolescence with headache: A case-control study. *Cephalalgia*. 1997;17:492–498.

Gilman, DK, Palermo, TM, Kabbouche, MA, Hershey, AD, Powers , SW. Primary headaches and sleep disturbances in adolescents. *Headache*. 2007;47: 1189–1194.

Guilleminault C, Eldridge FL, Simmons FB, Dement WC. Sleep apnea in eight children. *Pediatrics*. 1976;58:23–30.

Hill, W. On some causes of backwardness and stupidity in children. *BMJ*. 1889;ii:711–712.

Loh NK, Dinner DS, Foldvary N, Skobieranda F, Yew WW. Do patients with obstructive sleep apnea wake up with headaches? *Arch Intern Med*. 1999;159:1765–1768.

Luc ME, Gupta A, Birnberg JM, Reddick D, Johrman MH. Characterization of symptoms of sleep disorders in children with headache. *Ped Neurol*. 2006;34:7–12.

52

A Stroke of Bad Luck

MAHA ALATTAR, MD

JOYCE LEE-IANNOTTI, MD

Case History

Ralph was a 50-year-old, right-handed man who presented to the sleep center with complaints of excessive daytime sleepiness (EDS) and difficulty initiating and maintaining sleep. His symptoms began 1 year prior, following a left middle cerebral artery territory ischemic stroke. Prior to the stroke, he slept 6 hours per night, which was adequate and refreshing. After the stroke, his sleep became restless and he could not sleep for more than 4 hours a night. He woke up an average of 6 to 7 times nightly and often had difficulty resuming sleep. At the time of initial consultation, he was going to bed by 9 p.m., but it took him 2 hours to fall asleep. He usually got out of bed at 5 a.m. and did not feel rested. On weekends, he would sleep in until 6 to 8 a.m. but still felt tired and sleepy. He endorsed bedtime anxiety and recurrent thoughts about not being able to have a restful night. He also had thoughts about his overall health, including the possibility of having another stroke. Sleeping in an unfamiliar environment had a more positive effect on his sleep quality. He knew of no reasons for his multiple nocturnal awakenings, although he woke himself up snoring a few times. Snoring was worse in the supine position, but he typically slept on his side. His wife denied witnessing apneic episodes. On days off, Ralph took a 30-minute nap that was refreshing. He denied falling asleep while driving or on the job, though his Epworth Sleepiness Scale (ESS) score was 16. His only caffeine consumption was an 8-oz cup of coffee each morning. He worked the first shift in an auto repair shop, from 6 a.m. to 2:30 p.m. He denied depression or anxiety, symptoms of restless legs, leg jerks during sleep, cataplexy, hypnagogic hallucinations, sleep paralysis, and dream enactment.

Ralph's stroke work-up included a brain MRI and MRA, neck MRA, cardiac evaluation (2-D echocardiogram, serial cardiac enzymes, electrocardiogram, telemetry), fasting lipid profile, vitamin B12 and folate levels, serum rapid plasma reagin, thyroid stimulating hormone, hemoglobin A1c, a hypercoagulable panel, and blood pressure measurements. Brain MRI demonstrated a small acute ischemic cortical infarct in the left middle cerebral artery territory (Figures 52.1, 52.2) MRA of the intracranial vessels revealed a normal circle of Willis. Neck MRA showed minimal irregularity in the carotid siphons bilaterally with a patent vertebrobasilar system. Bilateral carotid ultrasound showed no hemodynamically significant stenosis of the anterior of posterior circulations. Cardiac workup was normal. No obvious source for the stroke was found. Risk factor modification for secondary stroke prevention was implemented. Ralph's risk factors included hypertension, diabetes, obesity and hyperlipidemia. He was started on aspirin, statin therapy, antihypertensive therapy and dietary modification for diabetic control.

Ralph's medical history was otherwise remarkable for gastroesophageal reflux disease and a nasal fracture about 10 years prior. His family history was significant for coronary artery disease and diabetes mellitus. He took aspirin, ramipril, calcium, lipitor, and a multivitamin daily. He was a full-time car mechanic and an associate pastor at a local church. He lived with his wife and 2 teenage children. He denied tobacco, alcohol, or recreational drug use. He had a 20-lb weight gain over the past year that he attributed to inactivity.

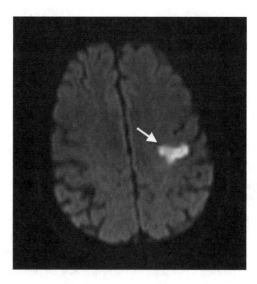

Figure 52.1 Axial diffusion-weighted image showing a focus of restricted diffusion compatible with a cortical infarction in the left precentral gyrus of the frontal lobe (arrow).

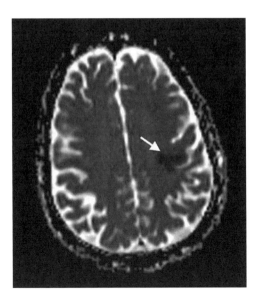

Figure 52.2 Axial apparent diffusion coefficient map demonstrating a defect in the left precentral gyrus (arrow) confirming the presence of an acute ischemic infarction.

Physical Examination

On examination, Ralph had a blood pressure of 113/74 mmHg, a heart rate of 80 beats per minute, and a respiratory rate of 14 breaths per minute. His neck circumference was 18 inches and his body mass index (BMI) was 30 kg/m². The head and neck examination revealed a nasal septal deviation to the right without congestion, a Grade II Friedman tongue position and a large, erythematous, and edematous uvula. The cardiac, respiratory and abdominal exams were normal. There were no jugular venous distension or lower extremity edema.

On neurological examination, Ralph had normal cognition, judgment, and insight. His speech was slightly dysarthric, but language functions were intact. His cranial nerves were normal. Motor testing revealed a right pronator drift with 4/5 strength in the right arm. Strength was 5/5 in all other muscle groups. Deep tendon reflexes were hyperactive with an extensor plantar reflex on the right. Sensory examination showed slight reduction in pinprick and temperature on the right arm compared to the left with intact vibratory, position sense, graphesthesia, and stereognosis. Rapid alternating movements were reduced on the right. The gait examination was normal.

Evaluation

Ralph underwent a polysomnogram (PSG) for evaluation of sleep apnea due to his BMI, large neck girth, and abnormal upper airway anatomy, and history of snoring and recurrent awakenings. His age and gender were additional risk factors. Sleep architecture was abnormal and showed a poor sleep efficiency of 43% with a total sleep time of 224 minutes. Sleep latency was 16 minutes; REM latency was 150 minutes. He had 8 awakenings and dozens of arousals, resulting in an arousal index of 28. Sleep staging was constituted by 21% stage 1, 55% stage 2 and 24% REM; no slow-wave sleep was recorded. He spent 63% of sleep time in the supine position. Snoring was present and the apnea-hypopnea index (AHI) was 22 with oxygen desaturations as low as 84% and 8% of total sleep time spent with an oxygen saturation less than 90%. The periodic limb movement index was 4. EKG tracing was normal.

Diagnoses

Moderate obstructive sleep apnea syndrome (OSAS).
Psychophysiological insomnia.
Left middle cerebral artery ischemic stroke.

Outcome

Ralph was treated with continuous positive airway pressure (CPAP) therapy following a successful titration study that revealed an optimal pressure of 10 cmH$_2$O with normalization of the AHI and consolidation of sleep architecture. The initial use of CPAP was a challenge, due to difficulty tolerating the mask, but desensitization sessions and a mask-refitting improved his compliance. He was able to use CPAP on a nightly basis for at least 6 hours. Follow-up ESS of 6 suggested improvement of his EDS. Insomnia, though improved with CPAP use, remained a problem, due to concerns about his health. He underwent cognitive behavioral therapy to discuss healthy coping mechanisms and stress reduction. Subsequent visits revealed significant improvement in his ability to initiate and maintain sleep. Bedtime anxiety and ruminating thoughts had resolved and his overall quality of life and daytime performance improved.

Discussion

Ralph's case illustrates the importance of recognizing sleep disorders in patients with cerebrovascular disease and sleep disordered breathing (SDB) as a risk factor for stroke. Stroke is a leading cause of disability and the third most common cause of mortality in the United States. Sleep-wake disorders are common in patients with stroke and can adversely affect functional outcome and recovery. Risk factors for strokes include systemic hypertension, tobacco abuse, obesity, hyperlipidemia, ischemic heart disease, and diabetes. There is growing evidence that SDB is also a stroke risk factor. The mechanisms linking SDB and stroke include hemodynamic changes such as sympathetic activation, endothelial damage, and inflammatory and coagulation abnormalities, all of which occur as a result of the respiratory disturbance and nocturnal hypoxemia. Strokes can also aggravate SDB. Besides the obstructive form of sleep apnea, stroke patients may have central sleep apnea with or without Cheyne Stokes respiration. Studies have shown the benefit of PAP therapy in this clinical setting. In one study, long-term CPAP treatment in moderate to severe OSA patients with ischemic stroke was associated with a reduction in mortality. Whether treatment of SDB confers a reduction in stroke risk remains unknown.

Sleep apnea screening is recommended in all stroke patients, particular in the presence of typical sleep apnea symptoms. Impaired dexterity, motor, and cognition pose challenges to patients, caretakers, and health care providers. Caretakers may need to aid in the application and maintenance of CPAP to optimize adherence. Close monitoring is required to customize treatment and address issues such as mask comfort, drooling, and air leaks that are common in patients with facial weakness. Other treatment options include oral appliances, weight control and positional therapy. If the presence of severe neurologic impairment precludes laboratory PSG, ambulatory monitoring or an autotitrating PAP device may be considered.

Patients with strokes also suffer from insomnia, EDS unrelated to SDB, fatigue, restless legs syndrome, and other sleep disturbances. Pain from spasticity, decreased functional (cognitive and physical) abilities, psychosocial stressors and mood disorders from disability contribute to poor sleep quality and quantity. Routine screening for insomnia in stroke patients is recommended. As in Ralph's case, a nonpharmacological approach to treatment is preferred. Effective methods include optimizing sleep habits by establishing routine bed and wake times, avoiding the use of stimulants such as caffeine, addressing mood disorders, and considering behavioral techniques such as biofeedback and progressive muscle relaxation. The patient should also be encouraged to engage in physical activity as permitted. Sedative-hypnotics should be used with caution due to the risk of increased cognitive dysfunction, falls and respiratory depression.

Recognition of sleep and wake disorders should be a routine part of the treatment of all stroke survivors. Improving sleep quality can lead to better daytime functioning, which can motivate patients to adhere to therapy and adopt healthy lifestyles, reducing the risk for recurrent strokes.

Bibliography

Bassetti CL, Milanova M, Gugger M. Sleep-disordered breathing and acute ischemic stroke: diagnosis, risk factors, treatment, evolution, and long-term clinical outcome. *Stroke.* 2006;37(4):967–72. Epub 2006 Mar 16.

Leppävuori A, Pohjasvaara T, Vataja R, Kaste M, Erkinjuntti T. Insomnia in ischemic stroke patients. *Cerebrovasc Dis.* 2002;14(2):90–97.

Martínez-García MA, Galiano-Blancart R, Román-Sánchez P, Soler-Cataluña JJ, Cabero-Salt L, Salcedo-Maiques E. Continuous positive airway pressure treatment in sleep apnea prevents new vascular events after ischemic stroke. *Chest.* 2005;128(4):2123–2129.

Martínez García MA, Galiano Blancart R, Cabero Salt L, Soler Cataluña JJ, Escamilla T, Román Sánchez P. Prevalence of sleep-disordered breathing in patients with acute ischemic stroke: Influence of onset time of stroke. *Arch Bronconeumol.* 2004;40(5):196–202.

Martínez-García MA, Soler-Cataluña JJ, Ejarque-Martínez L, Soriano Y, Román-Sánchez P, Illa FB, Canal JM, Durán-Cantolla J. Continuous positive airway pressure treatment reduces mortality in patients with ischemic stroke and obstructive sleep apnea: A 5-year follow-up study. *Am J Respir Crit Care Med.* 2009;180(1): 36–41. Epub 2009 Apr 30.

Yaggi HK, Concato J, Kernan WN, Lichtman JH, Brass LM, Mohsenin V. Obstructive sleep apnea as a risk factor for stroke and death. *NEJM.* 2005;353(19):2034–41.

Appendix I
Epworth Sleepiness Scale

How likely are you to doze off or fall asleep in the following situations, in contrast to just feeling tired?

This refers to your usual way of life in recent times.

Even if you have not done some of the things recently, try to work out how they would have affected you.

Use the following scale to choose **the most appropriate number** for each situation:

0 = would **never** doze
1 = **slight** chance of dozing
2 = **moderate** chance of dozing
3 = **high** chance of dozing

Situation	Chance of Dozing (0–3)
Sitting and reading..	_____
Watching TV	_____
Sitting inactive, in a public place (e.g. a theater or meeting)........	_____
As a passenger in a car for an hour without a break....................	_____
Lying down to rest in the afternoon when circumstances permit	_____
Sitting and talking to someone..	_____
Sitting quietly after a lunch without alcohol	_____
In a car, while stopped for a few minutes in traffic	_____

The responses are summed to derive a total score ranging from 0 to 24. A score of 10 and higher is indicative of daytime sleepiness.

Source: M. W. Johns, 1990

Appendix II
Insomnia Severity Index (ISI)

1. Please rate the current (i.e., last 2 weeks) **SEVERITY** of your insomnia problem(s).

	None	Mild	Moderate	Severe	Very Severe
a) Difficulty falling asleep	0	1	2	3	4
b) Difficulty staying asleep	0	1	2	3	4
c) Problem waking up too early	0	1	2	3	4

2. How satisfied/dissatisfied are you with your current sleep pattern?

Very Satisfied	Satisfied	Neutral	Dissatisfied	Very Dissatisfied
0	1	2	3	4

3. To what extent do you consider your sleep problem to interfere with your daily functioning (e.g., daytime fatigue, ability to function at work/daily chores, concentration, memory, mood, etc.)?

Not at all Interfering	A Little	Somewhat Interfering	Much	Very Much Interfering
0	1	2	3	4

4. How noticeable to others do you think your sleeping problem is in terms of impairing the quality of your life?

Not at all Noticeable	A little	Somewhat	Much	Very Much Noticeable
0	1	2	3	4

5. How worried/distressed are you about your current sleep problem?

Not at all Worried	A Little	Somewhat	Much	Very Much Worried
0	1	2	3	4

The responses are summed to derive a total score ranging from 0 to 28. The severity of insomnia is classified as follows:

0–7   No clinically significant insomnia
8–14   Subthreshold insomnia
15–21   Clinical insomnia (moderate severity)
22–28   Clinical insomnia (severe)

Source: C. M. Morin, 1993

Appendix III
The Fatigue Severity Scale

Read each statement and circle a number from 1 to 7, based on how accurately it reflects your condition during the past week and the extent to which you agree or disagree that the statement applies to you.

A low value (e.g. 1) indicates strong disagreement with the statement, whereas a high value (e.g. 7) indicates strong agreement.

It is important you circle a number (1 to 7) for every question.

	Disagree					Agree
1. My motivation is lower when I am fatigued	1	2	3	4	5	6	7
2. Exercise brings on my fatigue	1	2	3	4	5	6	7
3. I am easily fatigued	1	2	3	4	5	6	7
4. Fatigue interferes with my physical conditioning	1	2	3	4	5	6	7
5. Fatigue causes frequent problems for me	1	2	3	4	5	6	7
6. My fatigue prevents sustained physical functioning	1	2	3	4	5	6	7
7. Fatigue interferes with carrying out certain duties and responsibilities	1	2	3	4	5	6	7
8. Fatigue is among my 3 most disabling symptoms	1	2	3	4	5	6	7
9. Fatigue interferes with my work, family, or social life	1	2	3	4	5	6	7

The responses are tallied yielding a total score ranging from 7 to 63.

A total score of 36 or more suggests significant fatigue that may warrant further evaluation.

Source: Lauren B. Krupps

Appendix IV
Horne-Ostberg Morningness-Eveningness Scale

Select the most appropriate answer for each of the following 7 questions:

1. If you were entirely free to plan your evening and had no commitments the next day, at what time would you choose to go to bed?
    1. 2000hrs – 2100hrs.....5
    2. 2100hrs – 2215hrs.....4
    3. 2215hrs – 0030hrs.....3
    4. 0030hrs – 0145hrs.....2
    5. 0145hrs – 0300hrs.....1

2. You have to do 2 hours of physically hard work. If you were entirely free to plan your day, in which of the following periods would you choose to do the work?
    1. 0800hrs – 1000hrs.....4
    2. 1100hrs – 1300hrs.....3
    3. 1500hrs – 1700hrs.....2
    4. 1900hrs – 2100hrs.....1

3. For some reason you have gone to bed several hours later than normal, but there is no need to get up at a particular time the next morning. Which of the following is most likely to occur?
    1. Will wake up at the usual time and not fall asleep again.... 4
    2. Will wake up at the usual time and doze thereafter............ 3
    3. Will wake up at the usual time but will fall asleep again 2
    4. Will not wake up until later than usual.............................. 1

4. You have a 2 hour test to sit which you know will be mentally exhausting. If you were entirely free to choose, in which of the following periods would you choose to sit the test?
   1. 0800hrs – 1000hrs.....4
   2. 1100hrs – 1300hrs.....3
   3. 1500hrs – 1700hrs.....2
   4. 1900hrs – 2100hrs.....1

5. If you had no commitments the next day and were entirely free to plan your own day, what time would you get up?
   1. 0500hrs – 0630hrs.....5
   2. 0630hrs – 0745hrs.....4
   3. 0745hrs – 0945hrs.....3
   4. 0945hrs – 1100hrs.....2
   5. 1100hrs – 1200hrs.....1

6. A friend has asked you to join him twice a week for a workout in the gym. The best time for him is between 10 and 11 p.m. Bearing nothing else in mind other than how you normally feel in the evening, how do you think you would perform?
   1. Very well 1
   2. Reasonably well 2
   3. Poorly...........................3
   4. Very poorly 4

7. One hears about "morning" and "evening" types of people. Which of these types do you consider yourself to be?
   1. Definitely morning type.............................. 6
   2. More a morning than an evening type...... 4
   3. More an evening than a morning type...... 2
   4. Definitely an evening type 0

Responses to the 7 items are tallied yielding a total score ranging from 6 to 32. Based on the total score, a subject is assigned to one of the following categories:
   1. Definitely morning type........ 32 – 28
   2. Moderately morning type..... 27 – 23
   3. Neither type.......................... 22 – 16
   4. Moderately evening type....... 15 – 11
   5. Definitely evening type .... 10 – 6

Source: Horne JA, Ostberg O. A self-assessment questionnaire to determine morningness-eveningness in human circadian rhythms. *Int J Chronobiol.* 1976;4:97–110.

Appendix V
Patient Health Questionnaire (PHQ-9)

How often have you been bothered by any of the following problems?
Use the following scale to choose the most appropriate response for each situation.

Time period: Preceding 2 weeks

	Not at all	Several days	More than half the days	Nearly every day
1. Little interest or pleasure in doing things..	0	1	2	3
2. Feeling down, depressed, or hopeless	0	1	2	3
3. Trouble falling or staying asleep, or sleeping too much	0	1	2	3
4. Feeling tired or having little energy...........	0	1	2	3
5. Poor appetite or overeating........................	0	1	2	3
6. Feeling bad about yourself or that you are a failure or that you have let yourself or your family down	0	1	2	3
7. Trouble concentrating on things, such as reading the newspaper or watching TV	0	1	2	3
8. Moving or speaking so slowly that other people could have noticed, or the opposite, being so fidgety or restless that you have been moving around a lot more than usual	0	1	2	3
9. Thoughts that you would be better off dead or of hurting yourself in some way ..	0	1	2	3

10. If you checked off *any* problems, how *difficult* have these problems made it for you to do your work, take care of things at home, or get along with other people?

Not difficult at all _____
Somewhat difficult _____
Very difficult _____
Extremely difficult _____

The responses to items 1 through 9 are tallied and the total score interpreted as follows:

1–4   Minimal depression
5–9   Mild depression
10–14 Moderate depression
15–19 Moderately severe depression
20–27 Severe depression

Source: Spitzer R, Kroenke K, Williams J. Validation and utility of a self-report version of PRIME-MD: the PHQ Primary Care Study. *JAMA.* 1999; 282:1737–1744.

Appendix VI
International Restless Legs Syndrome Study Group (IRLS) Rating Scale (Investigator Version 2.2)

Have the patient rate his/her symptoms for the following ten questions. The patient and not the examiner should make the ratings, but the examiner should be available to clarify any misunderstandings the patient may have about the questions. The examiner should mark the patient's answers on the form.

In the past week...
(1) <u>Overall</u>, how would you rate the <u>RLS discomfort in your legs or arms</u>?

^{4}□ Very severe

^{3}□ Severe

^{2}□ Moderate

^{1}□ Mild

^{0}□ None

In the past week...
(2) <u>Overall</u>, how would you rate the <u>need to move</u> around because of your RLS symptoms?

^{4}□ Very severe

^{3}□ Severe

^{2}□ Moderate

^{1}□ Mild

^{0}□ None

In the past week…

(3) Overall, how much relief of your RLS arm or leg discomfort did you get from moving around?

- 4☐ No relief
- 3☐ Mild relief
- 2☐ Moderate relief
- 1☐ Either complete or almost complete relief
- 0☐ No RLS symptoms to be relieved

In the past week…

(4) How severe was your sleep disturbance due to your RLS symptoms?

- 4☐ Very severe
- 3☐ Severe
- 2☐ Moderate
- 1☐ Mild
- 0☐ None

In the past week…

(5) How severe was your tiredness or sleepiness during the day due to your RLS symptoms?

- 4☐ Very severe
- 3☐ Severe
- 2☐ Moderate
- 1☐ Mild
- 0☐ None

In the past week…

(6) How severe was your RLS as a whole?

- 4☐ Very severe
- 3☐ Severe
- 2☐ Moderate
- 1☐ Mild
- 0☐ None

In the past week…

(7) How often did you get RLS symptoms?

- 4☐ Very often (This means 6 to 7 days a week)
- 3☐ Often (This means 4 to 5 days a week)
- 2☐ Sometimes (This means 2 to 3 days a week)
- 1☐ Occasionally (This means 1 day a week)
- 0☐ Never

In the past week…

(8) When you had RLS symptoms, how severe were they on average?

    ⁴□ Very severe (This means 8 hours or more per 24 hour day)

    ³□ Severe (This means 3 to 8 hours per 24 hour day)

    ²□ Moderate (This means 1 to 3 hours per 24 hour day)

    ¹□ Mild (This means less than 1 hour per 24 hour day)

    ⁰□ None

In the past week…

(9) Overall, how severe was the impact of your RLS symptoms on your ability to carry out your <u>daily affairs</u>, for example carrying out a satisfactory family, home, social, school or work life?

    ⁴□ Very severe

    ³□ Severe

    ²□ Moderate

    ¹□ Mild

    ⁰□ None

In the past week…

(10) How severe was your <u>mood disturbance</u> due to your RLS symptoms - for example angry, depressed, sad, anxious or irritable?

    ⁴□ Very severe

    ³□ Severe

    ²□ Moderate

    ¹□ Mild

    ⁰□ None

Responses to the 10 questions are tallied yielding a total score ranging from 0 to 40. The severity of RLS is as follows:

Mild: 1–10

Moderate: 11–20

Severe: 21–30

Very severe: 31–40

Source: Walters AS, LeBrocq C, Dhar A, Hening W, Rosen R, Allen RP, Trenkwalder C; International Restless Legs Syndrome Study Group. Validation of the International Restless Legs Syndrome Study Group rating scale for restless legs syndrome. *Sleep Med.* 2003 Mar;4(2):121–32.

Appendix VII
International Classification of Sleep Disorders, 2nd edition

Insomnias

1. Adjustment insomnia (acute insomnia)
2. Psychophysiological insomnia
3. Paradoxical insomnia
4. Idiopathic insomnia
5. Insomnia due to mental disorder
6. Inadequate sleep hygiene
7. Behavioral insomnia of childhood
8. Insomnia due to drug or substance
9. Insomnia due to medical condition
10. Insomnia not due to substance or known physiological condition, unspecified (nonorganic insomnia, NOS)
11. Physiological (organic) insomnia, unspecified

Sleep related breathing disorders

A. Central sleep apnea syndromes
   1. Primary central sleep apnea
   2. Central sleep apnea due to Cheyne Stokes breathing pattern
   3. Central sleep apnea due to high altitude periodic breathing
   4. Central sleep apnea due to medical condition not Cheyne Stokes
   5. Central sleep apnea due to drug or substance
   6. Primary sleep apnea of infancy (formerly primary sleep apnea of newborn)

B. Obstructive sleep apnea syndromes
1. Obstructive sleep apnea, adult
2. Obstructive sleep apnea, pediatric
C. Sleep related hypoventilation/hypoxemic syndromes
1. Sleep related nonobstructive alveolar hypoventilation, idiopathic
2. Congenital central alveolar hypoventilation syndrome
D. Sleep related hypoventilation/hypoxemia due to medical condition
1. Sleep related hypoventilation/hypoxemia due to pulmonary parenchymal or vascular pathology
2. Sleep related hypoventilation/hypoxemia due to lower airways obstruction
3. Sleep related hypoventilation/hypoxemia due to neuromuscular and chest wall disorders
E. Other sleep related breathing disorder
1. Sleep apnea/sleep related breathing disorder, unspecified

Hypersomnias of central origin: Not due to a circadian rhythm sleep disorder, sleep related breathing disorder, or other cause of disturbed nocturnal sleep

1. Narcolepsy with cataplexy
2. Narcolepsy without cataplexy
3. Narcolepsy due to medical condition
4. Narcolepsy, unspecified
5. Recurrent hypersomnia
   - Kleine-Levin syndrome
   - Menstrual-related hypersomnia
6. Idiopathic hypersomnia with long sleep time
7. Idiopathic hypersomnia without long sleep time
8. Behaviorally induced insufficient sleep syndrome
9. Hypersomnia due to medical condition
10. Hypersomnia due to drug or substance
11. Hypersomnia not due to substance or known physiological condition (nonorganic hypersomnia, NOS)
12. Physiologic (organic) hypersomnia, unspecified (organic hypersomnia, NOS)

Circadian rhythm sleep disorders

1. Circadian rhythm sleep disorder, delayed sleep phase type (delayed sleep phase disorder)

2. Circadian rhythm sleep disorder, advanced sleep phase type (advanced sleep phase disorder)
3. Circadian rhythm sleep disorder, irregular sleep-wake type (irregular sleep-wake rhythm)
4. Circadian rhythm sleep disorder, free-running type (nonentrained type)
5. Circadian rhythm sleep disorder, jet lag type (jet lag disorder)
6. Circadian rhythm sleep disorder, shift work type (shift work disorder)
7. Circadian rhythm sleep disorder due to medical condition
8. Other circadian rhythm sleep disorder (circadian rhythm disorder, NOS)
9. Other circadian rhythm sleep disorder due to drug or substance

Parasomnias

A. Disorders of arousal (from NREM sleep)
   1. Confusional arousals
   2. Sleepwalking
   3. Sleep terrors
B. Parasomnias usually associated with REM sleep
   1. REM sleep behavior disorder (including parasomnia overlap disorder and status dissociatus)
   2. Recurrent isolated sleep paralysis
   3. Nightmare disorder
C. Other parasomnias
   1. Sleep related dissociative disorders
   2. Sleep enuresis
   3. Sleep related groaning (catathrenia)
   4. Exploding head syndrome
   5. Sleep related hallucinations
   6. Sleep related eating disorder
   7. Parasomnia, unspecified
   8. Parasomnia due to drug or substance
   9. Parasomnia due to medical condition

Sleep related movement disorders

1. Restless legs syndrome
2. Periodic limb movement disorder
3. Sleep related leg cramps
4. Sleep related bruxism
5. Sleep related rhythmic movement disorder
6. Sleep related movement disorder, unspecified

7. Sleep related movement disorder due to drug or substance
8. Sleep related movement disorder due to medical condition

Isolated symptoms, apparently normal variants and unresolved issues

1. Long sleeper
2. Short sleeper
3. Snoring
4. Sleep talking
5. Sleep starts (hypnic jerks)
6. Benign sleep myoclonus of infancy
7. Hypnagogic foot tremor and alternating leg muscle activation during sleep
8. Propriospinal myoclonus at sleep onset
9. Excessive fragmentary myoclonus

Other sleep disorders

1. Other physiological (organic) sleep disorder
2. Other sleep disorder not due to substance or known physiological condition
3. Environmental sleep disorder

Glossary

Actigraph: A wristwatch like biomedical device that is used in measuring body movement. The data from the device is used to determine approximate sleep and wake times.

Advanced sleep phase disorder (ASPD): A circadian rhythm sleep disorder. Phases of the daily sleep-wake cycle are advanced with respect to clock time. The sleep phase occurs ahead of conventional bedtime and the tendency is to wake up too early. It is more commonly seen in the elderly.

Apnea: Polysomnogram terminology. A respiratory event characterized by 90% or greater reduction in oro-nasal airflow in sleep lasting at least 10 seconds. There are 3 types of apneas: obstructive, central and mixed.

Arousal: Polysomnogram terminology. An abrupt change in EEG to a higher frequency lasting at least 3 seconds and preceded by at least 10 seconds of uninterrupted sleep. A simultaneous increase in chin EMG at least 1 second in duration is necessary to score an arousal in REM.

Body mass index (BMI): Body mass index is derived from weight and height measurements and expressed as kg/m^2 units.

Bright-light therapy: Bright, broad-spectrum light exposure used in the treatment of circadian rhythm sleep disorders and seasonal affective disorder. The timing of light exposure can shift the sleep period in the desired direction, delaying or advancing.

Bruxism: Grinding or clenching of the teeth during sleep.

Cataplexy: Loss of muscle tone precipitated by strong emotion, such as laughter, anger or excitement, that leads to weakness and/or loss of voluntary muscle control. Cataplexy is characteristic of narcolepsy.

Central sleep apnea: A type of sleep apnea in which the upper airway is patent and respiratory effort is absent.

Cheyne Stokes breathing: A pattern of breathing characterized by gradual increase followed by gradual decrease in breathing (crescendo-decrescendo pattern) punctuated by central apneas or hypopneas. This is often seen in patients with heart failure, kidney failure and central nervous system disorders.

Chronotherapy: A treatment for circadian rhythm sleep disorders. The bedtime is systematically adjusted over several days until the desired sleep-wake schedule is achieved.

Circadian rhythms: Biological rhythms under the control of the suprachiasmatic nucleus (also known as the "internal clock") that influences the timing and duration of sleep as well as other physiological functions, including body temperature and secretion of certain hormones.

Cognitive behavioral therapy (CBT): A psychological therapy that is aimed at identifying and correcting maladaptive thoughts and beliefs. Relaxation is a key component of behavioral therapy. CBT is often used in the treatment of insomnia.

Continuous positive airway pressure (CPAP): A treatment for sleep apnea that delivers air at a fixed pressure to prevent collapse of the airway when asleep.

Delayed sleep phase disorder (DSPD): A circadian rhythm sleep disorder. Phases of the daily sleep-wake cycle are delayed with respect to clock time. The sleep phase occurs beyond the conventional bedtime and the tendency is to wake up late in the morning or early afternoon. It is more commonly seen in adolescents and young adults.

Delta sleep: Also known as slow-wave sleep or deep sleep, it is Stage N3 of NREM sleep.

Friedman staging: Friedman staging system (I through IV) is based upon tongue position, tonsil size, and body mass index. It is often used to predict success of upper airway surgery in patients with obstructive sleep apnea.

Gamma-aminobutyric acid (GABA): An amino acid and neurotransmitter in the central nervous system that regulates various physiological functions, including sleep.

Hypnagogic hallucinations: Hallucinations occurring during transition from wakefulness to sleep or at sleep onset. These are most common in people with narcolepsy.

Hypnogram: A pictorial representation of sleep stages and sleep cycles.

Hypnopompic hallucinations: Hallucinations occurring during transition from sleep to wakefulness or at sleep offset. These are most common in people with narcolepsy.

Hypopnea: Polysomnogram terminology. A respiratory event in sleep characterized by a reduction in oro-nasal airflow associated with continued efforts to breathe based upon chest and abdominal effort signals and a desaturation and/or EEG arousal. Definitions vary for adult and pediatric events.

Insomnia: Difficulty with falling asleep, staying asleep, early morning awakening, or nonrestorative sleep, despite adequate opportunity to sleep.

Jet lag: A clinical condition resulting when travel across time zones leaves a person feeling "out of sync" with local time at destination.

K-complex: Polysomnogram terminology. A high amplitude biphasic wave (sharp negative wave followed by a positive wave) lasting for at least 0.5 seconds. One of the hallmark features of Stage N2 sleep.

Maintenance of wakefulness test (MWT): A daytime sleep test that measures the ability to remain awake in a non-stimulating environment. It is comprised of 4 nap trials performed at 2-hour intervals.

Mean sleep latency (MSL): The time from "lights out" to sleep onset, measured in minutes, and averaged over the nap trials of the MSLT or MWT. In adults, a MSL of 10 minutes or greater is normal while a MSL of less than 10 minutes signifies daytime sleepiness on the MSLT.

Multiple sleep latency test (MSLT): A daytime sleep test that measures the ability to fall asleep in a sleep-promoting environment. It is comprised of 5 nap trials performed at 2-hour intervals.

Melatonin: A neuro-hormone produced by the pineal gland that is involved in the regulation of circadian rhythms.

Mixed apnea: Polysomnogram terminology. An apnea characterized by absent inspiratory effort in the initial portion of the event, followed by resumption of inspiratory effort in the second portion of the event.

Narcolepsy: A sleep disorder characterized by severe daytime sleepiness, cataplexy, sleep paralysis, and hypnagogic/hypnopompic hallucinations.

Nightmare: A terrifying dream.

Nonrapid eye movement (NREM) sleep: One of the 2 basic states of sleep. It comprises Stages N1 and N2 (light sleep), and N3 (deep sleep).

Obstructive sleep apnea (OSA): Sleep apnea caused by a blockage of the upper airway. It is the most common form of sleep apnea.

Overbite: A vertical measure of the overlap of the upper incisors with the lower incisors.

Overjet: A horizontal measure of the position of the upper incisors relative to the lower incisors.

Parasomnia: Abnormal behavior or experience that occurs during sleep or in transition to or from sleep. These disorders can interrupt sleep and result in insomnia, excessive daytime sleepiness, and other daytime impairments.

Periodic limb movement disorder (PLMD): A disorder in which rhythmic jerking of the legs interrupts sleep, causing insomnia and/or excessive daytime sleepiness and daytime impairments.

Periodic limb movements in sleep (PLMS): Polysomnogram terminology. A series of at least four stereotyped limb movements each lasting for at least 0.5 seconds but less than 10 seconds and occurring consecutively at intervals of 5 to 90 seconds.

Polysomnography (PSG): A sleep test that records sleep architecture and a variety of other body functions during sleep, including breathing patterns, heart rhythms, and limb movements.

Progressive muscle relaxation (PMR): A technique that involves tensing and relaxing muscles of the body in a particular order (usually starting at the toes and moving upward toward the head), ultimately to achieve relaxation of the whole body. It is often used in the treatment of insomnia.

Rapid eye movement (REM) sleep: One of the 2 basic states of sleep. Also known as "dream sleep," it is characterized by rapid eye movements, atonia of skeletal muscles, and more irregular breathing and heart rate compared to NREM sleep.

Rebound insomnia: Insomnia that is worse than before treatment with sedative substances.

REM latency: Polysomnogram terminology. The time in minutes from sleep onset to the first epoch of REM sleep.

Respiratory inductance plethysmography (RIP): A method of quantifying thoracoabdominal respiratory effort.

Restless legs syndrome (RLS): A condition characterized by an irresistible urge to move the legs usually accompanied by unpleasant sensations. Symptoms start or worsen at rest, and they decrease when legs are moved/stretched. They are usually worse in the evening, especially when lying down, and may interfere with sleep onset. Most people with RLS also have leg jerks while asleep.

Sexsomnia: A type of parasomnia characterized by sexual behaviors usually towards the bed partner without the patient's awareness.

Sleep architecture: The structure of sleep, generally comprising a cyclical pattern of the NREM and REM sleep stages.

Sleep apnea: A sleep disorder that occurs when a person's breathing is interrupted during sleep.

Sleep cycle: A sequence of sleep stages that usually begins with a period of NREM sleep followed by REM sleep. Each cycle lasts for approximately 80 to 110 minutes in adults and is repeated 4 to 6 times per night. Similar rhythms are seen in children with a different cyclicity based upon maturity.

Sleep deprivation: Lack of sleep over a period of time resulting in physical or psychiatric symptoms affecting daytime functions.

Sleep efficiency: Polysomnogram terminology. Total sleep time divided by total time in bed, expressed as a percentage.

Sleep enuresis (bed wetting): Urination during sleep most often seen in children.

Sleep hygiene: A set of practices, habits, and environmental factors that are important for getting a good night's sleep.

Sleep latency: Polysomnogram terminology. It is the time in minutes from "lights out" to the first 30-second epoch of sleep.

Sleep onset: The transition from wakefulness to sleep.

Sleep onset REM period (SOREMP): Onset of REM sleep within 15 minutes after sleep onset. This terminology is used in the MSLT.

Sleep paralysis: A temporary inability to move or speak while falling asleep or waking up, often seen in narcolepsy, but also seen after sleep deprivation and as an isolated sleep disorder.

Sleep spindle: Polysomnogram terminology. Spindle-shaped 12-14 Hz EEG waves lasting for 0.5 to 1.5 seconds best seen over the vertex region. One of the hallmark patterns of Stage N2 sleep.

Sleep stages: Divided into NREM (N1, N2 and N3) and REM stages based upon American Academy of Sleep Medicine scoring guidlines.

Sleep talking (somniloquy): A parasomnia characterized by talking in sleep. It originates from NREM sleep.

Sleep terror: A sleep disorder characterized by abrupt awakenings from deep NREM sleep associated with screaming and prominent autonomic activation without awareness or recollection. This is typically observed in children.

Somnambulism (sleepwalking): A parasomnia characterized by walking in sleep. Often seen in children, it originates from NREM sleep.

Suprachiasmatic nucleus (SCN): A structure in the human brain that is also known as the "internal clock." It regulates sleep and wakefulness in addition to various other physiological functions.

Index

Note: Page numbers followed by "*f*" and "*t*" denote figures and tables, respectively.

A

Acetazolamide, 331, 370
Actigraphy, 23, 30, 58, 60*f*, 106, 240, 242*f*,
    243, 397
Adaptive servo-ventilation (ASV), 21, 73,
    74*f*, 77, 81, 84, 95, 96*f*, 98*f*, 99,
    154–55, 155*t*, 340
Adenoidectomy, 132, 160, 165, 186, 240
Adenoid hypertrophy, 131
Adjustment disorder not otherwise
    specified, 54
Adjustment insomnia, 31, 48
Advanced sleep phase disorder (ASPD), 397
Alcohol, 41, 185, 194, 197, 198, 214, 230,
    240, 259, 273, 276, 298, 310
Alcohol and Drug Rehabilitation Center, 229
Alpha delta sleep, 69
Alternating leg muscle activation (ALMA),
    326, 327*f*, 328–29
Alzheimer's disease, 28, 273, 368
American Academy of Sleep Medicine
    (AASM), 14, 15, 17, 23, 106, 401
American Society of Anesthesiology Difficult
    Airway Algorithm, 119
Amytriptyline, 33
Angles classification, Type I, II, III, 170
Anticholinergics, 185
Anticonvulsants, 308, 314, 317
Antiepileptic drug, 6, 259
Anxiety, 48
Apnea, 17, 397
Apnea-hypopnea index (AHI), 20
Armodafinil, 199*t*, 200

Arousal, 397
Aryepiglottoplasty, 139, 142, 143
Attention deficit disorder, 165, 170
Augmentation, 306, 308–10
Auto-titrating device, 21, 73, 103–4, 111,
    121, 154–55, 157

B

Barbiturates, 32
Bariatric surgery, 117–21
Bedwetting. *See* Sleep enuresis (bedwetting)
Behavioral insomnia of childhood, 8, 51,
    52*t*, 53, 54–55, 267–71
    limit-setting type, 8
    sleep onset association type, 8
Behaviorally induced insufficient sleep
    syndrome, 198, 212, 219, 222–26,
    230, 236, 249
Benzodiazepine receptor agonists
    (BZRAs), 32–33
Benzodiazepines, 32, 57, 62–63, 76,
    119, 259, 276, 290, 292, 308,
    314, 324
Bi-level PAP, 72, 73, 77, 81, 84, 88, 110–11,
    113–14, 148, 152
Body mass index (BMI), 7, 397
Body position monitoring, 15, 21
Brain natriuretic peptide (BNP), 79, 82
Brainstem glioma, 85, 87
Bright light/blue light therapy. *See* Light
    therapy
Bruxism, 86, 240, 301, 302, 397
Bupropion, 34, 41, 43, 48, 222, 295, 298

C

Caffeine, 5, 6, 9, 22, 35, 101, 197, 198, 226, 251, 276, 285, 298, 310, 324, 379

Canadian Continuous Positive Airway Pressure for Patients with Central Sleep Apnea and Heart Failure Trial (CANPAP), 83–84

Cannabinoids, 228, 229

Capnometry, 20, 24, 187

Carbamazepine, 213, 302, 308, 331, 337

Cataplexy, 194–202, 206, 397
pharmacotherapy, 200t

Catathrenia (sleep related expiratory groaning), 301–2

Centers for Medicare and Medicaid Services (CMS), 21, 106

Central sleep apnea (CSA), 397
due to Cheyne Stokes breathing pattern, 80–83
due to medical condition (brainstem glioma) not Cheyne Stokes, 87

Cephalometric analysis, 123, 128, 166f, 170
SNA in, 124, 166f
SNB in, 124, 166f

Chemosensitivity, 75

Cheyne Stokes breathing pattern, 71, 74, 76, 77, 80, 82–83, 87, 99, 398

Chronic daily headache (CDH), 370–73

Chronic headache, 35, 369. See also Chronic daily headache

Chronic obstructive pulmonary disease (COPD), 177, 180, 183–84

Chronotherapy, 241, 372, 398

Circadian rhythms, 398

Circadian rhythm sleep disorder (CRSD), 393–94
delayed sleep phase type, 235–38, 240–45, 367–68
jet lag type, 253–56
shift work type, 247–51

Clomipramine, 201, 200t

Clonazepam, 57, 259, 275, 276, 282, 292, 302, 317, 324, 331, 349, 360, 363

Cluster headaches, 371

Cognitive behavioral therapy (CBT), 398

Cognitive Behavioral Therapy for Insomnia (CBTi), 29, 35, 37, 41, 45–46, 62

Cognitive impairment, 275, 352, 367

Cognitive therapy, 39

Complex sleep apnea, 91, 94–95, 96–98, 152–59

Concussion/closed head injury, 258, 259, 331, 365

Cone beam computed tomography scan (CBCT), 169, 170

Confusional arousals, 259–65, 269, 270, 289–92

Continuous positive airway pressure (CPAP), 44, 72–73, 77, 81, 83–84, 93, 95, 100, 109–10, 115, 123, 139, 151, 153–54, 162, 165, 171, 179, 181, 184–85, 289, 322–23, 357, 378, 398

Continuous spike waves during NREM sleep (CSWS), 352–55

Controller gain, 75, 76

Core body temperature, 250, 250f

Counter-stimulation, 308

CPAP. See Continuous positive airway pressure (CPAP)

Craniopharyngiomas, 204–5f

D

Daytime sleepiness, 6, 100, 326

Deep brain stimulation (DBS), 361, 361f, 363

Delayed sleep phase disorder (DSPD; DSPS), 87, 89, 198, 235–38, 370, 372, 398

Delta sleep, 398

Dementia, 367

Depression, 48, 170, 319

Desipramine, 200t

Dextroamphetamine, 165, 168, 199t, 200–201, 240

Diagnostic and Statistical Manual of Mental Disorders, 4th Edition (DSM-IV), 53

Diaphragmatic breathing, 112f, 113–14

Differentiation of arousal disorders and seizures, 264

Diffuse Lewy body disease, 275

Diffusion capacity, 174, 181

Diphenhydramine hydrochloride, 33

Disorder of arousal during NREM sleep–sleepwalking and confusional arousals, 259–65, 281, 338

Dopaminergic agents, 297, 298, 308, 309, 310, 314

Doxylamine
citrate, 33
succinate, 33

Doxylamine succinate, 33

Dream enactment, 260, 263, 274f, 282, 363

Drowsy driving, signs and symptoms of, 224t

Dysembryoplastic neuroepithelial tumor (DNET), 259, 260*f*
Dyspnea, 141, 173

E
Echocardiogram, 71, 78, 148, 174, 176, 177, 181
Ekbom's disease, 307
Electrocardiogram (ECG), 15, 148, 274
Electroencephalogram (EEG), 15, 16, 17, 210, 268, 299, 333*f*, 335, 338, 342, 343–44*f*, 345, 350, 353*f*, 355
in arousal disorders, 262, 264
Electromyogram (EMG), 15, 18, 279, 282, 314
Electro-oculogram (EOG), 15
End tidal CO_2 ($EtCO_2$), 20, 78, 145, 181, 186
Enuresis, 9, 150, 284–86
overweight children and, 285
Epilepsy, 259, 337, 339, 347, 354
Epileptiform activity, 264, 268, 279, 301
Epworth Sleepiness Scale (ESS), 10, 381
Esophageal pH channel, 20
Estazolam, 32
Eszopiclone, 32*t*, 33, 57, 320
Excessive daytime sleepiness (EDS), 27, 91, 92, 101, 104, 123, 151, 165, 191, 194–95, 198–201, 215, 221, 222, 225, 233, 236–37, 239, 252, 320, 339, 357, 375, 378
signs and symptoms of, 224*t*

F
Fatigue Severity Scale (FSS), 11, 384
Febrile seizure, 258, 259, 331, 345, 376
Ferritin, 306, 312, 314, 316–17, 323
Fetal alcohol syndrome, 147, 149
Fiberoptic laryngoscopy (FFL), 131, 132, 137
Flexible laryngoscopy, 124
Fluoxetine, 200*t*, 201
Flurazepam, 32
Focal (partial) seizures, 291, 339, 344*f*, 345
Folate deficiency, 317–18
Food and Drug Administration (FDA), 32*t*, 69, 200, 201, 251, 324, 346
Forced expiratory volume in 1 second (FEV1), 181, 187
Forced vital capacity (FVC), 181, 187
Freidman tongue position, classification, 29, 45, 58, 65, 247, 398
Frontal lobe epilepsy (FLE), 261, 270, 332–38

Frontal Lobe Epilepsy and Parasomnias (FLEP) Scale, 262, 263*t*
Fujita classification – Type I, II, III, 127–28
Functional hemispherectomy, 354, 355
Functional Outcome Sleep Questionnaire (FOSQ), 10, 11
Functional residual capacity (FRC), 119, 179

G
Gabapentin, 34, 213, 259, 302, 306, 308, 318, 319, 324, 370
Gamma-aminobutyric acid (GABA), 398
Gamma-aminobutyric acid-benzodiazepine (GABA-BDZ), 32
Gastric banding, 117, 118*f*
Gastroesophageal reflux disease (GERD), 92, 140, 143, 173, 176, 180, 297, 357, 376
Generalized anxiety disorder (GAD), 31, 36, 43, 48
Generalized seizures, 339, 352
Global Initiative for Obstructive Lung Disease (GOLD) guidelines, 185
GTPase-activating protein (GAP), 90

H
Headache. *See also* Migraine
excessive daytime somnolence and, 371
insomnia and, 370, 373
from medication overuse, 370
narcolepsy, and, 371
obstructive sleep apnea (OSA) and, 373
sleep disturbances and, 371
Heart failure, 7, 74, 78, 80, 177
Horne-Ostberg morningness-eveningness Scale, 11, 238, 385–86
Human leukocyte antigen (HLA), 195, 207
Hyperphagia, 213
Hypersomnia, 145, 202, 207, 362, 393
due to drug or substance (abuse), 212, 219, 228–31
due to medical condition, 212, 219, 362
due to mental disorders, 230
Hypnagogic foot tremor (HFT), 326, 328–29, 327*f*
Hypnagogic hallucinations, 70, 92, 130, 194, 197, 201, 216, 222, 227, 230, 258, 273, 288, 358, 375, 398
Hypnic headaches, 371, 373
Hypnogram, 20, 398
Hypnopompic hallucinations, 197, 216, 398
Hypocretin, 195
Hypocretin-1 in cerebral spinal fluid (CSF), 195

Hypopneas, 17–18, 398
Hypoventilation, 9, 91, 184, 188, 189, 190
Hypoxia-hypoventilation syndromes, 83, 91

I
ICSD-2. *See* International Classification of Sleep Disorders (ICSD-2)
Ictal EEG, 262, 332, 335, 370*f*, 345, 379*f*
Idiopathic hypersomnia, 198, 212, 230
    with long sleep time, 219
    management of, 219
    without long sleep time, 68, 217–19, 236, 237–38
        differential diagnosis of, 225
Idiopathic insomnia, 31, 62, 249
Idiopathic pulmonary hypertension, 176
Imagery rehearsal therapy, 45, 46
Imiprame, 200*t*
Injury, parasomnias, 275, 363
Insomnia, 31, 34, 43, 48, 392, 399
    due to drug, alcohol or substance, 41
    due to medical condition, 66, 67–68, 335–38, 359–63, 360*t*
        chronic daily headache (CDH), 370–73
    due to mental disorders, 30–31, 41, 45, 47*t*, 68
Insomnia Severity Index (ISI), 10, 36, 44, 382–83
Inspired PCO$_2$, 76
International 10–20 Electrode System, 15, 16*f*, 20, 264
International Classification of Sleep Disorders, 2nd Edition (ICSD-2), 3, 12, 392–95
    behaviorally induced insufficient sleep syndrome diagnostic criteria, 223*t*
    hypersomnia due to drug or substance diagnostic criteria, 229*t*
    idiopathic hypersomnia without long sleep time diagnostic criteria, 218*t*
    narcolepsy with cataplexy diagnostic criteria, 195*t*
    narcolepsy due to medical condition diagnostic criteria, 206*t*
    recurrent hypersomnia diagnostic criteria, 212*t*
    sleep related hypoventilation/hypoxemia due to neuromuscular and chest wall disorders diagnostic criteria, 189*t*
    sleep terrors diagnostic criteria, 269*t*

International Restless Legs Syndrome Study Group (IRLSSG) rating scale, 12, 305, 312, 389–91
Intracranial EEG, 332, 337, 338
Intracranial neoplasms, sleep related manifestations of, 91
Iron, 313, 314, 316, 317
Iron deficiency, 314, 316–18

J
Jet lag disorder, 399

K
K-complex, 24, 399
Kleine-Levin syndrome, 198, 212–14, 297
    differential diagnosis of, 212
    increased sexual drive and sexual disinhibition in, 213
    pathophysiology of, 213
    pharmacologic treatment in, 213–14

L
Laryngomalacia, 139–43
    anatomy of, 142*f*
    clinical findings in, 141
    treatment of, 142–43
Larynx, normal anatomy of, 141*f*
Le Fort I maxillary osteotomy, 125
Light therapy, 244–45, 255, 397
Lithium, 57, 214
Loop gain, 97

M
Magnetic resonance angiography (MRA), 167–70, 168*t*, 171, 376
Magnetic resonance imaging (MRI), 259, 316, 331, 342, 370
Maintenance of wakefulness test (MWT), 22–23, 201, 237, 399
Major depressive disorder (MDD), 31, 43, 48, 222
Malformation of cortical development, 332, 334*f*, 335, 353*f*, 354
Mallampati grading, 71, 187
Mandibular osteotomy, bilateral saggital split, 125
Mandibular repositioning appliance/device, 167, 169–71, 376
Marijuana, 229
    signs and symptoms of abuse, 231*t*
Maxillary and mandibular hypoplasia, 123, 125–28
Maxillomandibular advancement (MMA) surgery, 125–28

Maxillomandibular insufficiency, 127
Mean sleep latency (MSL), 193, 197, 211*f*, 230, 237, 260, 399
Melatonin, 33, 236, 241, 244, 245, 255, 276, 324, 367, 368, 370, 399
Menstrual-related hypersomnia, 212
Mesial temporal sclerosis, 345
Methamphetamine, 199*t*, 200–201
Methylphenidates, 194, 199*t*, 200, 206, 219, 240
Migraines, 36, 240, 371–73
Milnacipran, 69
Mini Mental Status Exam, 273
Mirtazapine, 33, 57
Mixed apnea, 9, 17, 399
Modafinil, 194, 199–200, 217, 219, 236, 240, 248, 251, 357, 358, 361
Morbid obesity, 116, 161
Mueller maneuver, 124, 131
Multiple sleep latency test (MSLT), 10, 22–23, 25, 87, 91, 145, 194*f*, 197–98, 205, 211, 216, 228, 234, 236, 237, 399
  for narcolepsy, 192, 197
Multiple system atrophy, 207, 276, 363

N
Narcolepsy, 9, 23, 192, 212, 218, 219, 230, 399
  with cataplexy, 194–202, 207
    management of patients with, 198
    scheduled naps in, 198
  without cataplexy, 198, 218, 225, 237
  due to craniopharyngioma resection, 206
  impact on quality of life, 197
  nocturnal sleep disruption, 197
  pharmacotherapy for, 199*t*
  precipitating factors, 195
Nasal pressure transducer, 15, 17
National Highway Traffic Safety Administration (NHTSA), 225
National Institutes of Health (NIH), 48, 308*t*
National Survey on Drug and Health, 230
Neurofibromatosis Type 1 (NF1), 85
  clinical features of, 90
Neurofibromin, 90
Neuronal nicotinic acetylcholine receptor, 337
Neuropsychological testing, 274, 332, 342
New York Heart Association Functional Class, 173
NF-1. *See* Neurofibromatosis Type 1 (NF1)
Night eating syndrome (NES), 296, 297
Nightmares, 43–44, 269–70, 399

Nocturnal frontal lobe epilepsy (NFLE), 261, 270, 332–38
Nocturnal oximetry, 179
Nocturnal oxygenation, 183, 185
Nocturnal paroxysmal dystonia (NPD), 337
Nocturnal penile tumescence test (NPT), 24
Nocturnal polysomnogram. *See* Polysomnogram (PSG)
Nocturnal seizures, 263, 276, 281
Nonrapid eye movement (NREM) sleep, 17, 66, 69, 259–60, 301, 338, 352–55, 399
  parasomnias, 269, 270, 276, 281, 283, 289*f*, 290

O
Obesity, pediatric OSA and, 163–64
Obstructive sleep apnea syndrome (OSA/ OSAS), 44, 68, 80, 81, 82, 93, 100–107, 109–10, 115–16, 123, 125–28, 130–35, 145, 151, 166–71, 188–89, 236, 253–56, 276, 279–82, 284–86, 289, 321–24, 326–29, 342–47, 359–63, 399
  pediatric, 8–9, 147–49, 161–64
    adenotonsillectomy in, 148, 149, 164, 284, 285
    enuresis in, 150, 285–86
    ICSD-2 criteria for, 147*t*
    PAP therapy in, 164
    and Pompe disease, 190
    postoperative pulmonary edema in, 149
    treatment with aryepiglottoplasty, 139, 143
Olanzapine, 33, 57
Opioids, 308, 314, 318, 324
Overbite, 399
Overjet, 399
Overlap syndrome (COPD and OSAS), 184
Oxygen, 7, 82, 83, 102*f*

P
Panic attacks, 27, 270
PAP. *See* Positive airway pressure (PAP)
Paradoxical insomnia, 30, 58, 61, 62
Parasomnia, 222, 261, 262, 264, 268–69, 290–91, 394, 399
  nocturnal seizures masquerading as, 270
  safety concerns in, 271
Parkinson's disease, 207, 276, 357, 358, 359, 361, 363
  and insomnia, 362

Patient Health Questionnaire-9 (PHQ-9), 11, 273, 294, 387–88
Pediatric OSA. *See* Obstructive sleep apnea, pediatric
Periodic limb movement disorder (PLMD), 276, 321–24, 329, 373, 399
Periodic limb movements in sleep (PLMS), 234, 289, 304, 314, 321, 323, 326, 329, 357, 399
Periodic limb movements in wakefulness (PLMW), 304, 314
Perioperative airway management, 119–20
Perioperative pain management, 120–21
Peripheral arterial tonometry (PAT), 24, 50
Peripheral neuropathy, 312, 314, 318–19
Phenytoin, 213, 330
Phototherapy, 235–36
Physical examination, 7–8, 145
Polysomnogram (PSG), 14, 400
    in children, 20
    event scoring in, 17–20. *See also* Scoring
    portable, 20–21, 102*f*
    sleep terror in, 269*f*
    special situations, 20
Pompe disease, 190
    and hypoventilation, 188
    and obstructive sleep apnea, pediatric, 190
    and restrictive lung disease, 186
Portable devices, types of, 20–21
Portable monitoring (PM), 101, 105–7
Positive airway pressure (PAP), 21–22, 72, 91, 155–56
    adherence, 156, 157
    complications, 158*t*
    download, 73, 95, 154, 155*t*, 162
    interfaces, 156
Positron emission tomography (PET), 316, 332
Posterior airway space (PAS), 124*f*, 125, 127*f*, 128
Post traumatic stress disorder (PTSD), 46–47
Precipitants of arousal disorders, 262*f*
Pregabalin, 33, 67, 69, 308, 318, 319
Pregnancy, 317
Pre-induction and maintenance positive end-expiratory pressure (PEEP), 119
Primary central sleep apnea, 72–77
Progressive muscle relaxation (PMR), 29, 295, 379, 400
Protriptyline, 200*t*, 201
Prozac eyes, 25
Pseudo-RBD, 282
Psychophysiological insomnia, 29, 30–31, 34–36, 39, 41, 61, 68, 247–51, 289, 295, 378–79

Pulmonary function test, 174, 174*t*, 181, 187, 188–89
Pulmonary hypertension (PH), 9, 89, 117, 141, 148, 177, 189
Pulse oximetry, 15, 102*f*
Pulse transit time (PTT), 24

Q
Quazepam, 32
Quetiapine, 33, 57, 258

R
Radiotherapy, 90
Ramelteon, 32*t*, 33, 57
Rapid eye movement. *See* REM sleep
RBD. *See* REM sleep behavior disorder (RBD)
Rebound, 309–10, 400
Recurrent hypersomnia. *See* Kleine-Levin syndrome
Refractory epilepsy, 332
Relaxation training, 39, 41, 45, 46, 67
REM latency, 66, 79, 87, 187, 216, 222, 234, 378, 400
REM parasomnias, 270
REM sleep, 17, 18, 72, 76, 79, 175, 187, 193, 197, 231, 237, 274, 400
    without atonia, 275, 282, 358, 359*f*
REM sleep behavior disorder (RBD), 260, 261, 262, 269, 275–77, 281, 359–63
Residual volume (RV), 181
Respiratory biofeedback, 113–14
Respiratory effort related arousal (RERA), 20
Respiratory inductance plethsmography (RIP), 15, 17, 400
Responsive Neurostimulator System Study (NeuroPace, Inc.), 343
Restless legs syndrome (RLS), 6, 173, 176, 222, 306–10, 312–19, 326–29, 400
    primary (idiopathic), 307, 308, 313
Reverse Tredelenburg position (RTP), 119
Right heart catheterization, 174, 175*t*, 177
Risperidone, 33
Ropinirole, 304, 305, 306, 314, 316, 322, 324, 348, 361
Rotigotine, 305, 306
Roux-en-Y gastric bypass (RYGB) surgery, 116, 117, 118*f*

S
Safety measures for parasomnias and seizures, 271
Scoring
    apnea, 17

arousal, 18
hypopnea, 17–18
periodic limb movement (PLM), 18
sleep stages, 17–18, 18t
Secondary narcolepsy, 91, 206
with cataplexy, conditions that cause, 207
Selective serotonin reuptake inhibitors
(SSRIs), 6, 200t, 201, 231, 276,
297, 314, 319, 323
Serotonin-norepinephrine reuptake
inhibitor, 276
Sexsomnia, 290–91, 400
Single photon emission computed
tomography (SPECT), 316, 332
6-minute walk test, 174, 176, 177
Sleep apnea, 400
Sleep architecture, 8, 25, 400
Sleep cycle, 400
Sleep deprivation, 62, 225–26, 270, 400
Sleep diary, 37, 222, 247
Sleep drunkenness, 236, 238
Sleep efficiency (SE), 35, 37, 46, 400
Sleep enuresis (bedwetting), 145–47, 150,
283, 400
causes and associations for, 285
secondary type, 284–86
Sleep hygiene, 41, 66, 400
Sleep latency (SL), 23, 401
Sleep log, 23, 28f, 38t, 39, 41, 58, 59f, 217f,
223f, 234, 235f, 240, 241, 248
Sleep misperception disorder, 30
Sleep onset, 5, 8, 401
Sleep onset REM periods (SOREMPs), 23,
193, 205, 211, 217, 228, 234, 401
Sleep paralysis, 194, 197, 401
Sleep related breathing disorders, 392–93
Sleep related dissociative disorders, 261,
263–64
Sleep related eating disorder (SRED), 295–98
Sleep related headaches, 370–73
Sleep related hypoventilation/hypoxemia,
83, 91
differential diagnosis of, 189
due to neuromuscular and chest wall
disorders, 188–89
treatment of, 189–90
Sleep related hypoxemia
due to lower airway obstruction
(moderate chronic obstructive
pulmonary disease), 181–83
due to pulmonary parenchymal or
vascular pathology, 176
Sleep related movement disorders, 394–95
Sleep restriction, 37–39
Sleep spindle, 18, 401

Sleep talking (somniloquy), 5, 401
Sleep terrors, 261, 267–71, 276,
281–82, 401
differential diagnosis of, 269–70
Sleepwalking (somnambulism),
259–65, 262t, 269, 276, 281–82,
296, 401
Slow-wave sleep arousals, 264
Sodium oxybate, 69, 194–95, 199t, 200t,
201, 202
Somatoform disorder, 370
Somnambulism. See Sleepwalking
(somnambulism)
Split-night study, 21, 117f, 153f, 340
Stereotypy, 5, 263, 281, 332
Stimulus control, 41, 63
STOP Questionnaire, 10, 104, 105
Stridor, 136, 137, 139, 140, 143, 302
Stroke, 151, 152, 375, 379–80
Subthalamic nucleus, 361, 363
Suggested immobilization test (SIT), 24
Sundowning, 367–68
Suprachiasmatic nucleus, 244, 368, 401
Synucleinopathies, 276, 363

T
Temazepam, 32, 57, 317, 324, 357
Temporal lobe epilepsy (TLE), 342–47
Temporomandibular joint (TMJ), 166
Tension-type headaches (TTH), 371, 372
10–20 electrode placement, 15, 16f, 20, 264
Thermistor, 15
Thyroid stimulating hormone, 79, 234, 273,
306, 358
Time in bed (TIB), 35, 37
Titration. See Positive airway pressure (PAP)
Tongue position grade, 29, 45, 58, 65, 247
Tonsillar hypertrophy, 131
Tonsils, grading, 7, 8, 29, 36, 45, 65, 93,
131, 132, 174, 192, 204, 258,
288, 358
Topiramate, 295, 297, 331, 370
Total iron binding capacity, 332
Total lung capacity (TLC), 181
Total sleep time (TST), 20, 37, 42, 46, 58,
79, 87, 93, 181, 183, 215, 216,
219, 225
Transcutaneous CO_2 (TcpCO$_2$), 20, 187,
188f, 189
Trazodone, 33, 34, 57, 302, 312, 319, 320
Triazolam, 32, 73, 76
Tricyclic antidepressants (TCAs), 6, 200t,
201, 271, 276, 314, 319, 323
Turbinate hypertrophy, 7, 131, 145, 160,
258, 284

U

Upper airway resistance syndrome (UARS),
     20, 236
Uremia, 318
Urine toxicology screen, 48, 198, 228,
     231, 238
Uvulopalatopharyngoplasty (UPPP), 101,
     131, 132, 133–34, 135

V

Vagus nerve stimulation (VNS), 339, 340,
     341f, 342, 346–47
Valproate (valproic acid), 57, 213, 292, 331,
     349, 355

Venlafaxine, 36, 57, 200t, 201–2
Ventilation perfusion scan, 174
Video EEG (VEEG) monitoring, 259, 331, 350
Video monitoring, 15
Vulnerable child syndrome, 90

W

Wake time after sleep onset (WASO), 37, 62,
     58, 326

Z

Zaleplon, 32t, 33, 57, 70
Zolpidem, 29, 32t, 33, 34, 43, 57, 76, 296,
     320, 357